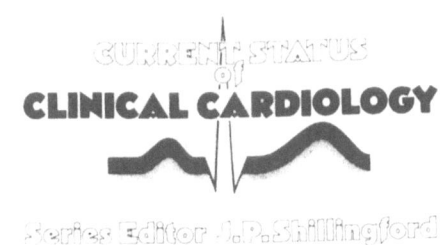

CURRENT STATUS
OF
CLINICAL CARDIOLOGY

Series Editor J.P.Shillingford

CLINICAL ASPECTS OF CARDIAC ARRHYTHMIAS

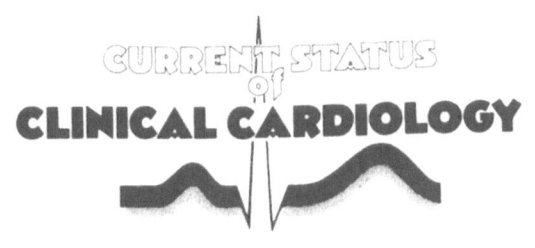

CURRENT STATUS
of
CLINICAL CARDIOLOGY

Series Editor J.P. Shillingford

CLINICAL ASPECTS OF CARDIAC ARRHYTHMIAS

Edited by
A. John Camm
Department of Cardiological Sciences
St. George's Hospital Medical School
Cranmer Terrace
London

and
David E. Ward
St. George's Hospital
Blackshaw Road
London

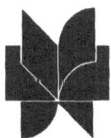

KLUWER ACADEMIC PUBLISHERS

DORDRECHT - BOSTON - LONDON

Distributors

for the United States and Canada: Kluwer Academic Publishers, PO Box 358, Accord Station, Hingham, MA 02018–0358, USA
for all other countries: Kluwer Academic Publishers Group, Distribution Center, PO Box 322, 3300 AH Dordrecht, The Netherlands

British Library Cataloguing in Publication Data

Clinical aspects of cardiac arrhythmias.
  1. Man. Heart. Arrhythmia
  I. Camm, A. John   II. Ward, David E.
  III. Series
616.1'28

Library of Congress Cataloging-in-Publication Data

Clinical aspects of cardiac arrhythmias.
  (Current status of clinical cardiology)
  Includes bibliographies and index.
  1. Arrhythmia. I. Camm, A. John. II. Ward, David E.
  III. Series. [DNLM: 1. Arrhythmia—physiopathology.
  2. Electrocardiography. 3. Electrophysiology.
WG 330 C6405]
RC685.A65C54 1988   616.1'28   88–12801

ISBN-13:978-94-010-7073-7   e-ISBN-13:978-94-009-1289-2
DOI:10.1007/978-94-009-1289-2

Published in the United Kingdom by Kluwer Academic Publishers, PO Box 55, Lancaster, UK.

Kluwer Academic Publishers BV incorporates the publishing programmes of D. Reidel, Martinus Nijhoff, Dr W. Junk and MTP Press.

Contents

CONTENTS

Current Status of Clinical Cardiology Series

Drugs in the Management of Heart Disease
Edited by A. Breckenridge

Heart Muscle Disease
Edited by J. F. Goodwin

Congenital Heart Disease
Edited by F. J. Macartney

Ischaemic Heart Disease
Edited by K. M. Fox

Immunology and Molecular Biology of Cardiovascular Diseases
Edited by C. J. F. Spry

Clinical Aspects of Cardiac Arrhythmias
Edited by A. J. Camm and D. E. Ward

Preface

We were particularly pleased to compile this volume entitled 'Clinical Aspects of Cardiac Arrhythmias'. Recent years have seen the publication of many textbooks on cardiac arrhythmias, some of which concentrate on one particular aspect such as drug management, electrocardiographic appearances, electrophysiological evaluation etc; and others of which are the collated reports of symposia, often dealing with detailed considerations of highly specialised problems. Most of the larger more comprehensive texts have devoted a substantial proportion to basic considerations and experimental observations, far removed from the clinical arena. When asked to contribute to the series 'Current Status of Clinical Cardiology' we felt that the clinical aspects of cardiac arrhythmias should be emphasized, and that the text should be as comprehensive as possible within the limitations of a single volume in this series. This comprehensive but clinical approach has necessitated the inclusion of certain subjects such as the mechanisms of tachycardia, metabolic aspects of cardiac arrhythmias and reperfusion arrhythmias, which are not directly or exclusively clinical. However, the rapid advances in these areas in recent years are likely to have increasingly important clinical consequences.

Although the epidemiology of clinical arrhythmias is difficult to discover, it is widely appreciated that arrhythmias are commonplace. For example, the Wolff–Parkinson–White pattern is found in one in 500 live births, sudden unexpected cardiac death occurs in approximately one per 1000 of the population each year; atrial fibrillation is the predominant rhythm in 10% of the elderly population, and about 1% of the total population has significant paroxysmal supraventricular tachycardia. The high prevalence of disabling or life threatening arrhythmias has encouraged the development of many sophisticated techniques for their investigation.

Each year many new anti-arrhythmic drugs, implantable devices and anti-arrhythmic ablative procedures are introduced and described. The investigation and treatment of cardiac arrhythmias have spawned an enormous literature which constitutes one of the largest in cardiological journals. Those concerned with the management of cardiac arrhythmias are, therefore, faced with an almost impossible task of keeping up to date. We, therefore, asked the twenty-eight contributors, each working in the United Kingdom, to provide current and comprehensive reviews. In this multi-authored text we have tried to maintain consistent presentation, whilst preserving the individual approach.

Although written predominantly for physicians, we hope that this book will interest all those involved in the care of patients with cardiac arrhythmias.

A. John Camm
David E. Ward
London 1988

Series Editor's Note

The last few decades have seen an explosion in our knowledge of cardiovascular disease as a result of research in many disciplines. The tempo of research is ever increasing, so that it is becoming more and more difficult for one person to encompass the whole spectrum of the advances taking place on many fronts.

Even more difficult is to include the advances as they affect clinical practice in one textbook of cardiovascular disease. Fifty years ago all that was known about cardiology could be included in one textbook of moderate size and at that time there was little research so that a textbook remained up to date for several years. Today all this has changed, and books have to be updated at frequent intervals to keep up with the results of research and changing fashions.

The present series has been designed to cover the field of cardio-vascular medicine in a series of, initially, eight volumes which can be updated at regular intervals and at the same time give a sound basis of practice for doctors looking after patients.

The volumes include the following subjects: heart muscle disease; congenital heart disease, invasive and non-invasive diagnosis; ischaemic heart disease; immunology and molecular biology of the heart in health and disease; irregularities of the heart beat; and each is edited by a distinguished British author with an international reputation, together with an international panel of contributors.

The series will be mainly designed for the consultant cardiologist as reference books to assist him in his day-to-day practice and keep him up to date in the various fields of cardiovascular medicine at the same time as being of manageable size.

J. P. Shillingford
British Heart Foundation

List of Contributors

R. S. Bexton
Department of Cardiology
Freeman Hospital
Freeman Road
Newcastle-upon-Tyne NE7 7DN
UK

E. Boyd
Cardiac Department
Guy's Hospital
St Thomas Street
London SE1 9RT
UK

A. K. Brown
Royal Lancaster Infirmary
Ashton Broad
Lancaster LA1 4RP
UK

G. S. Butrous
Department of Cardiological
    Sciences
St. George's Hospital Medical
    School
Cranmer Terrace
Tooting
London SW17 0RE
UK

A. J. Camm
Department of Cardiovascular
    Sciences
St George's Hospital Medical
    School
Cranmer Terrace
Tooting
London SW17 0RE
UK

R. W. F. Campbell
Department of Academic
    Cardiology
Freeman Hospital
Newcastle-upon-Tyne NE7 7DN
UK

S. M. Cobbe
Department of Medical
    Cardiology
University of Glasgow
Royal Infirmary
Glasgow G31 2ER
UK

J. C. P. Crick
Royal Postgraduate Medical
    School
Hammersmith Hospital
London
UK

D. W. Davies
Department of Cardiology
St Bartholomew's Hospital
West Smithfield
London EC1A 7BE
UK

M. J. Davies
BHF Cardiovascular Pathology
  Unit
St George's Hospital Medical
  School
Cranmer Terrace
Tooting
London W17 0RE
UK

N. A. Flores
Department of Cardiology
St Mary's Hospital Medical
  School
Norfolk Place
London W2 1PG
UK

C. Garratt
Department of Cardiovascular
  Sciences
St George's Hospital Medical
  School
Cranmer Terrace
Tooting
London SW17 0RE
UK

R. Hayward
Department of Cardiology
The Middlesex Hospital
Mortimer Street
London
UK

P. Holt
Cardiac Department
Guy's Hospital
St Thomas Street
London SE1 9RT
UK

G. G. Kaye
Department of Cardiology
Leeds General Infirmary
Great George Street
Leeds LS1 3EX
UK

A. Martin
Department of Medicine
The General Hospital
St Helier
Jersey
Channel Islands

D. Mehta
Department of Cardiological
  Sciences
St George's Hospital Medical
  School
Cranmer Terrace
Tooting
London SW17 0RE
UK

A. W. Nathan
Department of Cardiology
St Bartholomew's Hospital
West Smithfield
London EC1A 7BE
UK

D. B. O'Keeffe
Cardiac Unit
Belfast City Hospital
Lisburn Road
Belfast BT9 7AB
Northern Ireland

E. J. Perrins
Department of Medical
  Cardiology
General Infirmary
Great George Street
Leeds LS1 3EX
UK

E. Rowland
Cardiothoracic Institute
University of London
London
UK

D. C. Russell
Cardiovascular Research Unit
University of Edinburgh
High Robson Building
George Square
Edinburgh EH8 9XF
UK

D. J. Sheridan
Department of Cardiology
St. Mary's Hospital Medical
 School
Norfolk Place
London W2 1PG
UK

J. A. Till
Department of Paediatric
 Cardiology
Brompton Hospital
Fulham Road
London SW3 6HP
UK

W. D. Toff
Department of Cardiovascular
 Sciences
St George's Hospital Medical
 School
Cranmer Terrace
Tooting
London SW17 0RE
UK

R. Vincent
Cardiac Department
Royal Sussex County Hospital
Eastern Road
Brighton
Sussex BN2 5BE
UK

D. E. Ward
Regional Cardiothoracic Unit
St George's Hospital
Blackshaw Road
London W17 0QT
UK

D. A. Zideman
Department of Anaesthetics
Royal Postgraduate Medical
 School
Hammersmith Hospital
Du Cane Road
London W12 0HS
UK

1
Mechanisms of tachycardia in the experimental setting and their possible clinical importance

S. M. COBBE

INTRODUCTION

Our knowledge of the basic mechanisms underlying clinical cardiac arrhythmias arises from an enormous experimental literature describing the normal and abnormal electrophysiology of the heart. Although the concepts derived from experimental electrophysiology are fundamental to the understanding of cardiac arrhythmias, extrapolation from the experimental to the clinical setting is often fraught with difficulty. This brief review will first describe the fundamental mechanisms of tachycardia, and then evaluate the evidence for their participation in various cardiac arrhythmias.

FUNDAMENTAL MECHANISMS OF ARRHYTHMIA

The mechanisms of generation of abnormal beats, whether single or sustained, are indicated in Table 1.1. A subdivision is possible into mechanisms which can occur within a single cell, and those which require intercellular interaction.

Enhanced automaticity

The term automaticity is used to describe the ability of a cardiac cell to depolarize spontaneously to its threshold, and thus initiate an action potential. This is of course a normal property of sinoatrial and atrioventricular nodal cells, and confers pacemaker properties on these areas. Purkinje fibres show a slow rate of spontaneous depolarization *in vitro*, while isolated preparations of normal atrial and ventricular myocardial cells are virtually quiescent. The rate of spontaneous discharge of Purkinje fibres may be enhanced by mechanical interference such as stretching, or by the administration of catecholamines or ouabain (Figure 1.1a).

1

Table 1.1 Fundamental mechanisms of arrhythmia

Unicellular
  Enhanced automaticity
  Triggered activity – early afterdepolarizations
                          delayed afterdepolarizations
Multicellular
  Re-entry
  Electrotonic interaction
  Mechano–electrical coupling

Automatic activity is independent of external stimulation, and cannot therefore be initiated or terminated by pacing.

Triggered activity

The term 'triggered activity' was introduced by Cranefield[1] to describe the phenomenon of repetitive activity of the heart arising from depolarizing afterpotentials. The essential distinction between triggered activity and automaticity is that a cell capable of triggered activity may remain quiescent for prolonged periods, and requires an extrinsic depolarization to initiate afterpotentials which may then lead to repetitive activity. Microelectrode studies have distinguished between early afterdepolarizations which interrupt the repolarization phase of the action potential, and delayed afterdepolarizations, which occur after full repolarization has occurred, and are preceded by a transient hyperpolarization (Figures 1.1b, c). Both forms of afterdepolarizations may initiate a non-driven action potential. This itself may be followed by an afterdepolarization, and hence a repetitive discharge ensues. The last action potential of the sequence is usually followed by one or more oscillatory afterpotentials. Experimentally, triggered activity has been identified in Purkinje fibres, muscle fibres inserted into the atrial margin of the mitral valve, and cells in the proximal coronary sinus. Agents which predispose to the initiation of triggered activity include barium and caesium salts, cardiac glycosides, veratrine, hypoxia, stretch or exposure to sodium-free, calcium-rich solutions. Oscillatory afterpotentials are associated with mechanical aftercontractions, and are attributable to oscillations in intracellular calcium activity. Organic or inorganic antagonists of slow inward current (e.g. verapamil, manganese salts) inhibit the amplitude of afterdepolarizations and abolish triggered activity.

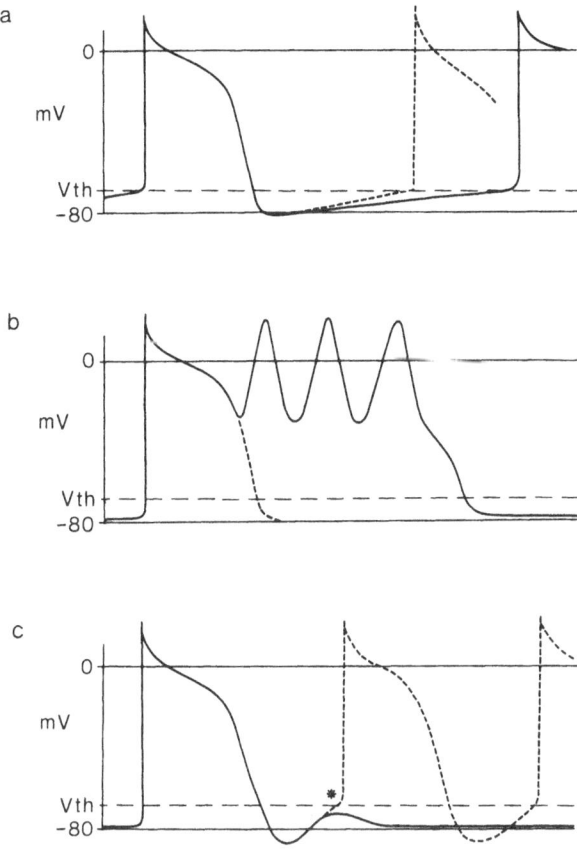

Figure 1.1 Mechanism of spontaneous automaticity and triggered activity. Each panel represents a schematic Purkinje fibre action potential. The zero-potential, normal resting membrane potential ($-80\,mV$) and threshold potential for normal depolarization (V_{th}) are illustrated. **Panel A** After completion of the first action potential and full repolarization, a slow spontaneous (phase 4) depolarization occurs towards the threshold potential. Once the threshold potential is reached, a propagated action potential is initiated. Enhancement of diastolic depolarization by catecholamines (dashed line) shortens the interval to the appearance of the next action potential. **Panel B** Appearance of early afterdepolarizations following a stimulated action potential. Repolarization is interrupted by repetitive firing of the cell, which arises at a low membrane potential. **Panel C** Mechanism of triggered activity associated with delayed afterdepolarizations. Note full repolarization after initial action potential, followed by transient hyperpolarization and delayed afterdepolarization (*). If this reaches threshold, a propagated action potential occurs. This may be followed by another delayed afterdepolarization, thus allowing sustained discharge of the cell

3

Table 1.2 Characteristics of re-entry

Potential circuit with anatomically or functionally inexcitable centre

Unidirectional block

Slow conduction – conduction time in circuit exceeds refractory period of normal myocardium

Division of circuit terminates re-entry activity

Re-entry

The mechanism of 'circus movement' tachycardia, or re-entry, was first postulated by Mines in 1913[2]. The fundamental requirements for re-entry are listed in Table 1.2. The size of a potential re-entry circuit is determined by the effective conduction velocity, since it is a prerequisite of re-entrant excitation that the conduction time in the circuit exceeds the refractory period of the myocardium which is to be re-excited. If conduction velocity is only moderately depressed, the re-entrant circuit must be several centimetres in length (macro re-entry). However, Wit, Cranefield and Hoffman[3] showed that localized hyperkalaemia caused a depression of effective conduction velocity to $0.02–0.08 \, m, s^{-1}$, which permitted re-entry in circuits of only 12–35 mm in length (micro re-entry). The property of unidirectional block is usually a function of incomplete recovery of excitability following a preceding beat. Further delay while the impulse traverses the circuit allows recovery of the initially blocked area, thus allowing conduction in the retrograde direction and completion of the re-entrant circuit. The likelihood of incomplete recovery of excitability leading to unidirectional block in part of a potential re-entry circuit is greater at higher heart rates or following premature beats. This property is utilized in experimental and clinical studies, where premature stimulation is used to initiate re-entry.

Premature stimulation may also be utilized to terminate a re-entry tachycardia. Premature stimulation of the normal myocardium before arrival of the re-entrant wavefront will render the tissue refractory and thus result in extinction of the circuit. However, the premature stimulus may itself generate conditions appropriate to the continuation of re-entry.

A further mechanism akin to re-entry is that of reflection, where an impulse enters an area of depressed conduction, and may return along the pathway by which it entered, thus re-exciting the normal myocardium.

Electrotonic interaction

It has been suggested that the current of injury flowing at the boundary between normal and ischaemic myocardium may result in the genesis of ectopic beats by electrotonic interaction[4]. Direct current flow occurs as a result of the depolarization of ischaemic cells, and may be enhanced by the delay in conduction in the ischaemic area which results in the action potential in that same area continuing after completion of repolarization in the normal myocardium. Experimental studies have shown that depolarization caused by exposure of a remote tissue site to high extracellular potassium concentration may initiate automatic activity.

Mechano-electrical interaction

The role of stretching Purkinje fibres in the initiation of automaticity and triggered activity has already been mentioned. Experimental mechanical perturbations of ventricular muscle cells have been shown to initiate afterdepolarizations which may reach threshold potential and trigger extrasystoles[5]. It is postulated that mechanical effects of this nature might occur as a result of incoordinated contraction and relaxation in acute ischaemia, or in dyskinetic segments secondary to previous myocardial infarction.

MECHANISMS OF CLINICAL ARRHYTHMIAS

The above discussion has illustrated several potential mechanisms for the generation of clinical arrhythmias. Unfortunately it is rarely possible to infer the mechanism of clinical arrhythmia directly from the surface electrocardiogram. However, careful study of the mechanism of spontaneous initiation and termination of the arrhythmia, along with knowledge of the anatomical and pathophysiological substrate, may permit reasonable inference of the mechanism. Further precision is provided by intracardiac electrophysiological investigation, which permits localization of the site of origin of the arrhythmia, the pathways by which it is conducted, and further study of the mode of initiation and termination. Even with the benefit of invasive investigation, however, it may be impossible to distinguish between certain mechanisms of arrhythmia, in particular between triggered activity and micro re-entry.

Automaticity

The characteristic electrocardiographic feature of an automatic tachycardia is the lack of a constant coupling interval with the preceding normal beat. Instead, appearance of the tachycardia is related principally to the underlying heart rate. Thus automatic tachycardias are not *initiated* by a premature beat, nor can they be induced or terminated by electrical stimulation. The electrocardiographic pattern of parasystole may indicate an automatic focus. Automatic atrial tachycardia is a relatively rare but well recognized arrhythmia which fulfils the above criteria. The rate of an automatic focus may be variable, the principal influence being the level of sympathetic tone.

5

There is uncertainty concerning the possible role of enhanced automaticity in the generation of arrhythmias after myocardial infarction. Experimental coronary ligation results in an early phase of arrhythmias whose origin is considered to be re-entry (see below). A phase of quiescence is then followed, at 24–48 hours, by a period of enhanced ventricular automaticity. Microelectrode studies of surviving subendocardial fibres at this stage have shown accelerated diastolic depolarization. Although automatic ventricular arrhythmias are not a prominent feature of myocardial infarction in man as they are in the dog, the behaviour of certain post-infarction arrhythmias, particularly accelerated idioventricular rhythm, suggests an automatic basis.

Triggered activity

Considerable interest has centred on the possible role of triggered activity in the genesis of clinical arrhythmias since its identification *in vitro*. The experimental conditions under which triggered activity may be initiated include hypoxia, and the presence of high concentrations of cardiac glycosides and catecholamines. It is, therefore, reasonable to suggest that some, if not all of the arrhythmias associated with digitalis toxicity may be mediated by triggered activity. The presence of early afterdepolarizations associated with gross lengthening of action potential duration has been noted in cells exposed to high concentrations of Class III antiarrhythmic agents. This mechanism may trigger repetitive firing, although the mechanism of the characteristic *torsade de pointes* ventricular tachycardia is still controversial (see below). Experimental studies of subendocardial fibres from dogs 24–28 h after coronary ligation have suggested that triggered activity as well as enhanced automaticity may underlie the 'automatic' ventricular tachyarrhythmias seen at that time. It is not known whether a clinical counterpart to these arrhythmias exists. Identification of fibres capable of triggered activity inserted into the atrial margin of the mitral valve in canine and simian hearts has led to speculation that the arrhythmias associated with mitral valve prolapse may have a triggered basis. Finally, experimental observation that the transient inward current responsible for the development of afterpotentials is sensitive to calcium antagonists has led to the suggestion that some tachycardias susceptible to verapamil may have a triggered basis. Examples include multifocal atrial tachycardia, commonly seen in the presence of severe hypoxaemia, and fascicular ventricular tachycardia.

Having listed a variety of arrhythmias in which a triggered mechanism is at least plausible, it is important to emphasize that it is virtually impossible to prove the existence of the mechanism in a clinical context. Catheter or intraoperative mapping may identify a focal origin of the tachycardia, but in view of the fact that micro re-entry may occur within an area of a few square centimetres, the distinction between focal triggered activity and re-entry cannot be made with conventional tech-

Table 1.3   Proposed features distinguishing triggered activity from re-entry

	Re-entry	Triggered activity
Initiation/termination by premature beat	+	+
Termination by overdrive	+	rate related
Overdrive acceleration	?	+
Inverse relationship between coupling interval of premature beat and interval to first tachycardia beat	+	−
Suppression by verapamil	?	+

niques. The relationships between the underlying cycle length, coupling interval of the first ectopic and the subsequent interectopic interval has been analysed in depth to try to clarify the uncertainty. A series of characteristic features has been suggested (Table 1.3) on the basis of the behaviour of triggered activity *in vitro*[6]. Using these criteria, examples of triggered activity have been proposed, for example accelerated junctional escape rhythm. However, the sensitivity and specificity of these

Table 1.4   Clinical re-entry arrhythmias

Sinus node re-entry tachycardia

Atrial flutter

Atrial fibrillation

AV nodal re-entry tachycardia

Atrioventricular reciprocating tachycardia (WPW syndrome)

Pacemaker-mediated (endless loop) tachycardia

Ventricular tachycardia secondary to previous myocardial infarction

Polymorphic ventricular tachycardia secondary to QT-interval prolongation

Ventricular fibrillation

indirect criteria cannot be assessed in the absence of direct evidence for or against triggered activity *in vivo*. Recently, recording of after-potentials by electrode catheters *in vivo* has been achieved[7], and raises the hope that the role of triggered activity in clinical arrhythmias may be more effectively evaluated.

Re-entry

Available evidence suggests that the majority of clinically important tachyarrhythmias have a re-entry basis. Examples for which evidence is most convincing are listed in Table 1.4. A characteristic feature of re-

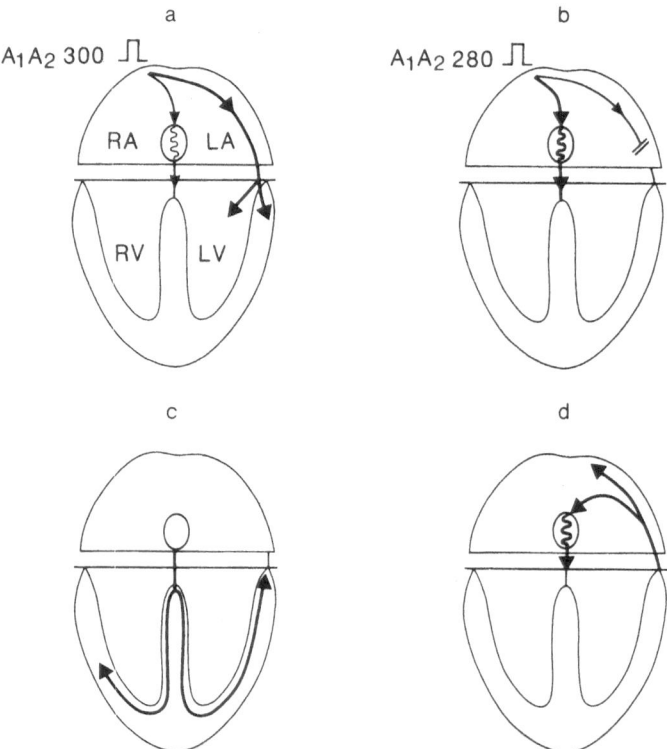

Figure 1.2 Reciprocating tachycardia in Wolff–Parkinson–White syndrome – an example of macro re-entry. Schematic diagram of effects of premature stimulation of the right atrium (stimulus artefact) on conduction through AV node and His–Purkinje system, and through a left-sided bypass tract. Bold lines illustrate predominant direction of activation. **Panel A** illustrates a premature atrial depolarization at a coupling interval of 300 ms. This is conducted through both bypass tract and AV node. In view of the conduction delay in the AV node, however, the ventricles are predominantly activated via the bypass. A more premature impulse at 280 ms (**Panel B**) falls within the refractory period of the bypass, and is blocked. It encounters further delay in the AV node, but is conducted to the ventricles via the His–Purkinje system (**Panel C**). The bypass tract, which has now recovered excitability, conducts the impulse in a retrograde direction, thus re-exciting the atria. The AV node has by this time partially recovered, and can conduct the impulse, with delay, back to the ventricles, thus continuing the tachycardia (**Panel D**). Note the participation of large areas of the heart in the re-entry circuit, which has a 'ring' configuration. Opportunities for interrupting the circuit exist either at the AV node/His bundle or at the site of the bypass tract

entry arrhythmias is the ability to initiate and terminate the arrhythmia by premature stimulation. The best-understood example of the induction of re-entry associated with premature stimulation is seen in the Wolff–Parkinson–White syndrome (Figure 1.2). Progressively premature atrial stimuli are conducted with increasing degrees of pre-excitation via the bypass tract. When the coupling interval of the stimulus is brought within the effective refractory period of the bypass, antegrade conduction block occurs. The atrial impulse is conducted, with delay, via the atrioventricular node and His–Purkinje system to the ventricle. The impulse reaches the distal site of insertion of the bypass tract after a sufficient delay to permit retrograde conduction and re-excitation of the atria. A reciprocating tachycardia then ensues. The involvement of a macro re-entry circuit in this tachycardia is demonstrated by three features: (1) the increase in tachycardia cycle length which occurs if bundle branch block develops on the ipsilateral side of a free wall bypass, (2) by the increase in tachycardia cycle length achieved by drugs slowing conduction either in the atrioventricular node or in the bypass tract, and (3) the abolition of the tachycardia by ablation either of the His bundle or the bypass tract.

Recurrent ventricular tachycardia after previous myocardial infarction is another clinically important arrhythmia for which strong evidence of a re-entry mechanism exists[8]. Ventricular tachycardia may be reproducibly initiated and terminated by premature stimuli. There is an inverse relationship between the coupling interval of the premature beat inducing tachycardia and the interval to the first non-stimulated beat. Intra-operative mapping has enabled localization of the site of origin of the tachycardia, normally on the endocardium at the boundary between normal and scarred myocardium. Occasionally a macro re-entry circuit can be demonstrated, with continuous electrical activation circulating around a non-excitable core, analogous to the 'ring' model of re-entry (Figure 1.2). More commonly, the tachycardia appears to originate from a circumscribed area of a few square centimetres (micro re-entry). High-density mapping of this area has confirmed the existence of a re-entry circuit, usually of the 'figure 8' variety (Figure 1.3). These results correspond closely to those obtained in mapping studies performed in chronically infarcted canine hearts. The basis of slow conduction and re-entry in 'scar-related' ventricular tachycardia has been investigated histologically and electrophysiologically in tissues which have been identified by mapping studies as forming part of the re-entry circuit. Although individual muscle fibres may appear histologically normal, a characteristic feature is the interspersion of strands of fibrous tissue which divide the myocardial cells into functionally discrete bundles. This results in a loss of the syncytial fibre arrangement which normally ensures uniform conduction within the heart, and also results in marked differences in conduction velocity according to whether conduction is parallel or perpendicular to fibre orientation. Electrophysiological recording demonstrates some cells with depressed action potentials and abnormal prolongation of refractory period. Such cells can readily be the source of unidirectional block and slow conduction. Even if cells appear to have normal action potential characteristics, impaired intercellular communication may cause slow conduction and a high risk of block.

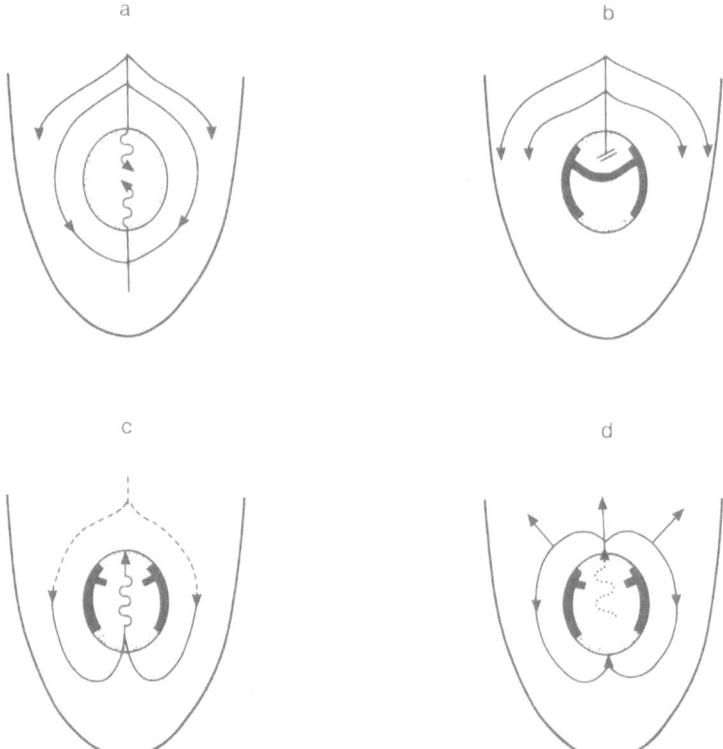

Figure 1.3 Initiation of ventricular tachycardia at a site of acute or prior ischaemic damage – an example of micro re-entry. The diagram schematically represents an area of ischaemic damage (shaded) within the left ventricle. In **Panel A**, the activation sequence during sinus rhythm is illustrated. Although slow conduction is seen within the ischaemic area (wavy lines), no conduction block develops, and extinction of the impulse results, with no arrhythmia initiated. Note that conduction within the depressed area occurs preferentially in the base–apex axis. A premature beat (**Panel B**) occurs before recovery of the depressed area and encounters a broad front of conduction block in the anterograde direction (heavy line). The impulse skirts the perimeter of the depressed area to the apical edge. The depressed area has by now recovered enough to allow very slow conduction in a retrograde direction (**Panel C**). Sufficient conduction delay occurs in the ischaemic area to permit recovery of excitability in the normal myocardium, with re-initiation of the wavefronts circulating around the edges of the depressed area (**Panel D**). The re-entry circuit thus comprises two wavefronts circulating in opposite directions, with a common front of severely depressed conduction within a restricted area. The overall pattern thus resembles a figure 8 on its side. Interruption of the circuit can only take place by blockade of the slowly conducting common wavefront, which may occur within a very localized area

Arrhythmias in acute myocardial ischaemia and infarction

The clinical examples of re-entry described above lend themselves to study because of the stability of the underlying pathophysiological and anatomical substrate. Although recurrent ventricular tachycardia is a common clinical arrhythmia, its frequency and importance is far exceeded by that of ventricular fibrillation secondary to acute myocardial ischaemia and infarction. The majority of deaths from acute myocardial ischaemia occur suddenly as a result of ventricular fibrillation, usually before medical help is sought or arrives, and before transport to hospital. By its nature, therefore, the underlying mechanism of ventricular fibrillation secondary to acute coronary occlusion cannot readily be studied in man.

Extensive animal studies of the electrophysiological effects of acute myocardial ischaemia have clearly identified re-entry as the mechanism for the development of ventricular fibrillation. The critical biochemical changes occurring in ischaemic myocardium include tissue hypoxia, acidosis, elevation of extracellular potassium concentration and sympathetic stimulation. Intracellular recordings in acutely ischaemic cells demonstrate a reduction in membrane potential, action potential upstroke velocity and conduction velocity, and shortening of action potential duration. The effective refractory period may shorten initially, but in severely ischaemic cells there is a depression of excitability which results in an increase of refractory period to values in excess of action potential duration (post-repolarization refractoriness). The majority of the electrophysiological changes in ischaemia may be simulated by exposing cells to an elevated extracellular potassium concentration of $12–14\,mmol\,l^{-1}$, values which have been recorded in ischaemic myocardium. Ischaemic cells are, however, depressed to a greater degree than can be attributed to extracellular hyperkalaemia.

These electrophysiological changes provide the critical substrate for re-entry, namely the presence of slowed conduction with the possibility of inexcitability and rate-dependent conduction block (Figure 1.3). Heterogeneity in the biochemical severity of ischaemia will result in the presence of areas with varying degrees of slowed conduction and alteration in refractoriness, thus providing ideal conditions for re-entry. Multielectrode mapping studies in experimental coronary occlusion have identified re-entry circuits as the basis for ventricular ectopics and tachycardia, while ventricular fibrillation is characterized by degeneration of cardiac conduction into a series of uncoordinated micro re-entry circuits.

Reperfusion arrhythmias

Although there is a wide acceptance of the relevance of experimental models of acute ischaemia in explaining the development of ventricular fibrillation after acute coronary occlusion, the paradoxical situation with regard to reperfusion arrhythmias emphasizes the importance of caution in extrapolation from experimental to clinical arrhythmias. Reperfusion after periods of coronary occlusion up to 2 hours in open-chested dogs results in an extremely high incidence of ventricular fibrillation within the first 2 min. Electrophysiological studies have identified a rapid but uneven resolution of areas of slow conduction and the development of gross action potential shortening secondary to reperfusion damage as mechanisms for the development of re-entry at this stage. On the basis of experimental work, it would be predicted that therapeutic coronary reperfusion in man would likewise be associated with a very high incidence of ventricular fibrillation. Clinical experience has not confirmed this supposition, and reperfusion arrhythmias have been confined in the majority of patients to frequent ventricular ectopic activity or the development of accelerated idioventricular rhythm.

The difference between experimental and clinical reperfusion arrhythmias is not fully explained. The duration of coronary occlusion in man is more commonly 4–6 hours prior to reperfusion, but sufficient experience exists in very early clinical reperfusion to suggest that the duration of occlusion is not the critical factor. The presence of enhanced sympathetic activity in experimental animals may be a possible factor, as may be the difference between abrupt reperfusion occurring by release of a ligature, and gradual reperfusion as lysis of an intracoronary thrombus occurs.

Arrhythmias associated with QT-interval prolongation

The association between lengthening of the QT-interval of the surface electrocardiogram and the development of arrhythmias is well recognized in a number of congenital and acquired conditions. The characteristic arrhythmia is a polymorphic ventricular tachycardia – *torsade de pointes*. The electrocardiographic pattern of this arrhythmia, with a constantly changing electrical axis, could be explained either on the basis of multiple re-entry circuits or by a single re-entry circuit or focus of triggered activity with variable exit into the normal myocardium. QT-interval lengthening may be produced in a number of ways, some of which may be arrhythmogenic, and others antiarrhythmic. QT-interval prolongation secondary to a lengthening of action potential duration in all cardiac cells, as a result of Class III antiarrhythmic drug therapy or hypothyroidism, should be antiarrhythmic, provided that the effect is uniform and equal. In contrast, non-homogeneous lengthening of action potential duration in certain areas of the ventricle as a result of imbalanced sympathetic innervation is regarded as the underlying mechanism in the congenital long-QT syndromes. The development of *torsade de pointes* as an arrhythmogenic response to Class 1a antiarrhythmic agents such as quinidine, procainamide and disopyramide is facilitated both by the prolongation of repolarization and slowed conduction caused by these drugs.

Clinical electrophysiological studies of patients with *torsade de pointes* have not resulted in reproducible initiation of the arrhythmia, and have led to the suggestion that a re-entrant mechanism is not responsible. Experimental studies have been undertaken in a simple canine model in which dispersion of action potential duration is achieved by perfusing part of the myocardium with blood at a different temperature from the rest[9]. No conduction delay was induced by this technique, and no spontaneous arrhythmia occurred. However, it was found that premature stimulation could induce a critical degree of dispersion of repolarization (mean 111 ms) which led to the development of sustained arrhythmia. The site of stimulation was critical. Arrhythmias could not be initiated by stimulation in areas with 'long' action potentials, but could be reproducibly induced in areas with 'short' action potentials. These observations suggest that some of the difficulty in inducing *torsade de pointes* in the clinical electrophysiology laboratory may relate to the site of stimulation.

The above experimental model does not, of course, explain the genesis of the initial triggering premature beat in episodes of spontaneous arrhythmia. Experimental studies of agents causing gross lengthening of action potential duration and QT-interval, such as caesium chloride or toxic concentrations of sotalol, have demonstrated the presence of early afterdepolarizations which may reach threshold and initiate triggered activity. It is not certain whether re-entry or triggered activity is responsible for the maintenance of the arrhythmia thus produced.

It is clear that the experimental evidence regarding the mechanisms of initiation and maintenance of *torsade de pointes* in long QT-interval syndromes is at present incomplete and conflicting. It remains entirely feasible that, as in the case of other arrhythmias, multiple mechanisms may be responsible for an apparently uniform electrocardiographic appearance.

Electrotonic interaction

Although this mechanism is a plausible cause for the development of ectopic beats in acute myocardial ischaemia, there is as yet no direct clinical evidence of its role in arrhythmogenesis.

Mechano–electrical coupling

As in the case of electrotonic interaction, this mechanism is a possible but unproven source of ectopic activity. As well as its possible association with areas of dyskinesis, mechano–electrical coupling may be implicated in the genesis of arrhythmias associated with mitral valve prolapse. The only arrhythmias in which the mechanism is definitely implicated are those associated with mechanical disturbance of the heart by intracardiac catheters or pacing electrodes.

CONCLUSIONS

It is clear from the examples cited above that considerable gaps in our understanding of clinical arrhythmias and their mechanisms still exist. Further progress in this field is inevitably dependent on a two-way interaction between clinical and experimental electrophysiologists. A clear understanding of the basic mechanisms of arrhythmia initiation, maintenance and termination is essential for optimal clinical practice. Experimental workers must for their part continue to develop models of arrhythmia which have direct clinical relevance.

References

1. Cranefield, P. F. (1977). Action potentials, after potentials and arrhythmias. *Circ. Res.*, **41**, 415–23
2. Mines, G. R. (1913). On dynamic equilibrium in the heart. *J. Physiol.*, **46**, 350–83
3. Wit, A. L., Cranefield, P. F. and Hoffman, B. F. (1972). Slow conduction and re-entry in the ventricular conducting system. ii. Single and sustained circus movement in networks of canine and bovine Purkinje fibres. *Circ. Res.*, **30**, 11–22
4. Janse, M. J. and van Capelle, F. J. L. (1982). Electrotonic interaction across an inexcitable region as a cause of ectopic activity in acute regional myocardial ischaemia. A study in intact porcine and canine hearts and computer models. *Circ. Res.*, **50**, 527–37
5. Lab, M. J. (1982). Contraction–excitation feedback in myocardium. Physiological basis and clinical relevance. *Circ. Res.*, **50**, 757–66
6. Wellens, H. J. J., Brugada, P., Vanagt, E. D. G. M., Ross, D. J. and Bar, F. W. (1981). New studies with triggered automaticity. In Harrison, D. C. (ed.) *Cardiac Arrhythmias, A Decade of Progress.* pp. 601–10. (Boston: G. K. Hall)
7. Levine, J. H., Spear, J. F., Guarnieri, T., Weisfeldt, M. L., De Langen, C. D. J., Becker, L. C. and Moore, E. N. (1985). Cesium chloride-induced long QT syndrome: demonstration of afterdepolarizations and triggered activity *in vivo*. *Circulation*, **72**, 1092–1103
8. Josephson, M. E., Buxton, A. E., Marchlinski, F. E., Doherty, J. U., Cassidy, D. M., Kienzle, M. G., Vassallo, J. A., Miller, J. M., Almendral, J. and Grogan, W. (1985). Sustained ventricular tachycardia in coronary artery disease – evidence for a re-entrant medianism. In Zipes, D. P. and Jalife, J. (eds.) *Cardiac Electrophysiology and Arrhythmias.* pp. 409–18. (Orlando: Grune and Stratton)
9. Kuo, C. S., Munakata, K., Reddy, C. P. and Surawicz, B. (1983). Characteristics and possible mechanism of ventricular arrhythmia dependent on the dispersion of action potential durations. *Circulation*, **67**, 1356–67

2
Metabolic factors in the genesis of ventricular arrhythmias

D. C. RUSSELL

INTRODUCTION

A wide range of metabolic factors and biochemical derangements within the heart have been implicated in the pathogenesis of ventricular arrhythmias[1-8]. Much is based however on experimental observations, and the exact role of metabolic influences in initiating or modulating arrhythmogenesis in a clinical setting remains largely ill-defined. Many metabolic effects are interdependent and several responses which might have electrophysiological effects may operate at any one time. In addition metabolic changes often coexist with other potential arrhythmogenic influences, including abnormal neurogenic stimulation of the heart, ventricular dysfunction and coronary reperfusion[9]. This brief review will confine itself to an overview of the spectrum of metabolic factors which might contribute to the pathogenesis of ventricular arrhythmias specifically associated with acute myocardial ischaemia or infarction. The mechanisms of reperfusion arrhythmias and their possible metabolic basis are discussed in Chapter 3.

Recent advances have occurred in two main areas: first, concerning the relation of fluctuations in circulating levels of hormones, electrolytes and myocardial substrates to arrhythmogenesis during acute myocardial infarction; and second concerning the specific biochemical and metabolic changes within cardiac tissue which might have adverse electrophysiological effects and promote arrhythmogenesis. These latter studies are by necessity experimental and have focussed primarily on the biochemical mechanisms underlying arrhythmogenesis during very early ischaemia which is of relevance to the clinical problem of sudden cardiac death. However, it must be recognized that the electrophysiological mechanisms of these very early arrhythmias, occurring within minutes of a coronary occlusive event, differ from those occurring some hours later during evolving infarction. Accordingly any evidence

15

implicating metabolic or biochemical derangements in their pathogenesis cannot necessarily be extrapolated from one to the other.

Metabolic influences on arrhythmogenesis during acute myocardial infarction

Acute myocardial infarction is accompanied by a marked generalized
stress reaction[10] with activation of cardiosympathetic and sympatho-
adrenal reflexes[11] and neuroendocrine and peripheral metabolic changes
any of which singly or in combination might modulate myocardial
vulnerability to arrhythmogenesis. Plasma catecholamines are elevated
within the first 15 minutes of coronary occlusion[12] and both peripheral
and intramyocardial lipolysis are stimulated causing a 3- or 4-fold
elevation in plasma levels of free fatty acids and a corresponding increase
in myocardial oxygen consumption[13]. Plasma glucose is also elevated
due to the enhanced hepatic mobilization of glucose, α-adrenergic suppression of insulin release and increased plasma levels of cortisol, glu-
cagon and growth hormone possibly resulting in hypokalaemia and
hypomagnesaemia[14,15], attributable, at least in part, to β_2 adrenoceptor
mediated effects of catecholamines[16,17].

To disentangle which of these varied responses might contribute to
arrhythmogenesis poses some difficulties. Myocardial ischaemic injury
itself might promote arrhythmogenesis regardless of extracardiac
factors. In addition it is well established that cardiac sympathetic stimulation and autonomic neural imbalances can be powerfully arrhythmogenic under certain conditions[11,18]. To what extent therefore alterations in circulating plasma catecholamines, electrolyte shifts or enhanced
supply of the myocardial substrates glucose and free fatty acids might
modulate electrophysiological responses, either directly or more indirectly, by enhancing the rate of progression of ischaemic injury, is a
subject of current controversy.

Are circulating catecholamines arrhythmogenic?

Both plasma levels and urinary excretion of catecholamines can be
markedly elevated within the first 24 hours of onset of myocardial
infarction[19]. Moreover, these changes roughly parallel the severity of
infarction and the incidence of complications including serious ventricular arrhythmias[19]. The question has arisen, therefore, as to whether
clinical correlations between elevated circulating levels of catecholamines and arrhythmias might be more a reflection of the extent of
infarction and associated sympatho-adrenal stimulation than any direct
arrhythmogenic effect of circulating catecholamines themselves.

However, distinction must be made between the possible arrhythmogenic effects of adrenaline and of noradrenaline. Most studies have
demonstrated higher plasma noradrenaline than adrenaline levels during
the early hours of acute infarction[20-22]. Moreover, these elevations of

plasma noradrenaline are likely in large part to represent neural spillover from associated enhanced sympathetic activity[23] and might not therefore exert significant additional arrythmogenic effects. Plasma adrenaline by contrast is largely derived by secretion from the adrenal medulla. Although plasma levels are lower than those of noradrenaline during acute infarction, adrenaline has 10 times the potency of noradrenaline and even small fluctuations in plasma levels might exert haemodynamic, metabolic or electrophysiological effects which could be powerful stimuli to arrhythmogenesis[23].

A practical difficulty in answering this question has been the imprecision of earlier methods for assaying catecholamines – now largely resolved with the advent of a sensitive radioenzymatic technique[24]. This may account, for example, for the failure of some earlier studies to demonstrate a correlation between total catecholamine levels and arrhythmogenesis during the early hours of acute myocardial infarction[12]. It is of interest, therefore, that using these improved assay techniques Bertel et al. have reported a significant correlation between plasma adrenaline, but not plasma noradrenaline, and the severity of ventricular arrhythmias during the early hours of acute myocardial infarction in a series of 41 patients. Moreover, these changes were unrelated to differences in left ventricular dysfunction[22] (see Figure 2.1). Perhaps not surprisingly, however, both adrenaline and noradrenaline levels have been found to be markedly elevated in patients developing ventricular fibrillation[22,25].

Elevations in plasma catecholamines may be transient, and isolated estimations without reference to the time of onset of arrhythmias may thus be misleading. Spontaneous fluctuations of plasma adrenaline levels (as much as 15 fold) have been observed over periods of less than 30 minutes in association with episodes of chest pain[21], and similar but smaller fluctuations in both plasma adrenaline and noradrenaline have been observed in 9 of 27 patients studied in our own Coronary Care Unit again during the early hours of acute myocardial infarction[26] (an example is shown in Figure 2.2). In neither study was sufficient data obtained to directly relate the timing of these fluctuations to arrhythmogenesis. However, experimental evidence indicates that exposure of ischaemic tissue to catecholamine fluctuations of such an order of magnitude could induce enhanced automaticity, ameliorate conduction blocks and increase dispersion of refractoriness thus enhancing ventricular vulnerability to arrhythmogenesis[27].

Are free fatty acids arrhythmogenic?

That intracellular accumulation of free fatty acids or their derivatives might be arrhythmogenic was first proposed by Kurien and Oliver in 1970 in their much quoted 'free fatty acid hypothesis'[1]. This hypothesis was based on the findings of a crude, but positive, relationship between the incidence of ventricular fibrillation and elevated plasma levels of free

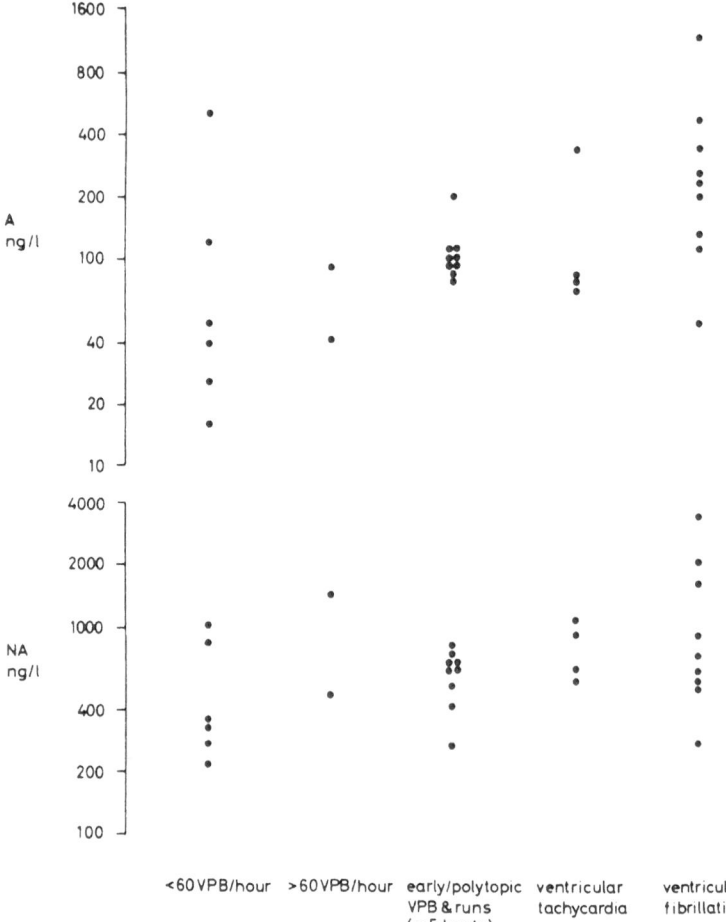

Figure 2.1 The relationship between plasma catecholamine concentrations and progressive severity of ventricular arrhythmias during acute myocardial infarction. A significant trend is demonstrated between adrenaline but not noradrenaline levels and arrhythmias. (Reproduced with permission from reference 22)

fatty acids in patients within the first 24 hours after onset of symptoms of acute myocardial infarction. However, plasma catecholamines were not assayed, and it could not, therefore, be established to what extent plasma free fatty acid elevations were causally related to arrhythmias, were a consequence of sympatho–adrenal activation, or acted synergistically with effects of adrenergic stimulation which itself might be arrhythmogenic.

Although several subsequent studies failed to confirm a similar association, several could be criticized on methodological grounds for assaying plasma free fatty acids after treatment with heparin – this releases the

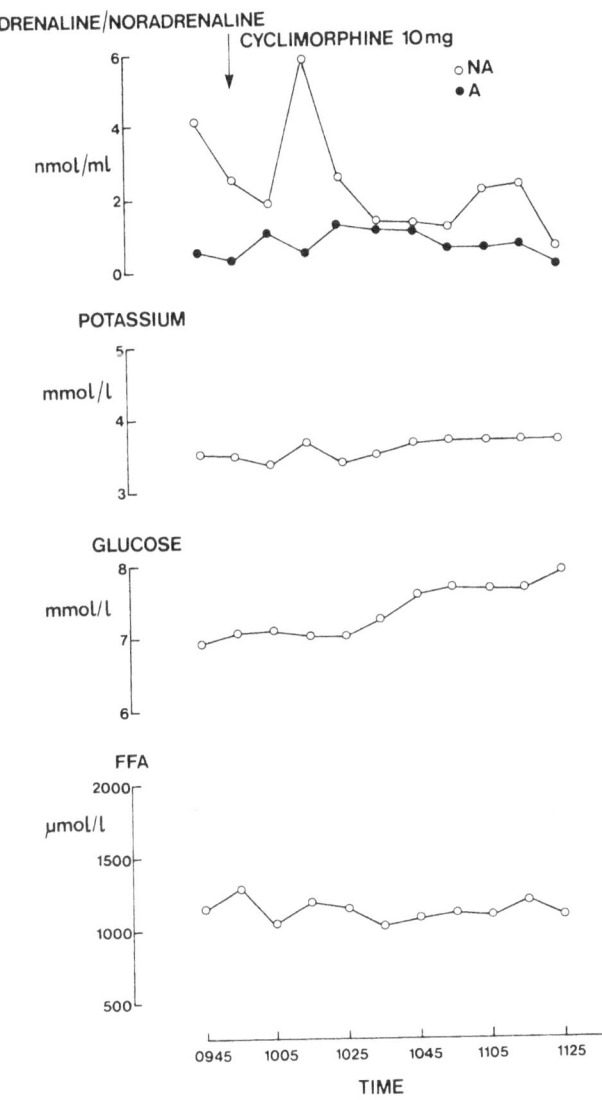

Figure 2.2 Spontaneous fluctuations in plasma catecholamines, potassium, glucose and free fatty acid in association with an episode of chest pain in a patient studied 6–8 hours after onset of symptoms of myocardial infarction

enzyme lipoprotein lipase from endothelium and so enhances *in vitro* lipolysis giving spuriously high plasma free fatty acid levels[27]. More recently Tansey and Opie have confirmed such an association, and have demonstrated a better correlation between mean rather than peak plasma free fatty acid levels and ventricular arrhythmias during the first

Table 2.1 Incidence of ventricular tachycardia during acute myocardial infarction

Delay from onset (h)	3–12	Nicotinic acid analogue within 5	5–12
FFA levels			
>50% fall in 4 h <800 μmol/1 for 20 h	42%	0%**	70%
<50% fall in 4 h >800 μmol/l	70%	29%	77%

*p <0.01   **p <0.003
Reproduced with permission from Reference 30.

12 hours of acute myocardial infarction[28]. Plasma catecholamines again were not assayed and their independent predictive value not assessed. Nevertheless these and other observations have led to an additional proposal that elevated levels of plasma free fatty acids could contribute to arrythmogenesis by initiating a vicious cycle of increasing myocardial metabolic demand, hence increasing ischaemic injury and increasing sympatho-adrenal activation leading in turn to further stimulation of lipolysis, elevation of plasma free fatty acid levels and further enhancement of ischaemic injury[29].

Perhaps the best supportive evidence for an independent arrhythmogenic effect of free fatty acids still derives from the early study of Rowe et al., which demonstrated a significant reduction in the incidence of ventricular tachycardias in patients during the early hours of acute myocardial infarction following administration of the antilipolytic agent 5-fluoronicotinic acid[30]. This effect was only apparent in those patients showing a rapid normalization of plasma free fatty acid levels, and was unrelated to alterations in haemodynamics or plasma catecholamines (see Table 2.1). Antilipolytic agents, however, have the action not only to suppress peripheral lipolysis but also to inhibit intramyocardial lipolysis which in turn may be greatly accelerated by both sympathetic neural stimulation and myocardial ischaemic injury[2,31]. Indeed enhanced intramyocardial lipolysis can account for up to 45% of increased myocardial oxygen consumption in the catecholamine stimulated human heart, and can be further enhanced by elevated plasma free fatty acid levels and increased myocardial free fatty acid uptake[31]. It seems probable, therefore, that these antiarrhythmic effects of inhibition of lipolysis may be more a reflection of intramyocardial metabolic changes than a direct response to reduced plasma levels of free fatty acids.

More indirect supportive evidence for a independent arrhythmogenic role of free fatty acids derives from the effects of glucose–insulin–potassium infusions in myocardial infarction. Using one such regime Rogers et al. observed a 50% reduction in the incidence of ventricular tachycardia[32], but found that this effect was only apparent in patients in whom suppression of lipolysis and marked reduction of plasma free fatty acid levels was achieved.

The original suggestion that intracellular accumulation of free 'unbound' fatty acids within ischaemic tissue may have toxic electrophysiological effects now seems untenable, as direct measurements of absolute levels show these to be extremely low[33]. Experimental evidence indicates, however, that the progressive accumulation during ischaemia of lipid derivatives such as long chain acyl carnitine or lysophosphoglycerides, derived by hydrolysis of membrane phospholipid, could fulfil this role[3,34]. It may also be relevant that intracellular lipid deposits have been observed within the cytoplasm of Purkinje fibres, demonstrating enhanced automatic activity, taken experimentally from hearts within the first 24 hours of experimental infarction and which are no longer present some weeks later when automatic arrhythmias have resolved[35].

Hypokalaemia and ventricular arrhythmias

Several studies have shown a clear association between hypokalaemia and arrhythmias during the early hours of acute myocardial infarction[36-39]. It still remains to be established to what extent lowering of plasma potassium is an independent risk factor for arrhythmogenesis rather than a marker of associated enhanced sympathetic activity, increased circulating levels of catecholamines or of poor left ventricular function requiring diuretic therapy, each of which themselves may enhance the risk of arrhythmogenesis.

Perhaps arguing against an independent role of hypokalaemia are the observations of a lack of association between hypokalaemia and ventricular arrhythmias arising later than 8 hours after onset of symptoms of infarction[14], and that as many as two thirds of hypokalaemic patients have received diuretic therapy for cardiac failure and left ventricular dysfunction[40]. Many patients have also received digitalis, which may itself provoke arrhythmias particularly in the presence of low potassium levels. It is now established that, at least in normal subjects, infusion of adrenaline concentrations similar to those pertaining during acute myocardial infarction can induce an abrupt fall in potassium levels, and that this effect is inhibited by β_2-adrenoceptor blockade[16,17]. Such a mechanism might account for the 22% of patients, in one series of 106 patients admitted within the first 4 hours of onset of symptoms, with hypokalaemia unassociated with diuretic therapy. Furthermore, observations that similar elevations in plasma potassium followed treatment with a non-selective β-adrenoceptor blocking agent in both diuretic and non-diuretic treated patients suggest that catecholamine induced hypokalaemia could operate whether or not patients were receiving diuretics[15,40]. In our own small series of 27 patients studied during the first 12 hours of the onset of symptoms of myocardial infarction, transient spontaneous fluctuations of plasma potassium of up to 0.7 mmol/l were detected within 2 hour sampling periods which showed no apparent relation to associated fluctuations in plasma adrenaline levels[25] (see

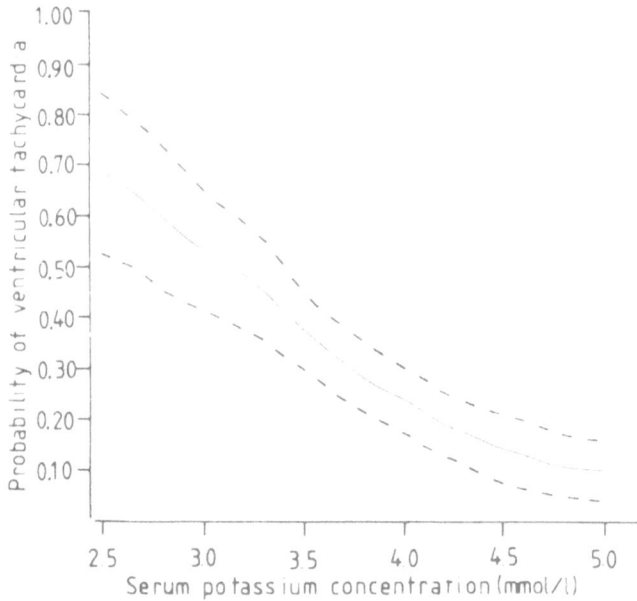

Figure 2.3   The probability of ventricular tachycardia in relation to serum potassium concentration. (Reproduced with permission from reference 38)

Figure 2.3). It is possible, therefore, that additional mechanisms may contribute to potassium shifts at this time, and that transient cardiac electrophysiological effects of hypokalaemia could occur independent of catecholamines.

Further arguing in favour of some arrhythmogenic effect of hypo-kalaemia independent of catecholamines are those observations of a higher incidence of ventricular fibrillation during acute myocardial infarction in hypokalaemic patients treated with a selective rather than non-cardioselective β-adrenoceptor blocker[15]. There is no doubt that decreased potassium levels *per se* can induce electrocardiographic changes and will exert cellular electrophysiological effects. In addition, Nordrehaug *et al.* have described a higher incidence of ventricular fib-rillation in hypokalaemic patients with acute myocardial infarction – in 93 of 1074 such patients developing ventricular fibrillation 17.2% were hypokalaemic compared with 7.5% who were normokalaemic[36,40]. More recently the same group report an inverse relationship between serum potassium and both the frequency of ventricular premature beats and of non-sustained tachycardia independent of several other risk factors[38], although plasma catecholamine estimations were not included. Data based on their regression analyses are shown in Figure 2.3. As cate-cholamine levels have not to my knowledge been determined in any clinical study correlating plasma potassium to arrhythmogenesis during acute myocardial infarction it cannot yet be concluded to what extent hypokalaemia is an independent arrhythmogenic factor. At least one other large prospective study failed to show a significant association between hypokalaemia and arrhythmias during acute myocardial infarction, although a weak trend was present[41].

Hypomagnesaemia

An inverse relation has also been demonstrated between serum magnesium and ventricular tachycardia during acute myocardial infarction, although correlations are less strong than for potassium[38]. Interestingly, the hypomagnesaemia associated with acute myocardial infarction could also be a consequence of catecholamine stimulation; it can be induced by adrenaline infusions in normal subjects[15]. In addition, in a series of 24 patients mean plasma magnesium levels have been found to rise from 0.9 to 1.03 mmol/l between the second and seventh days post-infarction, presumably in association with falling plasma catecholamine levels[15]. Certainly hypomagnesaemia can enhance automatic activity experimentally and could be an additional arrhythmogenic influence.

Myocardial metabolic factors and the genesis of early ischaemic ventricular arrhythmias

A number of controversial hypotheses have been proposed over the last few years linking the biochemical changes associated with acute myocardial ischaemia to the pathogenesis of ventricular arrhythmias and ventricular fibrillation[1–5,8]. The most important of these relate to the possible roles of altered cellular energy metabolism, the intracellular accumulation of electrophysiologically active lipid metabolites and derangements of catecholamine and prostanoid metabolism (see Table 2.2).

Prior to discussion of the evidence relating to these hypotheses some brief consideration of the intracellular biochemical response to acute myocardial ischaemia is perhaps in order. This is more comprehensively reviewed elsewhere[42].

The immediate effect of coronary occlusion is to restrict coronary blood flow and hence oxygen and substrate supply to the myocardium. Tissue oxygen tension rapidly falls and regional cyanosis and contraction abnormalities appear within 5 seconds. By 1 minute of ischaemia high energy phosphate levels have fallen, initially creatine phosphate and then ATP, and intracellular and extracellular acidosis progressively develops. At the same time a major shift in cellular energy metabolism occurs away from the normal oxidation of free fatty acids towards the aerobic and anaerobic metabolism of glucose. Glycogenolysis is greatly stimulated to provide a limited supply of ATP through glycolysis. Moreover, this may be transiently stimulated by as much as 20 or 30 fold within the first 5 minutes of ischaemia. Potassium, lactate, adenosine and inosine leak into the extracellular space, their extracellular accumulation

Table 2.2 Possible metabolic influences on arrhythmogenesis during early myocardial ischaemia

---

1. *Ionic shifts*
      Increased extracellular potassium
      Acidosis

2. *Electrophysiologically active metabolites*
      Lactate
      Long chain acyl carnitine
      Lysophosphoglycerides
      Lipid peroxidation products
      Free oxygen radicals

3. *Abnormal adrenergic mechanisms*
      Local noradrenaline release
      Enhanced α-adrenergic responsiveness
      Impaired neurotransmission
      Impaired adenylate cyclase activity
      Cyclic AMP

4. *Cellular energy status*
      ATP, ADP, AMP, creatine phosphate
      Myocardial glycogen stores

5. *Others*
      Prostanoids
      Histamine
      Linoleic acid

---

being enhanced by impaired coronary venous flow. Meanwhile various lipid metabolites accumulate within the cell, including long chain acyl carnitines and lysophosphoglycerides. Neuronal noradrenaline release may also be initially impaired, but later massive release may occur into the myocardium as energy dependent transport mechanisms fail.

The relation of these various effects to arrhythmogenesis will be considered.

Ionic imbalances

It has been suggested that elevations in extracellular potassium and inhomogeneities in its distribution might account for the majority of observed electrophysiological inhomogeneities of conduction and refractoriness preceding ventricular fibrillation during early ischaemia. Extracellular potassium sensitive electrode recordings demonstrate that tissue levels can rise to between 12 and 15 mmol/l within the first 5 minutes following coronary occlusion[43,44]. Changes of this order would be expected to cause partial depolarization and alterations in action potential morphology similar to those of ischaemia. Recently, however, Kleber et al.[45] have compared the effects of increasing extracellular potassium on conduction velocities in isolated porcine hearts with effects recorded during regional ischaemia. Potassium shifts alone could only account for about one half of the conduction changes during ischaemia in both longitudinal and transverse fibre orientations. The inference, therefore, is that other metabolic changes must mediate some electrophysiological responses.

Associated tissue acidosis, which can attain levels of pH 6.7 or less within 5 minutes of ischaemia, could further modulate responses, as acidosis can independently depress conduction velocity and impair cell-to-cell conduction in isolated tissue.

'Arrhythmogenic' metabolites

Several compounds have been identified which accumulate within ischaemic tissues, and also exert toxic electrophysiological effects similar to changes observed during ischaemia when superfused over isolated cardiac tissue. The most important of these include long chain acyl carnitine and lysophosphoglycerides derived from membrane phospholipid[3,34]. Corr and others[3] have argued that the electrophysiological effects of these compounds occur at tissue concentrations comparable to those found in ischaemia, and that they could be important mediators of many of the electrophysiological abnormalities of early myocardial ischaemia. Much dispute has arisen, however, concerning whether true tissue levels are much lower and whether some electrophysiological responses are merely non-specific detergent effects. Knabb et al.[46] have recently elegantly addressed this question with respect to long chain acyl carnitine. Quantitative electronmicroscopic autoradiography was used to determine the intracellular distribution of this compound in hypoxic neonatal rat myocytes. A 70-fold increase in the concentration of long chain acyl carnitine was found in sarcolemmal membranes in association with electrophysiological changes of loss of action potential amplitude and upstroke velocity, and these electrophysiological changes could be partially reversed by administration of an inhibitor of carnitine acyl transferase. However, the possibility was not excluded that some effects of this inhibitor were not mediated by stimulation of glycolytic activity as is found with the similar agent oxfenacine.

Accumulation of free oxygen radicals and lipid peroxidation products might also exert toxic electrophysiological effects and are currently under investigation.

Cyclic nucleotides

Podzuweit et al.[5] proposed the hypothesis, in 1976, that intracellular accumulation of cyclic AMP might be arrhythmogenic. This was supported by observations of elevated tissue levels of cyclic AMP immediately preceding ventricular fibrillation in coronary ligated baboon hearts. However, two recent papers have provided evidence which fails to confirm this hypothesis. First, administration of the drug forskolin, which greatly elevates tissue levels of cyclic AMP by stimulating adenylate cyclase, has been found to suppress arrhythmias in the coronary ligated rat heart as compared to the pro-arrhythmic effects of adrenaline at lower levels of tissue cyclic AMP[47]. In addition, in studies using a pig model of acute myocardial ischaemia administration of a β-adrenoceptor blocking agent was found to reduce the incidence of ventricular fibrillation in the presence of an increase in tissue cyclic AMP[48]. These authors still argue, however, that cyclic AMP may play a role in some forms of ischaemic arrhythmias.

Catecholamines

Both sympathetic neural stimulation and administration of catecholamines to the ischaemic heart can greatly enhance its vulnerability to the genesis of ventricular tachyarrhythmias[26]. That local release of noradrenaline within ischaemic tissue may also play a role has been suggested by the observations of Ebert and others[49] that chronic but not acute cardiac denervation can have antiarrhythmic effects. It has not yet been clearly established whether this mechanism operates as early as the first 5 minutes of ischaemic injury. Studies in the rat heart have demonstrated some impairment of sympathetic neurotransmission after 10 minutes of severe ischaemia, and a later massive noradrenaline release following failure of energy dependent transport mechanisms at the nerve terminals[50]. Electrophysiological responses may also be further modulated during ischaemia by impairment of adenylate cyclase activity or by enhanced α-adrenergic responsiveness. Given the metabolic heterogeneity of early ischaemia many of these effects could contribute to observed electrophysiological heterogeneities.

Prostanoids

Several prostanoids have been shown to have either proarrhythmic or antiarrhythmic effects[8]. In addition, the hypothesis has been proposed that the balance of local thromboxane A2 and prostacyclin release may be an important arrhythmogenic influence[8]. Inhibition of thromboxane A2 synthesis by low dose aspirin or doxaziben, pharmacological blockade of thromboxane A2 receptors and infusions of prostacyclin analogues can, for example, suppress early ischaemic arrhythmias in animal models. It remains unclear, however, whether these effects relate to alterations in vascular tone or platelet aggregation in the microcirculation.

Linoleic acid

The possibility that membrane linoleic acid might be an endogenous antiarrhythmic agent has been suggested by Lepran et al.[51]. Marked protection against early ischaemic ventricular fibrillation was found after the pretreatment of rats with a linoleic acid rich diet. Moreover, 'quinidine-like' changes were observed in isolated atrial tissue from these animals. Similar antiarrhythmic effects have been confirmed by others.

High energy phosphates

Adequate intracellular levels of ATP are necessary for the maintenance of several electrophysiological processes, including ionic pumping and slow inward channel activity which become deranged during ischaemia[52]. Moreoever, this ATP is derived largely from the anaerobic phase of glycolysis. It has, therefore, been suggested that regional inhomogeneities of ATP production within ischaemic myocardium might directly, or indirectly through effects on accumulation of metabolites or ionic shifts, influence abnormal patterns of impulse propagation resulting in ventricular fibrillation[53]. In support of this concept are our own findings in dogs of more marked heterogeneities, in not only tissue ATP but also cardiac glycogen and lactate, at the time of onset of early ischaemic ventricular fibrillation, in contrast to non-fibrillating hearts (Figure 2.4).

Myocardial glycogen

Enhancement of myocardial glycogen stores can ameliorate the metabolic response to ischaemia by providing added substrate to sustain aerobic and anaerobic glycolytic ATP production following coronary occlusion[54]. The possibility arises, therefore, that enhancement of myocardial glycogen stores might be protective against ischaemic arrhythmias. Our own biochemical mapping studies in dogs have demonstrated lower tissue glycogen levels in hearts which fibrillate than in hearts which do not, despite comparable levels of ATP and collateral perfusion to the ischaemic zone[55]. These findings have led to the hypothesis that prior myocardial glycogen depletion might predispose to ventricular fibrillation during early ischaemia by promoting more heterogeneous patterns of glycolytic activity and hence inhomogeneity of electrophysiological responses.

CLINICAL IMPLICATIONS

Many serious ventricular arrhythmias associated with acute myocardial ischaemia or infarction appear refractory to conventional anti-arrhythmic therapy. However, evidence is accumulating to suggest that many of these arrhythmias could derive from the electrophysiological effects of specific biochemical or metabolic changes within ischaemic myocardium and further, that the threshold for arrhythmogenesis may be modulated by exposure of ischaemic tissue to altered circulating levels of electrolytes, hormones and substrates of myocardial metabolism. Although the clinical relevance of many effects remains as yet incom-

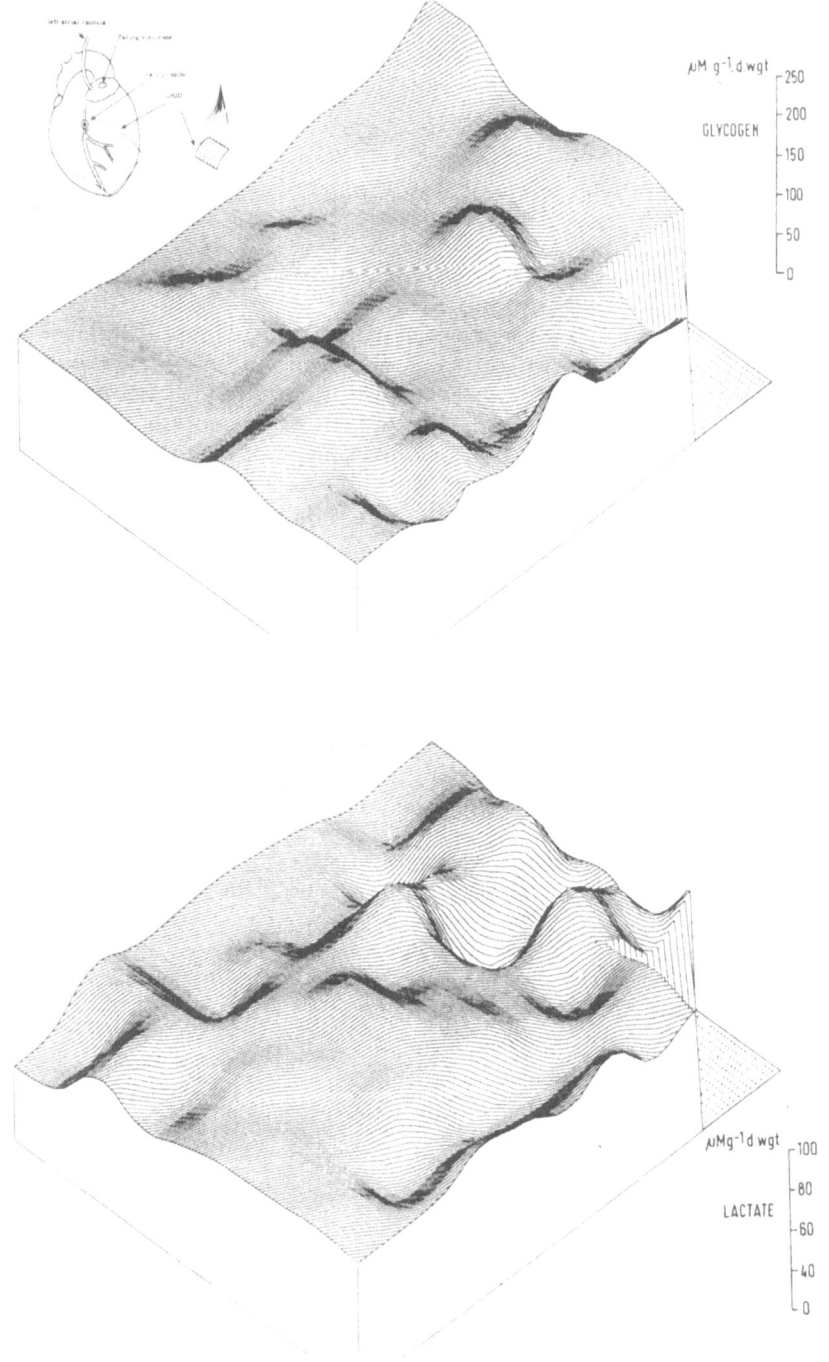

$\mu M \ g^{-1} \ d \ wgt$ — 250

GLYCOGEN — 200

— 150

— 100

— 50

— 0

$\mu M g^{-1} d \ wgt$ — 100

— 80

LACTATE — 60

— 40

— 0

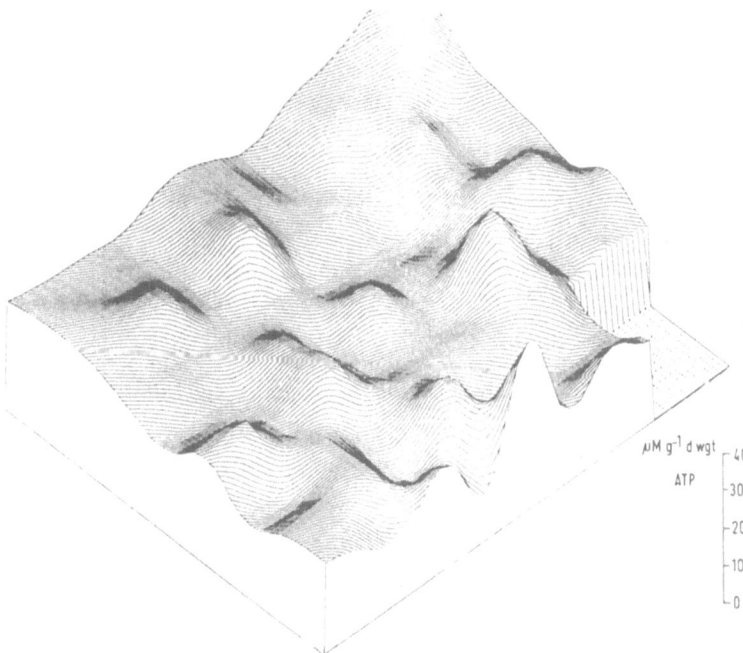

Figure 2.4 Maps of the patterns of distribution of glycogen, lactate and ATP within a 4 × 5 cm area of left ventricular dog epicardium at the time of onset of early ischaemic ventricular fibrillation. The area of interest is shown in the inset. Note the inhomogeneous distribution particularly of glycogen and ATP within ischaemic areas

pletely understood their better definition and diagnosis should provide a more rational basis for prophylaxis and management.

References

1. Kurien, V. A. and Oliver, M. F. (1970). A metabolic cause of arrhythmias during myocardial hypoxia. *Lancet*, **1**, 813–16
2. Russell, D. C. and Oliver, M. F. (1984). Free fatty acids, catecholamines and arrhythmias in man. In Ferrari, R., Katz, A. M., Shug, A. and Visioli, O. (eds.), *Myocardial Ischemia and Lipid Metabolism*. pp. 307–28 (NY, London: Plenum Press)
3. Corr, P. B. (1982). Potential arrhythmogenic role of biochemical factors in sudden cardiac death. In Sobel, B. E., Dingell, J. V. and Mock, M. B. (eds.) *Electrophysiological Mechanisms Underlying Sudden Cardiac Death*. pp. 105–30 (Mount Kisco, NY: Futura)
4. Opie, L. H. (1985). Products of myocardial ischemia and electrical instability of the heart. *J. Am. Coll. Cardiol.*, **5**, 162B–5B
5. Podzuweit, T., Lubbe, W. F. and Opie, L. H. (1976). Cyclic adenosine monophosphate, ventricular fibrillation and antiarrhythmic drugs. *Lancet*, **1**, 341–2
6. Helfant, R. H. (1986). Hypokalaemia and arrhythmias. *Am. J. Med.*, **80** (Supp. 4A), 13–22
7. Wolff, A. A. and Levi, R. (1986). Histamine and cardiac arrhythmias. *Circ. Res.*, **58**, 2–15
8. Coker, S. J. (1982). Early ventricular arrhythmias arising from acute myocardial

ischaemia; possible involvement of prostaglandins and thromboxanes. In Parrat, J. R. (ed.) *Early Arrhythmias Resulting from Myocardial Ischaemia.* pp. 219–38 (London: Macmillan Press)

9. Bigger, J. J., Dresdale, R. J., Heissenbuttel, J., Weld, F. M. and Wit, A. L. (1977). Ventricular arrhythmias in ischaemic heart disease: mechanism, prevalence, significance and management. *Progr. Cardiovasc. Dis.*, 19, 255–300

10. Vetter, N., Strange, R. C., Adams, W. and Oliver, M. F. (1974). Initial metabolic and hormonal response to acute myocardial infarction. *Lancet*, 1, 284–8

11. Robertson, D., Hollister, A. S., Forman, M. B. and Robertson, R. M. (1985). Reflexes unique to myocardial ischemia and infarction. *J. Am. Coll. Cardiol.*, 5, 99B-104B

12. Strange, R. C., Vetter, N., Rowe, M. J. and Oliver, M. F. (1974). Plasma cyclic AMP and total catecholamines during acute myocardial infarction in man. *Eur. J. Clin. Invest.*, 4, 115

13. Mjos, O. D. (1971). Effect of FFA on myocardial function and oxygen consumption in intact dogs. *J. Clin. Invest*, 50, 1386

14. Nordrehaug, J. E. (1985). Hypokalaemia, arrhythmias and early prognosis in acute myocardial infarction. *Acta Med. Scand.*, 217, 219

15. Johansson, B. W. (1986). Effect of beta blockade on ventricular fibrillation and ventricular tachycardia induced circulatory arrest in acute myocardial infarction. *Am. J. Cardiol.*, 51, 34F–7F

16. Brown, M. J., Brown, D. C. and Murphy, M. B. (1983). Hypokalaemia from beta2-receptor stimulation by circulating epinephrine. *N. Engl. J. Med.*, 309, 1414

17. Reid, J. L., Whyte, K. F. and Struthers, A. D. (1986). Epinephrine induced hypokalaemia: the role of beta adrenoceptors. *Am. J. Cardiol.*, 57, 23F–7F

18. Corr, P. B., Yamada, K. A. and Witkowski, F. X. (1986). Mechanisms controlling cardiac autonomic function and their relation to arrhythmogenesis. In Fozzard, H. A., Haber, E., Jennings, R. B., Katz, A. M. and Morgan, H. E. (eds.) *The Heart and Cardiovascular System*, pp. 1343–404 (New York: Raven Press)

19. Valori, C., Thomas, M. and Shillingford, J. P. (1967). Urinary excretion of free noradrenaline and adrenaline following acute myocardial infarction. *Lancet*, 1, 127

20. Mueller, H. S. and Ayres, S. M. (1978). Metabolic responses of the heart in acute myocardial infarction in man. *Am. J. Cardiol.*, 42, 363–71

21. Karlsberg, R. P., Cryer, P. E. and Roberts, R. (1981). Serial plasma catecholamine response early in the course of clinical acute myocardial infarction: relationship to infarct extent and mortality. *Am. Heart J.*, 102, 24–9

22. Bertel, O., Buhler, F. R., Baitsch, G., Ritz, R. and Burkart, F. (1982). Plasma adrenaline and noradrenaline in patients with acute myocardial infarction. Relationship to ventricular arrhythmias of varying severity. *Chest*, 82, 64–8

23. Cryer, P. E. (1980). Physiology and pathophysiology of the human sympathoadrenal neuroendocrine system. *N. Engl. J. Med.*, 303, 436–44

24. Da Prada, M. and Zurcher, G. (1976). Simultaneous radioenzymatic determination of plasma and tissue adrenaline, noradrenaline and dopamine within the femtomole range. *Life Sci.*, 19, 1161–74

25. Little, R. A., Frayn, K. N., Randall, P. E., Stoner, H. B., Yates, D. W., Laing, D. W., Kumar, S. and Banks, J. M. (1985). Plasma catecholamines in patients with acute myocardial infarction and in cardiac arrest. *Q. J. Med.*, 54, 133–40

26. McAreavey, D., Riemersma, R. A. and Russell, D. C. (1985). Transient metabolic changes during acute myocardial infarction. *Eur. Heart J.*, 6, 58 (Abs.)

27. Riemersma, R. A., Logan, R., Russell, D. C., Smith, H. J., Simpson, J. and Oliver, M. F. (1982). Effect of plasma free fatty acid concentration after acute myocardial infarction. *Br. Heart J.*, 48, 134–9

28. Tansey, M. J. B. and Opie, L. H. (1983). Relation between plasma free fatty acids and arrhythmias within the first 12 hours of acute myocardial infarction. *Lancet*, 2, 419–21

29. Opie, L. H., Tansey, M. J. and de Leiris, J. (1984). Clinical relevance of free fatty acid excess. In Ferrari, R., Katz, A. M., Shug, A. and Visioli, O. (eds.) *Myocardial Ischaemia and Lipid Metabolism*, pp. 283–95 (NY, London: Plenum Press)

30. Rowe, M. J., Neilson, J. M. M. and Oliver, M. F. (1975). Control of ventricular arrhythmias during myocardial infarction by antilipolytic treatment using a nicotinic acid analogue. *Lancet*, **1**, 295–302
31. Simonsen, S. and Kjekshus, J. K. (1978). The effect of free fatty acids on myocardial oxygen consumption during atrial pacing and catecholamine infusion in man. *Circulation*, **58**, 484–90
32. Rogers, W. J., Stanley, A. W., Breinig, J. B., Prather, J. W., McDaniel, A. G., Maraski, R. E., Mantle, J. A., Russell, R. O. and Ruckley, L. E. (1976). Reduction of hospital mortality rate of acute myocardial infarction with glucose-insulin-potassium infusion. *Am. Heart J.*, **92**, 441–54
33. Van der Vusse, G. J., Rueman, T. H., Prinzen, F. W., Coumons, W. A. and Reneman, R. S. (1982). Uptake and tissue content of fatty acids in dog myocardium under normoxic and ischaemic conditions. *Circ. Res.*, **50**, 538–47
34. Corr, P. B., Cain, M. E., Witkowski, F. X., Price, D. A. and Sobel, B. E. (1979). Potential arrhythmogenic electrophysiological derangements in canine Purkinje fibres induced by lysophosphoglycerides. *Circ. Res.*, **44**, 822–32
35. Friedman, P. L., Fenoglio, J. J. and Wit, A. L. (1975). Time course for reversal of electrophysiological and ultrastructural abnormalities in subendocardial Purkinje fibres surviving extensive myocardial infarction in dogs. *Circ. Res.*, **36**, 127–44
36. Nordrehaug, G. and Von der Lippe, G. (1983). Hypokalaemia and ventricular fibrillation in acute myocardial infarction. *Br. Heart J.*, **50**, 525
37. Cooper, W. D., Kuan, P., Rueben, S. R. and Van den Burg, M. J. (1984). Cardiac arrhythmias following acute myocardial infarction. Associations with serum potassium level and prior diuretic therapy. *Eur. Heart J.*, **5**, 464
38. Nordrehaug, J. E., Johannessen, K. A. and Von der Lippe, G. (1985). Serum potassium concentration as a risk factor of ventricular arrhythmias early in acute myocardial infarction. *Circulation*, **71**, 645–9
39. Solomon, R. J. and Cole, A. G. (1981). Importance of potassium in patients with acute myocardial infarction. *Acta Med. Scand.*, (*Suppl.*) **647**, 87–93
40. Nordrehaug, J. E. (1985). Malignant arrhythmias in relation to serum potassium in acute myocardial infarction. *Am. J. Cardiol.*, **56**, 20D–23D
41. Adams, P., Murray, A., Higham, D., Smith, A. C., Julian, D. G. and Campbell, R. W. F. (1984). Plasma potassium and VF in acute myocardial infarction: a prospective study. *Circulation*, **70**, (Suppl. II) 1243 (Abstr.)
42. Reimer, K. A. and Jennings, R. B. (1986). Myocardial ischaemia, hypoxia and infarction. In Fozzard, H. A., Haber, E., Jennings, R. B., Katz, A. M. and Morgan, H. E. (eds.) *The Heart and the Cardiovascular System.* pp. 1343–1404 (New York: Raven Press)
43. Hill, J. L. and Gettes, L. S. (1980). Effect of acute coronary artery occlusion on local myocardial extracellular K activity in swine. *Circulation*, **61**, 768–77
44. Hirche, H. J., Franz, C., Bos, F. L., Bissig, R., Lamg, R. and Schramm, M. (1980). Myocardial extracellular K^+ and H^+ increase and noradrenaline release during coronary occlusion in pigs. *J. Mol. Cell. Cardiol.*, **12**, 579–93
45. Kleber, A. G., Janse, M. J., Wilms-Schopman, F. J. G., Wilde, A. A. M. and Coronel, R. (1986). Changes in conduction velocity during ischaemia in the isolated porcine heart. *Circulation*, **73**, 189–98
46. Knabb, M. T., Saffitz, J. E., Corr, P. B. and Sobel, B. E. (1986). The dependence of electrophysiological derangements on accumulation of endogenous long-chain acyl carnitine in hypoxic neonatal rat myocytes. *Circ. Res.*, **58**, 230–40
47. Manning, A. S., Kinoshita, K., Buschmans, E., Coltart, D. J. and Hearse, D. J. (1985). The genesis of arrhythmias during myocardial ischaemia. Dissociation between changes in cyclic adenosine monophosphate and electrical instability in the rat. *Circ. Res.*, **57**, 669–75
48. Muller, C. A., Opie, L. H., Hamm, C. W., Peisach, M. and Gihwala, D. (1986). Prevention of ventricular fibrillation by metoprolol in a pig model of acute myocardial ischaemia: absence of a major arrhythmogenic role of cyclic AMP. *J. Mol. Cell. Cardiol.*, **18**, 375–87

49. Ebert, P. A., Allgood, R. J. and Sabiston, D. C. (1968). The antiarrhythmic effects of cardiac denervation. *Ann. Surg.*, **168**, 728–35
50. Schomig, A., Dart, A. M., Dietz, R., Kubler, W. and Mayer, E. (1985). Paradoxical role of neuronal uptake for the locally mediated release of endogenous noradrenaline in the ischaemic myocardium. *J. Cardiovasc. Pharmacol.*, **7** (Suppl. 5), S40–4
51. Lepran, I., Nemecz, G., Koltoi, M. and Szekeres, L. (1981). Effect of linoleic acid rich diet on the acute phase of coronary occlusion in conscious rats. Influence of indomethacin and aspirin. *Cardiovasc. Res.*, **3**, 847–53
52. McDonald, T. F. and McLeod, D. P. (1973). Metabolism and electrical activity of anoxic ventricular muscle. *J. Physiol.*, **229**, 559–82
53. Russell, D. C., Lawrie, J. S., Riemersma, R. A. and Oliver, M. F. (1981). Metabolic aspects of rhythm disturbances. *Acta Med. Scand.*, **230**, (Suppl. 2), 71–81
54. Scheuer, J. and Stezoski, S. W. (1970). Protective role of increased myocardial glycogen stores in cardiac anoxia in the rat. *Circ. Res.*, **27**, 835–49
55. Russell, D. C., Lawrie, J. S., Whipps, D. and Riemersma, R. A. (1986). Is myocardial glycogen protective against early ischaemic ventricular fibrillation? *J. Mol. Cell. Cardiol.*, **18** (Suppl. 2), 32 (Abstr.)

3
The electrophysiology of reperfusion-induced arrhythmias following acute myocardial ischaemia

N. A. FLORES AND D. J. SHERIDAN

INTRODUCTION

The observation that reperfusion of the ischaemic myocardium frequently leads to the development of ventricular arrhythmias has become well established from results obtained during experimental studies, and from clinical observations during reperfusion[1–3]. Much useful information has been obtained during the past decade; however, the precise mechanisms which induce these arrhythmias remain incompletely understood. Experimental studies have revealed for example that ventricular fibrillation may occur more frequently on reperfusion than during the preceding period of ischaemia[4,5], however the arrhythmogenic effects of reperfusion, although intense, are short lived and this has made it difficult to provide direct evidence of their involvement in sudden cardiac death. As a result almost all of our understanding of the electrophysiological changes which are associated with the development of ventricular arrhythmias during reperfusion is based on the use of animal models. This chapter will attempt to consolidate these findings, and provide an insight into the mechanisms responsible for the arrhythmogenic effects of reperfusion.

EXPERIMENTAL OBSERVATIONS

Electrophysiological changes which occur during acute myocardial ischaemia and reperfusion have been studied using a variety of techniques and animal models from different species. Arrhythmogenesis has been studied in isolated hearts[5–10], hearts *in situ*[8,11,12], in hearts subjected to regional ischaemia induced by coronary artery occlusion[7–14], and in hearts subjected to global ischaemia[5,6]. Species studied have included cats[11], dogs[10,12], pigs[7,10], rats[8,9] and guinea pigs[5,6], and reperfusion has been studied following periods of myocardial ischaemia lasting from 1

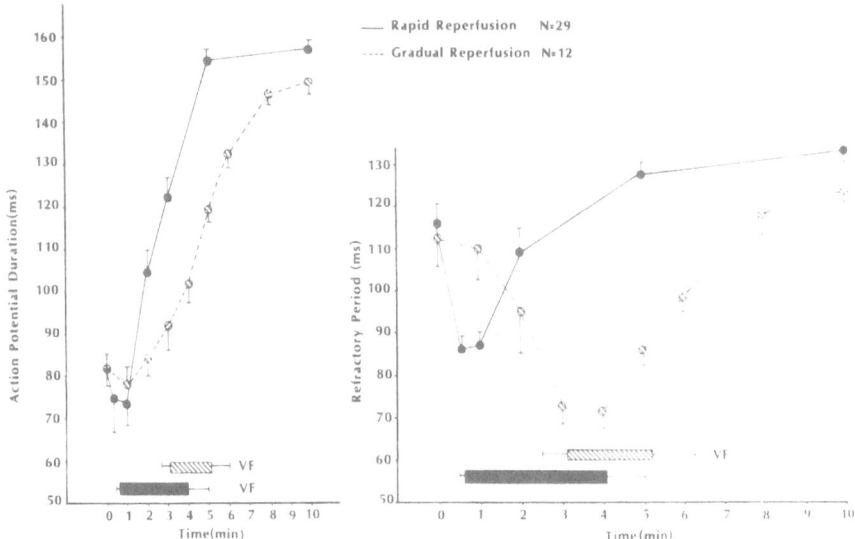

Figure 3.1 Electrophysiological changes during reperfusion. Changes in the duration of the action potential and the refractory period during rapid (●, $n = 29$) and gradual (○, $n = 12$) reperfusion of isolated perfused guinea-pig hearts. Note that reperfusion initially shortened and then lengthened the duration of the action potential and the refractory period in both groups. Ventricular fibrillation (VF) occurred in both groups to a similar extent, although the onset was delayed in the gradually reperfused hearts (horizontal bars)

to 90 minutes. Electrophysiological changes have been quantified from electrocardiograms alone[6,8,12], or in conjunction with intracellular and extracellular recordings[5,7,10]. Intracellular recordings have been made from single sites[5] and from multiple sites[7,10] to allow estimates of conduction velocity to be made in order to attempt to explain the mechanisms responsible for the initiation of the arrhythmias. These studies have enabled the effects of acute myocardial ischaemia on action potential characteristics, conduction and excitability to be examined at both the cellular and whole-heart levels.

Electrophysiology during reperfusion

Several groups have described a rapid recovery in action potential characteristics during reperfusion whether this reperfusion followed regional ischaemia[13,14] or global ischaemia[5]. The commencement of recovery invariably precedes the development of arrhythmias. To correlate the timing of electrophysiological events with the development of reperfusion arrhythmias we studied reperfusion following global ischaemia in the isolated guinea pig heart[5]. At the end of a 30 minute period of ischaemia action potential amplitude, V_{max}, and duration were all reduced. Recovery commenced within seconds of the onset of reperfusion and was complete by 15 minutes. The pattern of changes is illustrated in Figure 3.1, which shows the rapidity of recovery and its commencement well in advance of the occurrence of VF (onset time $= 81 \pm 12$ seconds). Interestingly, while recovery of action potential amplitude and V_{max} commenced immediately on reperfusion, action potential duration and refractory period underwent further transient shortening (Figure 3.1), and this appears to be a consistent precedent for the occurrence of VF on reperfusion, in that interventions which successfully prevent reperfusion VF also prevent or attenuate these changes in action potential duration and refractory period[15,16].

Understanding the factors which precipitate VF is complicated by the suddenness of the event and the complexity of electrical propagation changes associated with it. Attempts have been made to 'map' changes in propagation during the initiation of VF with considerable success[10], and there is little doubt that ventricular fibrillation is a manifestation of re-entry probably occurring at several sites within the heart simultaneously. The question remains however, as to whether the initiation of VF results from the occurrence of an ectopic beat (i.e. an automatic focus) or from re-entry following a beat which arose from the sinus node. Further work is needed to resolve this question. Certainly, attempts to prevent sudden death using antiarrhythmic drugs which alter the major determinants of re-entry (conduction and refractoriness) have been unsuccessful. It may be more important, therefore, to attend to the electrophysiological changes which destabilize the normal electro-physiological regulating mechanisms and precede the onset of VF. In other words successful prevention of VF is likely to depend more on preventing or modifying the electrophysiological effects of ischaemia and reperfusion rather than attempting to prevent its initiation in a vulnerable heart. Figure 3.2 illustrates the importance of this concept and shows electrophysiological and rhythm changes during reperfusion. In this heart, stable VT had been present for the last 3 minutes of ischaemia and was therefore present at the onset of reperfusion. As described above, electrophysiological recovery commenced immediately following the onset of reperfusion but with further shortening of action potential duration. In association with these changes, the VT which had been present at a steady rate for several minutes, accelerated and eventually degenerated into VF. The gradual acceleration in the rate of the VT indicates the crucial importance of the early electrophysiological changes on reperfusion and that the eventual conversion to VF is perhaps an inevitable, unavoidable and relatively late phenomenon. These findings suggest that in the context of ischaemic heart disease interventions targeted on the triggering of VF are less likely to be successful than prevention of the conditions which predispose to it.

CARDIAC ELECTROPHYSIOLOGY DURING MYOCARDIAL REPERFUSION

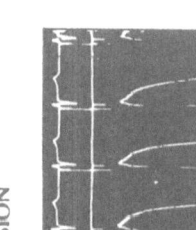

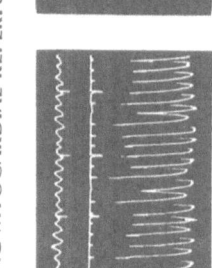

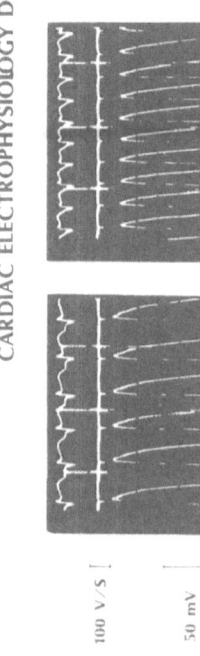

100 V/s

50 mV

0.15 minutes   0.5 minutes   1.5 minutes   9 minutes

Figure 3.2 Epicardial action potentials (lower traces), their first derivative, dV/dt (middle traces) and electrocardiograms (ECGs) recorded at various times after the onset of reperfusion following global ischaemia in an isolated guinea pig heart. Stable ventricular tachycardia had been present for several minutes at the end of the ischaemic period; with the onset of reperfusion it accelerated and led to the development of ventricular fibrillation. Coronary artery perfusion was continued (by the Langendorff technique) and a normal paced rhythm returned at 9 minutes
(Reproduced by kind permission from *Cardiovascular Research*)

FACTORS INFLUENCING THE INCIDENCE OF REPERFUSION-INDUCED ARRHYTHMIAS

Rate of reperfusion

It is often stated that abrupt reperfusion is an important prerequisite for the occurrence of arrhythmias. To study this we assessed electrophysiological changes and arrhythmias during reperfusion of abrupt or gradual onset following 30 minutes of ischaemia. Although gradual reperfusion was associated with delayed electrophysiological recovery and with a later onset of ventricular fibrillation, no difference was observed in the incidence of VT and VF (Figure 3.1). In addition the pattern of recovery was not altered qualitatively. Thus, transient reduction in action potential duration and refractory period occurred in both groups with an appropriate difference in the time course. Gradual reperfusion, therefore, modified the pattern of recovery following acute global ischaemia, but did not alter the incidence of arrhythmias.

The severity of ischaemia is likely to be an important determinant for the development of arrhythmias during subsequent reperfusion in the context of (1) degree of flow reduction, (2) amount of myocardium involved, and (3) the duration of ischaemia. A number of studies have shown that the incidence of reperfusion ventricular fibrillation is related to the duration of the preceding ischaemic period[5,17]. Reperfusion arrhythmias tend to occur most frequently following 20–30 minutes of ischaemia[5] and require a minimum period of 10–15 minutes. If the ischaemic period is prolonged for more than 60 minutes arrhythmias are less likely to occur[5] (Figure 3.3). Electrophysiological changes during reperfusion following varying periods of ischaemia are also illustrated in Figure 3.3. The reduction in arrhythmias following longer periods of ischaemia (60 min) was associated with slower and incomplete recovery. In contrast, recovery was most rapid following brief ischaemic episodes. When reperfusion followed 20–30 minutes of ischaemia and arrhythmias were most likely to occur, action potential duration underwent further transient shortening during reperfusion, in contrast to short (5 min) or long (60 min) preceding ischaemic episodes. While varying the duration of ischaemia had a substantial influence on reperfusion arrhythmias, varying the degree of flow reduction had little effect. Thus, reperfusion following zero flow ischaemia or low flow ischaemia (flow = 10% of control) produced arrhythmias to a similar extent[5]. These findings suggest that in the clinical setting of reperfusion by thrombolysis, the absence of arrhythmias on reperfusion may indicate poor myocardial recovery and, therefore, be an adverse prognostic sign.

Enhanced sympathetic activity

Increases in plasma and urine catecholamine levels are seen after myocardial infarction[18,19], and a rapid release of noradrenaline may follow periods of myocardial hypoxia or reperfusion[20]. These observations led

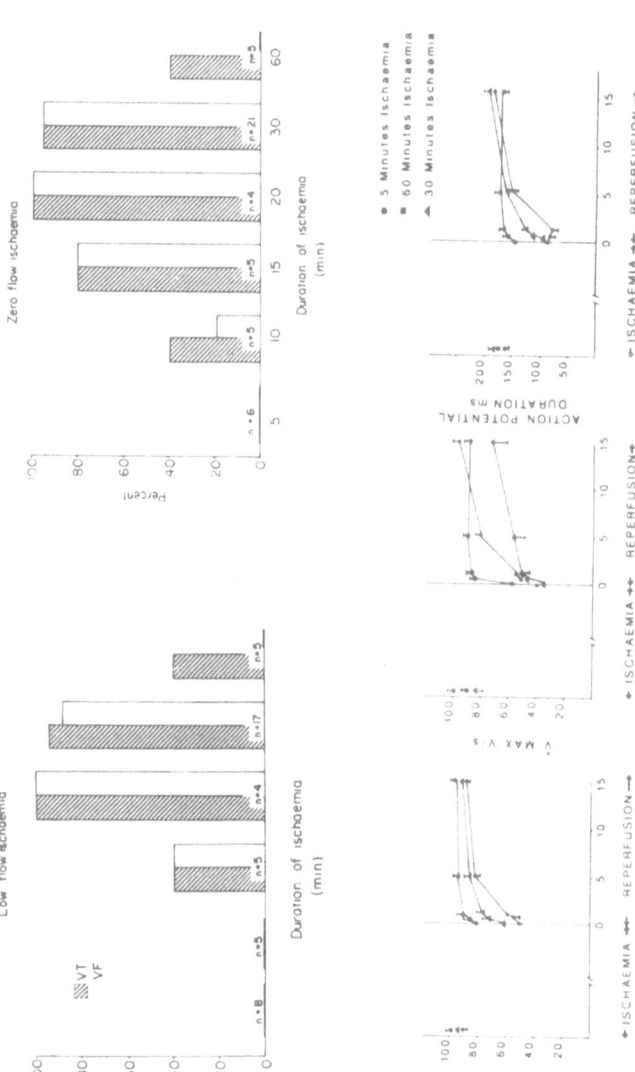

Figure 3.3 Influence of the duration of ischaemia on the percentage incidence of reperfusion-induced arrhythmias and the electrophysiology of reperfusion. A minimum of 15 and 10 min of low flow (10% of control – upper left panel) and zero flow (upper right panel) ischaemia, respectively was required for the subsequent development of reperfusion-induced arrhythmias. The incidence of both ventricular tachycardia (□) and ventricular fibrillation (▨) was maximal after 20 min of ischaemia, but fell after 60 min of ischaemia. Note that while altering the duration of ischaemia had a significant effect on the incidence of reperfusion-induced arrhythmias, the severity of the reduction of flow had little effect on their pattern. The changes in the amplitude, upstroke velocity and duration of the action potential during reperfusion after 5 (●), 30 (▲), and 60 (■) min of ischaemia are shown in the lower panel. Recovery of amplitude and upstroke velocity was most rapid after shorter periods of ischaemia. Note that the duration of the action potential was further reduced during reperfusion, but not after 5 or 60 min of ischaemia. (Data from reference 5) (Reproduced by kind permission from *Cardiovascular Research*)

to intense interest in the possibility that sympathetic activity may play an important role in the genesis of arrhythmias during ischaemia and reperfusion. Measurements during experimental ischaemia and reperfusion have demonstrated increased coronary arteriovenous noradrenaline differences at the time of onset of reperfusion arrhythmias[21], and several groups have shown that depletion of myocardial catecholamines with 6-hydroxydopamine[11,22] or reserpine[23] can prevent reperfusion-induced ventricular fibrillation. During 'normal' perfusion of the isolated guinea pig heart, myocardial catecholamine depletion prolonged action potential duration, refractory period, conduction time and QRS width, while action potential amplitude and V_{max} were unchanged[15]. The prevention of arrhythmias during ischaemia and reperfusion in these hearts was associated with the maintenance of longer action potentials and refractory periods during ischaemia, blunting of the ischaemia-induced reduction in action potential amplitude and V_{max}, and accentuation of the ischaemia-induced prolongation in conduction time and QRS width. Thus, at the onset of arrhythmias during ischaemia, control hearts had shorter action potentials, with higher V_{max} values, shorter refractory periods and more rapid conduction than depleted ones.

Antiarrhythmic effect of adrenergic blockade

Several investigators have studied the effect of α and β-adrenoceptor blockade on arrhythmias during ischaemia and reperfusion. Recent studies which examined the antiarrhythmic action of β-adrenoceptor antagonism during myocardial ischaemia without reperfusion have suggested that factors other than adrenoceptor blockade may be involved. Using a rat model of acute myocardial ischaemia induced by coronary artery ligation, both optical isomers of propranolol were equally effective in reducing the incidence of arrhythmias during ischaemia and atenolol had no antiarrhythmic action[8]. This led to the conclusion that β-adrenoceptors were not involved in the genesis of ventricular arrhythmias during ischaemia in this model. In pig hearts[24], although β-adrenoceptor blockade using metoprolol prevented ventricular fibrillation during ischaemia, propranolol and sotalol were ineffective. While adequate β-adrenoceptor antagonism was produced by all three agents, only metoprolol was antiarrhythmic, suggesting that this drug was effective by increasing blood flow which decreased the severity of ischaemia in the hearts studied[24]. Using the isolated guinea pig heart model, the effects of the β-adrenoceptor antagonist sotalol, on arrhythmias and electrophysiology during myocardial ischaemia and reperfusion were studied[25]. A concentration unlikely to be achieved therapeutically, (10^{-4} mol/l) was required to produce an antiarrhythmic effect. Increases in the number of β-adrenoceptors during ischaemia and reperfusion have been demonstrated[26], however the pathophysiological relevance of such changes remains unclear.

In the past decade, there has been considerable interest in the role of α-adrenoceptor stimulation and arrhythmias during ischaemia and reperfusion. Pretreatment with phentolamine has been shown to reduce the incidence of reperfusion-induced ventricular fibrillation[11,27,28], and this has been confirmed for a number of α-blocking agents in different animal models[11,16,29]. In addition, α-blockade was also effective when added just prior to the onset of reperfusion, suggesting that its anti-arrhythmic action is unlikely to result from a modification of the preceding ischaemic period. Phentolamine has been shown to reduce action potential V_{max} in isolated superfused myocardium[30] suggesting that its antiarrhythmic activity is related to direct myocardial action. However, its antiarrhythmic activity during ischaemia is associated with attenuation of action potential shortening and accentuation of ischaemia induced reduction in V_{max} and conduction[16]. Furthermore, when added to hearts depleted of endogenous catecholamines, phentolamine produced no additional electrophysiological effects[16]. It seems likely, therefore, that the antiarrhythmic action of drugs such as phentolamine is mediated via an adrenergic mechanism rather than through a direct myocardial electrophysiological action. The possibility of protection mediated by blockade of peripheral or coronary vascular α-adrenoceptors is also frequently put forward, although available evidence suggests that this is also unlikely, since no detectable changes in myocardial blood flow to ischaemic myocardium have been demonstrated in association with its antiarrhythmic action[11], and reversal of its haemodynamic effects does not attenuate its antiarrhythmic action[11].

Further evidence that the antiarrhythmic action of phentolamine and indoramin is due to α-adrenoceptor blockade rather than direct myocardial effects was provided by the observation that catecholamine depletion was equally effective in preventing arrhythmias and produced largely similar electrophysiological changes[15]. More importantly perhaps, the antiarrhythmic and electrophysiological actions of catecholamine depletion can be reversed by α-adrenoceptor stimulation by perfusion with methoxamine during ischaemia and reperfusion[31] (Figure 3.4). This arrhythmogenic effect of α-adrenoceptor stimulation was associated with several electrophysiological effects during ischaemia and reperfusion, namely shortening of action potential duration and refractory period (Figure 3.5), reduction in action potential amplitude and to a lesser extent, V_{max}, acceleration in conduction and reduction in QRS width, and a reduction in stimulation threshold[31]. In contrast to these changes, addition of methoxamine to normally perfused hearts had no arrhythmogenic and only minimal electrophysiological effects. Thus, α-adrenoceptor stimulation is arrhythmogenic, but only during myocardial ischaemia and reperfusion when myocardial sensitivity to its effects is increased.

Previous studies using isolated superfused myocardial preparations have demonstrated α-adrenoceptor mediated prolongation in action potential duration and refractory period, yet in isolated perfused hearts

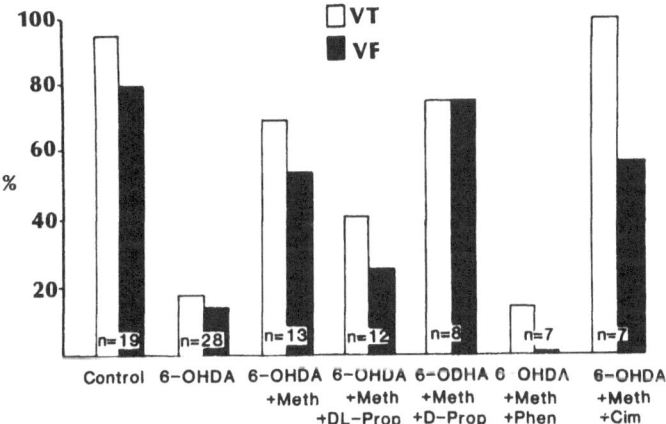

Figure 3.4 Incidence of VT and VF (■) during reperfusion in isolated Langendorff perfused guinea-pig hearts. Myocardial catecholamine depletion with 6-hydroxy-dopamine (6-OHDA) reduced VT and VF during ischaemia and reperfusion, but this was significantly reversed by the α-agonist, methoxamine (meth) independent of propranolol (prop) or H_2 receptor blockade with cimetidine (cim). In contrast, α-adrenoceptor blockade with phentolamine (phen) abolished the arrhythmogenic effect of methoxamine. (Data from reference 31)

α-adrenoceptor blockade and myocardial catecholamine depletion had similar effects. The basis for this apparent discrepancy is unclear. It may reflect a difference in the behaviour of superfused myocardial preparations and isolated perfused hearts, alternatively, it is possible that the presence of ischaemia modifies cardiac electrophysiological responses. Studies of changes in idioventricular rate during ischaemia and reperfusion support the latter explanation[11], although the mechanism responsible for enhanced sensitivity to α-adrenoceptor agonists during myocardial ischaemia and reperfusion still remains unclear. The possibility of a reversible increase in the number of α-adrenoceptors during ischaemia has been observed in the cat[32] but not in the rat[33] or guinea pig[34].

Other factors

The induction of myocardial ischaemia and its relief through reperfusion represents a complex pathophysiological picture and many other factors may be implicated in the genesis of arrhythmias in this situation. Alterations in lipid metabolism caused by myocardial ischaemia have been implicated as contributing to cell membrane dysfunction, cellular injury and arrhythmogenesis[35]. Release of prostanoids, accumulation of fatty acid esters, degradation of phospholipids and increases in lyso-phospholipids occurring during myocardial ischaemia and reperfusion have been demonstrated but proof of their direct involvement in the production of arrhythmias is still awaited. Possible arrhythmogenic effects of histamine have also come under scrutiny. Histamine has

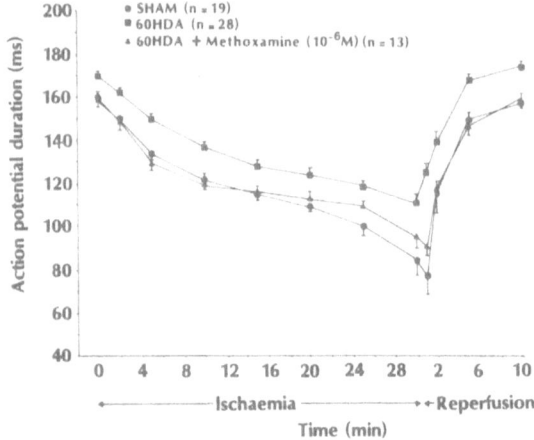

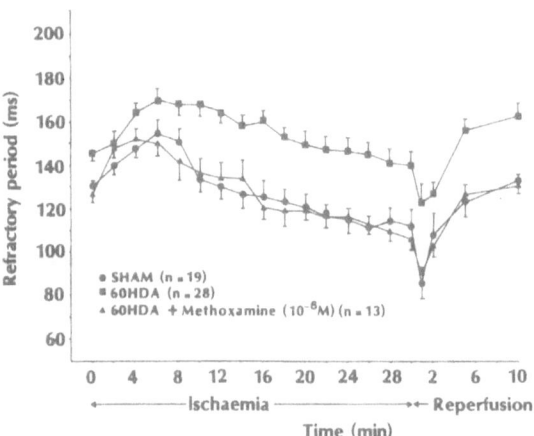

Figure 3.5 Changes in action potential duration (APD) [upper panel] and refractory period [lower panel] during ischaemia and reperfusion in isolated Langendorff perfused guinea pig hearts. APD was shortened during ischaemia in all groups. Myocardial catecholamine depletion by pretreatment with 6-hydroxydopamine (6-OHDA) prolonged APD and this effect was maintained throughout the ischaemic period. Perfusion with the α-agonist, methoxamine reversed this effect on APD, restoring values to control. Note that APD underwent further transient shortening during early reperfusion in control hearts; catecholamine depletion prevented this and methoxamine restored it. Refractory period shortened during ischaemia following initial lengthening. Catecholamine depletion prolonged refractory period and this effect was maintained throughout ischaemia and reperfusion periods; perfusion with the α-agonist, methoxamine reversed this. (Data from reference 31)

been shown to prolong atrioventricular conduction (mediated by H_1-receptors)[36] and to increase heart rate and ventricular automaticity (both mediated by H_2-receptors)[37,38] and enhanced sensitivity of ischaemic myocardium to the arrhythmogenic effects of histamine has been demonstrated in experimental preparations[39,40]. Thus, while there is some circumstantial evidence linking histamine and reperfusion arrhythmias, direct evidence of its involvement is not available.

Oxygen derived free radicals have recently been suggested as playing an important role in the genesis of reperfusion arrhythmias[41,42]. Inhibition of free radical formation or the rapid removal of formed free radicals has significant antiarrhythmic action, but the enhancement of free radical formation increases the incidence of reperfusion arrhythmias[42]. Further work is needed to identify and measure free radicals in the intact heart. Nevertheless, these observations may have considerable importance, and free radical production may provide an explanation for the reperfusion-induced injury noted in capillary endothelium and adjacent contractile cells which becomes especially prominent with reperfusion after prolonged periods of ischaemia.

Endogenous opioid peptides have also been suggested as contributing to arrhythmogenesis during myocardial ischaemia and reperfusion. This follows observations that naloxone inhibits arrhythmias during ischaemia and reperfusion in dogs[43] and that stereospecific antiarrhythmic effects of opioid receptor antagonists can be demonstrated during myocardial ischaemia in the rat[44]. The mechanism of this action has not yet been examined in detail and the evidence is, therefore, circumstantial. Central neural effects of these agents should also be considered before a link between opioid peptides and the occurrence of reperfusion arrhythmias is accepted.

CORRELATION WITH BIOCHEMICAL AND MORPHOLOGICAL CHANGES

Numerous studies have investigated the biochemical alterations which occur during the early stages of myocardial ischaemia (for review see reference 45). Interest in cyclic adenosine monophosphate (cAMP) arose because of its role in mediating adrenoceptor stimulation. Following the observation that levels of cAMP increase in the ischaemic heart, it was proposed that this increase might be a critical factor in the genesis of ventricular arrhythmias and fibrillation[46]. Indeed, several studies showed a close temporal correlation between cAMP levels and the development of ventricular fibrillation during ischaemia[47,48]. However, during reperfusion this correlation was less clear, and further recent studies question the validity of the correlation during myocardial ischaemia[9,24]. Furthermore, recent evidence suggests that increased levels of cAMP during ischaemia may not reflect levels of adrenoceptor activation, but rather a reduction in adenylate cyclase activity secondary to myocardial ischaemia[49].

The induction of acute myocardial ischaemia and its relief through reperfusion have major metabolic effects and the relationship of these to the incidence of arrhythmias has been investigated. Acute myocardial ischaemia characteristically produces depletion of high energy phosphates and accumulation of adenine nucleotide metabolites and lactate in addition to raising the levels of cAMP as described[46]. Electrical instability during reperfusion has, however, been shown not to be directly related to accumulation of lactate or increases in cAMP[6]. The energy requiring process involved in maintaining transmembrane ionic gradients would be affected by a mismatch in energy production and energy requirements resulting in alterations in intracellular and extracellular ionic concentrations. In support of this, increased potassium efflux has been demonstrated in ischaemic myocardium resulting in accumulation of extracellular potassium in areas of poor perfusion[6,50]. Such changes are likely to have an important influence on electrophysiology and arrhythmias during ischaemia and reperfusion. The situation during reperfusion, however, is further complicated by the effect of reflow and washout of accumulated products of ischaemia. A reduction towards normal extracellular potassium would be expected to occur during reperfusion, resulting in recovery in resting membrane potential and action potential amplitude and upstroke velocity. The importance of such recovery in the arrhythmogenic process is not clear, but it is likely to be important since incomplete recovery, which occurs following prolonged ischaemia, is associated with attenuation of reperfusion arrhythmias[5]. There is also evidence that calcium influx occurs during early reperfusion[51,52], and such changes could also contribute to the arrhythmogenic process by reducing refractoriness and promoting cell disruption.

The morphological changes in the coronary microcirculation and in myocardial cells which are a consequence of acute myocardial ischaemia and subsequent reperfusion have been examined in detail[53-55]. In the early stages of ischaemia, cellular changes occur which are essentially reversible, and following relief of ischaemia ultimately return to normal; however, if ischaemia is prolonged, irreversible cellular injury occurs. The time limit for reversibility appears to be 30–60 min, and subendocardial tissue appears to be more prone to injury than the subepicardium so that a wavefront of cell death progressing subepicardially has been described[56]. Morphological changes may be observed as early as 15 min after the induction of ischaemia, with margination of the nuclear chromatin and decreased cellular glycogen content. After 30–60 min of ischaemia, swelling of mitochondria occurs, associated with the appearance of amorphous bodies within them. Increased swelling of the mitochondria is followed by disruption of their cristae and outer membranes. Intracellular oedema becomes apparent with breaks in the sarcolemmal membrane which often lifts off the myofilaments. Reperfusion following prolonged ischaemia usually fails to reverse the morphological changes seen and frequently exacerbates the ultrastructural alterations, often producing marked further cellular swelling which may result in the 'no-reflow' phenomenon[55]. Following the observation of impeded reperfusion after myocardial ischaemia, attention has been directed to the changes which occur in myocardial capillaries. In the early stages of ischaemia loss of endothelial pinocytotic vesicles occurs followed by endothelial cell swelling and an increase in the numbers of intraluminal projections of the endothelial cell cytoplasm. Margination of the endothelial cell nuclear chromatin occurs, and following severe injury lasting more than 90 min, endothelial cell gaps and a general loss of integrity can be seen[55]. These changes occur later than those seen in the myocytes and generally are only evident after about 45 min of ischaemia. Attempted reperfusion at this time results in further damage to the capillary endothelium often producing such a loss of structural and functional integrity that microvascular haemorrhage occurs. An interesting observation is that areas of myocardial cell damage often occur without capillary damage, and yet damage to the microcirculation never occurs before the onset of myocardial cell damage[54]. This supports the current consensus that microvascular damage is not a primary cause of the development of irreversible ischaemic myocardial cell damage.

CONCLUSIONS

Reperfusion of ischaemic myocardium produces complex morphological, biochemical and electrophysiological events. The duration of preceding ischaemia is a major determinant of the severity of reperfusion arrhythmias. If the ischaemic period is short (< 10 minutes) arrhythmias are unlikely. Reversibility of the ischaemic process appears to be essential for the development of reperfusion arrhythmias which are uncommon following prolonged ischaemia (> 60 minutes).

Electrophysiological recovery precedes the development of reperfusion arrhythmias with further reduction in action potential duration and refractory period. Such changes may be associated with the occurrence of re-entry or automaticity, and the relative importance of each during reperfusion remains contentious. The most important events, however, are those which increase cardiac vulnerability prior to the onset of arrhythmias. There is considerable evidence linking adrenergic activity and reperfusion arrhythmias. Production of oxygen free radicals and intracellular accumulation of calcium ions may also be of considerable importance.

References

1. Rentrop, P., Blanke, H., Karsch, K.R., Kaiser, H., Kostering, H. and Leitz, K. (1981). Selective intracoronary thrombolysis in acute myocardial infarction and unstable angina pectoris. *Circulation*, 63, 307–14
2. Araki, H., Koirvaya, Y., Nakagalir, O. and Nakamura, H. (1983). Diurnal dis-

tribution of ST segment elevation and related arrhythmias in patients with variant angina: a study of ambulatory ECG monitoring. *Circulation*, **67**, 995–1000

3. Previtali, M., Klersky, C., Salerno, J. A., Chimienti, M., Panciroli, C., Marangoni, E., Specchia, G., Comolli, M. and Bobba, P. (1983). Ventricular tachyarrhythmias in Prinzmetal's variant angina: clinical significance and relation to the degree and time course of ST segment elevation. *Am. J. Cardiol.*, **52**, 19–25

4. Blumgart, H. L., Hoff, H. E., Landowne, M. and Schlesinger, M. J. (1937). Experimental studies of the effect of temporary occlusion of coronary arteries in producing persistent electrocardiographic changes. *Am. J. Med. Sci.*, **194**, 493–502

5. Penny, W. J. and Sheridan, D. J. (1983). Arrhythmias and cellular electrophysiological changes during myocardial "ischaemia" and reperfusion. *Cardiovasc. Res.*, **17**, 363–72

6. Dennis, S. C., Yellon, D. M., Frasch, F., Anderson, G. J. and Hearse, D. J. (1983). The effect of ischaemia on metabolism and arrhythmias. *Int. J. Cardiol.*, **2**, 461–76

7. Kleber, A. G., Janse, M. J., van Capelle, F. J. L. and Durrer, D. (1978). Mechanism and time course of S-T and T-Q segment changes during acute regional myocardial ischaemia in the pig heart determined by extracellular and intracellular recordings. *Circ. Res.*, **42**, 603–13

8. Daugherty, A., Frayn, K. N., Redfern, W. S. and Woodward, B. (1986). The role of catecholamines in the production of ischaemia-induced ventricular arrhythmias in the rat *in vivo* and *in vitro*. *Br. J. Pharmacol.*, **87**, 265–77

9. Manning, A. S., Rinoshita, K., Buschmans, E., Coltart, D. J. and Hearse, D. J. (1985). The genesis of arrhythmias during myocardial ischemia. Dissociation between changes in cyclic adenosine monophosphate and electrical instability in the rat. *Circ. Res.*, **57**, 668–75

10. Janse, M. J., van Capelle, F. J. L., Morsink, H., Kleber, A. G., Wilms-Schopman, F., Cardinal, R., Nauman D'Almoncourt, C. and Durrer, D. (1980). Flow of injury current and patterns of excitation during early ventricular arrhythmias in acute regional myocardial ischaemia in isolated porcine and canine hearts. *Circ. Res.*, **47**, 151–65

11. Sheridan, D. J., Penkoske, P. A., Sobel, B.E. and Corr, P.B. (1980). Alpha adrenergic contributions to dysrhythmia during myocardial ischemia and reperfusion in cats. *J. Clin. Invest.*, **65**, 161–71

12. Ebert, P.A., Vanderbeek, R.B., Allgood, R.J. and Sabiston, D.C. Jr. (1970). Effect of chronic cardiac denervation on arrythmias after coronary artery ligation. *Cardiovasc. Res.*, **4**, 141–7

13. Downar, E., Janse, M. J. and Durrer, D. (1977). The effect of acute coronary artery occlusion on sub-epicardial transmembrane potentials in the intact porcine heart. *Circulation*, **56**, 217–34

14. Kaplinsky, E., Ogawa, S., Michelson, E.L. and Dreifus, L. S. (1981). Instantaneous and delayed ventricular arrhythmias after reperfusion of acutely ischaemic myocardium: evidence of multiple mechanisms. *Circulation*, **63**, 333–40

15. Culling, W., Penny, W. J., Lewis, M. J., Middleton, K. and Sheridan, D. J. (1984). Effects of myocardial catecholamine depletion on cellular electrophysiology and arrhythmias during ischaemia and reperfusion. *Cardiovasc. Res.*, **18**, 675–82

16. Penny, W. J., Culling, W., Lewis, M. J. and Sheridan, D. J. (1985). Antiarrhythmic and electrophysiological effects of alpha adrenoceptor blockade during myocardial ischaemia and reperfusion in isolated guinea-pig heart. *J. Molec. Cell. Cardiol.*, **17**, 399–409

17. Balke, C. W., Kaplinsky, E., Nichelson, E.L., Naito, N. and Dreifus, L.S. (1981). Reperfusion ventricular tachyarrhythmias correlation with antecedent coronary artery occlusion, tachyarrhythmias and duration of myocardial ischaemia. *Am. Heart. J.*, **101**, 449–56

18. Nadeau, R. A. and de Champlain, J. (1979). Plasma catecholamines in acute myocardial infarction. *Am. Heart. J.*, **98**, 548–54

19. Strang, R. C., Vetter, N., Rowe, M. J. and Oliver, M. F. (1974). Plasma cyclic AMP and total catecholamines during acute myocardial infarction in man. *Eur. J. Clin. Invest.*, **4**, 115–19

20. Riemersma, R. A. (1982). Myocardial catecholamine release in acute myocardial ischaemia; relationship to cardiac arrhythmias. In Parratt, J.R. (ed.) *Early Arrhythmias Resulting from Myocardial Ischaemia: Mechanisms and Prevention by Drugs*, pp. 125–38. (London: Macmillan)

21. Hirche, J., Franz, C., Bos, L., Bissig, R., Lang, R. and Schramm, M. (1980). Myocardial extracellular K^+ and H^+ increase and noradrenaline release as possible cause of early arrhythmias following acute coronary artery occlusion in pigs. *J. Molec. Cell. Cardiol.*, **12**, 579–93

22. Sethi, V., Haider, B., Ahmed, S.S., Olderwurtel, H.A. and Regan, T.J. (1973). Influences of beta-blockade and chemical sympathectomy on myocardial function and arrhythmias in acute ischaemia. *Cardiovasc. Res.*, **7**, 740–7

23. Maling, H.M., Colm, V.M. and Highman, B. (1959). The effects of coronary occlusion in dogs treated with reserpine and in dogs treated with phenoxybenzamine. *J. Pharmacol. Exp. Ther.*, **127**, 229–35

24. Muller, C.A., Opie, L.H., Hamm, C.W., Peisach, M. and Gihwala, D. (1986). Prevention of ventricular fibrillation by metoprolol in a pig model of acute myocardial ischaemia: absence of a major arrhythmogenic role for cyclic AMP. *J. Molec. Cell. Cardiol.*, **18**, 375–87

25. Culling, W., Penny, W.J. and Sheridan, D.J. (1984). Effects of sotalol on arrhythmias and electrophysiology during myocardial ischaemia and reperfusion. *Cardiovasc. Res.*, **18**, 397–404

26. Mukherji, A., Wong, T.M., Buja, M., Lefkowitz, R.J. and Willerson, J.T. (1979). Beta-adrenergic and muscarinic cholinergic receptors in canine myocardium. *J. Clin. Invest.*, **64**, 1423–8

27. Stephenson, S.E., Cole, R.K., Parrish, T.F. *et al.* (1960). Ventricular fibrillation during and after coronary artery occlusion: incidence and protection afforded by various drugs. *Am. J. Cardiol.*, **5**, 77–85

28. Stewart, J.R., Burmeister, W.E., Burmeister, J. and Lucchesi, B.R. (1980). Electrophysiologic and antiarrhythmic effects of phentolamine in experimental coronary artery occlusion and reperfusion in the dog. *J. Cardiovasc. Pharmacol.*, **2**, 77–91

29. Sheridan, D.J. (1982). Myocardial alpha adrenoceptors and arrhythmias induced by myocardial ischaemia. In Parratt, J.R. (ed.) *Early Arrhythmias Resulting from Myocardial Ischaemia; Mechanisms and Prevention by Drugs*, pp. 317–28 (London: MacMillan)

30. Rosen, M.R., Gelband, H. and Hoffman, B.E. (1971). Effects of phentolamine on electrophysiological properties of isolated canine Purkinje fibres. *J. Pharmacol. Exp. Ther.*, **179**, 586–93

31. Culling, W., Penny, W.J., Cunliffe, G., Flores, N.A. and Sheridan, D.J. (1987). Arrhythmogenic and electrophysiological effects of alpha adrenoceptor stimulation during myocardial ischaemia and reperfusion. *J. Molec. Cell. Cardiol.*, **19**, 251–8

32. Corr, B., Shayman, J.A., Kramer, J.B. and Kipris, R.J. (1981). Increased alpha-adrenergic receptors in ischaemic cat myocardium. A potential mediator of electrophysiological derangements. *J. Clin. Invest.*, **67**, 1232–6

33. Crome, R., Hearse, D.J., Maguire, M.E. and Manning, A.S. (1985). Dissociation between reperfusion arrythmias and increases in ventricular $alpha_1$ receptor density in the anaesthetised rat. *Br. J. Pharmacol.*, **86**, 498 P

35. Broadley, K.J., Chess-Williams, R.G. and Sheridan, D.J. (1985). [^{3}H]-prazosin binding during ischaemia and reperfusion in the guinea pig Langendorff heart. *Br. J. Pharmacol.*, **86**, 759 P

35. Corr, P.B., Gross, R.W. and Sobel, B.E. (1984). Amphipathic metabolites and membrane dysfunction in ischaemic myocardium. *Circ. Res.*, **55**, 135–54

36. Flacke, W., Atanackovic, D., Gillis, R.A. and Alper, M.H. (1967). The actions of histamine on the mammalian heart. *J. Pharmacol. Exp. Ther.*, **155**, 271–8

37. Flynn, S.B., Gristwood, R.W. and Owen, D.A.A. (1978). Differentiation of the roles of histamine H_1- and H_2-receptors in the mediation of the effects of histamine in the isolated working heart of the guinea pig. *Br. J. Pharmacol.*, **65**, 127–37

38. Capurro, N. and Levi, R. (1975). The heart as a target organ in systemic allergic reactions. Comparison of cardiac anaphylaxis *in vivo* and *in vitro*. *Circ. Res.*, **36**, 520–8
39. Gaide, M. S., Altman, C. B., Cameron, J. S., Kaiser, C. J., Crevar, G., Myerburg, R. J. and Bassett, A. L. (1984). Histamine modification of spontaneous rate and rhythm in infarcted canine ventricle. *Agents Actions*, **15**, 488–93
40. Cameron, J. S., Gaide, M. S., Goad, P. L., Altman, C. B., Cuevas, J., Myerburg, R. J. and Bassett, A. L. (1985). Enhanced adverse electrophysiologic effects of histamine after myocardial infarction in guinea pigs. *J. Pharmacol. Exp. Ther.*, **232**, 480–4
41. Woodward, B. and Zakaria, M. V. M. (1985). Effect of some free radical scavengers on reperfusion induced arrhythmias in the isolated rat heart. *J. Molec. Cell. Cardiol.*, **17**, 485–93
42. Bernier, M., Hearse, D. J. and Manning, A. S. (1986). Reperfusion-induced arrhythmias and oxygen-derived free radicals. Studies with 'anti-free radical' interventions and a free radical-generating system in the isolated perfused rat heart. *Circ. Res.*, **58**, 331–40
43. Huang, X. D., Lee, A. Y. S., Wong, T. M., Zhan, C. Y. and Zhao, Y. Y. (1986). Naloxone inhibits arrhythmias induced by coronary artery occlusion and reperfusion in anaesthetised dogs. *Br. J. Pharmacol.*, **87**, 475–7
44. Parratt, J. R. and Sitsapesan, R. (1986). Stereospecific antiarrhythmic effect of opioid receptor antagonists in myocardial ischaemia. *Br. J. Pharmacol.*, **87**, 621–2
45. de Jong, J. W. (1979). Biochemistry of acutely ischemic myocardium. In Schaper, W. (ed.) *The Pathophysiology of Myocardial Perfusion*, pp. 719–50. (Amsterdam: Elsevier/North Holland Biomedical Press)
46. Lubbe, W. F., Bricknell, O. L., Podzuweit, T. and Opie, L. H. (1976). Cyclic AMP as a determinant of vulnerability to ventricular fibrillation in the isolated rat heart. *Cardiovasc. Res.*, **10**, 697–702
47. Corr, P. B., Witkowski, F. X. and Sobel, B. E. (1978). Mechanisms contributing to malignant dysrhythmias induced by ischaemia in the cat. *J. Clin. Invest.*, **61**, 109–19
48. Podzuweit, T., Dalby, A. J., Cherry, G. W. and Opie, L. H. (1978). Cyclic AMP levels in ischaemic and non-ischaemic myocardium following coronary artery ligation: relation to ventricular fibrillation. *J. Molec. Cell. Cardiol.*, **10**, 81–94
49. Drummond, R. W. and Sordahl, L. A. (1981). Temporal changes in adenylate cyclase activity in acutely ischaemic dog heart: evidence of functional subunit damage. *J. Molec. Cell. Cardiol.*, **13**, 323–30
50. Hill, J. L. and Gettes, L. S. (1980). Effects of acute coronary artery occlusion on local myocardial extracellular K^+ activity in swine. *Circulation*, **61**, 768–78
51. Bourdillon, P. D. V. and Poole-Wilson, P. A. (1981). Effects of ischaemia and reperfusion on calcium exchange and mechanical function in isolated rabbit myocardium. *Cardiovasc. Res.*, **15**, 121–30
52. Whalen, D. A., Hamilton, D. G., Ganote, C. E. and Jennings, R. B. (1974). Effects of a transient period of ischaemia on myocardial cells. I. Effects on cell volume regulation. *Am. J. Pathol.*, **74**, 381–97
53. Schaper, J. (1979). Ultrastructure of the myocardium in acute ischemia. In Schaper, W. (ed.) *The Pathophysiology of Myocardial Perfusion*, pp. 581–673. (Amsterdam: Elsevier/North Holland Biomedical Press)
54. Kloner, R. A. and Braunwald, E. (1980). Observations on experimental myocardial ischaemia. *Cardiovasc. Res.*, **14**, 371–95
55. Kloner, R. A. (1982). The coronary microvasculature and experimental ischemic injury. In Kalsner, S. (ed.) *The Coronary Artery*, pp. 621–43. (London: Croom Helm Ltd)
56. Reimer, K. A., Lowe, J. E., Rasmussen, M. M. and Jennings, R. B. (1977). The wavefront phenomenon of ischaemic cell death. 1. Myocardial infarct size vs. duration of coronary occlusion in dogs. *Circulation*, **56**, 786–94

4
Autonomic tone modulation of cardiac arrhythmias

G. S. BUTROUS

The heart is extensively innervated by both the sympathetic and para-sympathetic system. These nerves regulate both the electrical and mechanical functions of the heart and play a very important role in the stabilization of cardiac function. Disturbances in this regulatory mechanism may play an important role in the genesis of cardiac arrhythmias.

INNERVATION OF THE HEART

All levels of the central nervous system from the cortex to the spinal cord contribute to the control of the circulation; but the main centres are localized in the bulbar regions. There is considerable variation in the anatomical details of cardiac innervation among different species[1,2]. Recently Janes and his co-workers[1] described a detailed analysis of the anatomy of human extrinsic nerves by dissecting 23 cadavers. They found that all major sympathetic nerves arise from the stellate ganglia and the caudal halves of the cervical sympathetic trunk. The main sympathetic nerves are the right and left stellate cardiopulmonary nerves; right and left dorso-lateral cardiopulmonary nerves and right and left dorso-medial cardiopulmonary trunk. In addition there is the ventral cardiopulmonary nerve which arises from the left ventral ansa. The vagus supplies many branches to the heart from the recurrent laryngeal nerves and the thoracic vagi. The above nerves from both the right and left interconnect to form the cardiopulmonary plexuses which innervate different cardiac structures (Figure 4.1).

The sino-atrial node receives its main supply from the right stellate cardiopulmonary nerve[3]. The atrioventricular node receives innervation from both the left and right sympathetic ganglia[4]. Both atria and ventricles are extensively innervated by the sympathetic nerves. The atria are also supplied by parasympathetic innervation, but there is inhomo-geneity in the distribution of these nerves to the atria, i.e. the left atrium contains half that of the sino-atrial node. The right atrium is

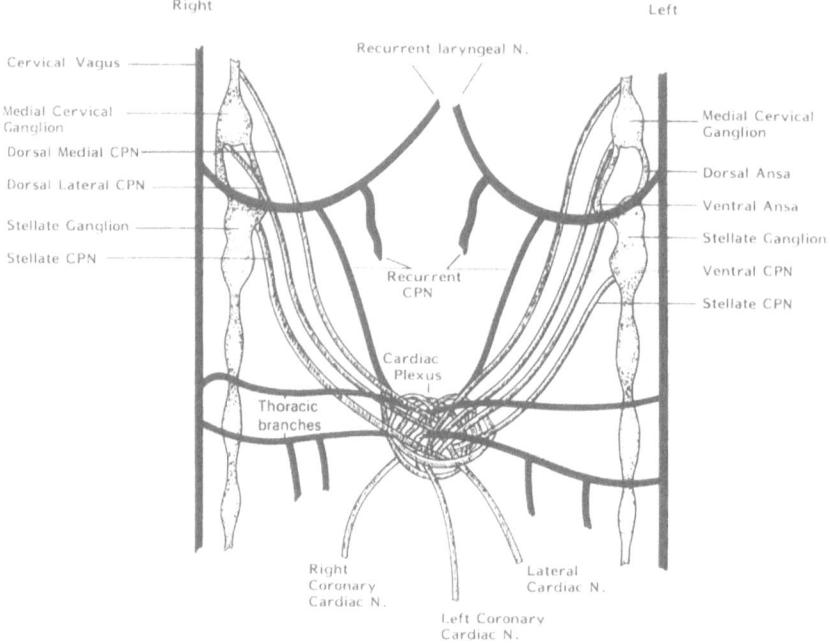

Figure 4.1 Diagrammatic representation of the sympathetic and parasympathetic nerves supply to the human heart (adapted from the description of Janes *et al.*, 1986[1]). CPN = cardiopulmonary nerve.

intermediate[5]. There is now good evidence that the vagus nerve also supplies the ventricles, particularly its basal part[6,7].

Generally, sympathetic effects oppose or antagonize the effects of parasympathetic tone in the cardiac tissue. There is, however, growing evidence that sympathetic–parasympathetic interaction plays a major role in the regulation of cardiac function. This interaction can be on several different levels, and shows different levels of antagonistic and agonistic effects. Disturbances in this interaction may facilitate cardiac arrhythmias[8,9].

AUTONOMIC TONE MODULATION OF ARRHYTHMIAS IN ISCHAEMIC HEART DISEASE

Both afferent and efferent sympathetic fibres are activated during myocardial ischaemia[10]. Adrenergic agonists do not significantly alter conduction velocity in normal myocardium but can speed conduction in the ischaemic myocardium[11]. Martins *et al.*[12] found that sympathetically denervated myocardium is more sensitive to noradrenaline infusion than in normal myocardium. This differential effect may increase the disparity in the electrical properties of the ventricles which facilitate the opportunity for arrhythmia. Sympathetic stimulation of ischaemic tissue is arrhythmogenic[13,14], but there are major differences between the effect of the β-agonist administered intravenously prior to coronary occlusion and the effect of sympathetic stimulation which occurs in the setting of acute ischaemia. Systemic administration of catecholamines produces global changes in the myocardium, whereas the effect of sympathetic neuronal stimulation may be regionally confined, largely to the ischaemic area[15]. Lombardi[16] found that sympathetic efferent activity increases significantly during coronary artery occlusion in dogs. This was associated with a decreased ventricular fibrillation threshold. However, with persistence of occlusion and myocardial ischaemia the vulnerability to fibrillation reverted to the preocclusion level and was associated with a decrease in sympathetic activity. After release of the occlusion (reperfusion phase) there was a second period of augmented vulnerability to fibrillation but no associated increase in sympathetic activity. The decrease in the ventricular fibrillation threshold during reperfusion has been associated with increased α-adrenergic receptors[17,18]. Alpha-adrenergic blockade can induce important antiarrhythmic effects during ischaemia and reperfusion, and may ultimately prove beneficial in the primary prevention of ventricular fibrillation in patients with ischaemic heart disease[17]. Thus α- and β-adrenergic receptors stimulation contribute to arrhythmogenesis during myocardial ischaemia. Blocking these receptors has a beneficial effect in reducing malignant ventricular arrhythmias in the experimental preparation[19]. These experiments have not yet been verified in the clinical situation.

Psychological stimuli or stress are well known in inducing disturbances of cardiac rhythm. Katz et al.[20] performed personality inventories on 102 patients undergoing 24 hour electrocardiograms. In their study they found a significant correlation between the presence of ventricular arrhythmias in the form of frequent ventricular premature beats (more than 30 per hour) and scores of anxiety, depression, social alienation and hysteria. Recently Tavazzi and his co-workers,[21] studied 19 patients with recent uncomplicated myocardial infarction using programmed ventricular stimulation at rest and during the stress of mental arithmetic. They showed that during mental stress there was a significant decrease in the ventricular refractory period and a significant increase in ventricular tachycardia induction by programmed stimulation. Ventricular fibrillation was provoked by double and triple extrastimuli during stress but not during the control period. These findings suggest the importance of stress in induction of ventricular arrhythmias in patients with acute myocardial infarction, and also the production of a significant electrophysiological modification which can be the substrate for ventricular arrhythmia.

Parasympathetic tone may possibly have a protective action in opposing the effect of sympathetic stimulation. There have been many studies on the role of baroreceptor reflexes in providing electrical stability in patients with myocardial infarction. Rowey and his co-workers[22] have shown that baroreceptor denervation significantly increases the pro-arrhythmic action of noradrenaline. Schwartz and his co-workers[23,24] have shown, by a series of experimental observations and prospective clinical studies, that in several post myocardial infarction patients baroreceptor sensitivity is transiently depressed. They suggested the possibility that depressed baroreflex sensitivity might be used for the early identification of a subgroup of post myocardial infarction patients at high risk for malignant arrhythmias. Ewing and his co-workers[25] have used 24 hour electrocardiograms to assess cardiac parasympathetic activity by measuring the incidence of large changes in successive RR intervals. They found that in normal subjects changes in successive RR intervals greater than 50 ms were 150–250 times higher during waking and 350–450 times higher during sleeping hours. This frequency of variation was extremely low in diabetics who were medically denervated and in heart transplant patients. This technique provides a valid and sensitive way of monitoring cardiac parasympathetic activity over prolonged periods. The use of this technique may be of value in assessing parasympathetic activity after myocardial infarction. This was shown by Magid and his co-workers[26] who found that a decreased heart rate variability, reflecting, at least in part, an increase in cardiac parasympathetic traffic, appears to characterize patients at proven high risk for sudden cardiac death.

The interaction between the two limbs of the autonomic nervous system may be important in the genesis of cardiac arrhythmias in ischaemic heart disease. In an intact animal vagal stimulation prolongs the right ventricular effective refractory period by antagonizing the prevailing sympathetic tone. However, the effect of vagal stimulation was abolished with propranolol[27]. Many multicentre trials have demonstrated that β-adrenoceptor blocking agents can significantly improve prognosis when given to survivors of acute myocardial infarction[28,29]. The fundamental mechanism by which the β-blocker modified prognosis is not well understood[30].

AUTONOMIC TONE MODULATION OF SINUS NODE FUNCTION

The intrinsic properties of the sinus node are highly regulated by autonomic tone. The importance of the role of autonomic tone has been shown by De Marneffe et al.[31] who demonstrated that the decrease in the intrinsic rate of the sinus node with age is balanced by the changes in the autonomic tone. Thus with age there is a progressive decrease in the parasympathetic activity so that basal properties of the sinus node appear stable throughout life. Many sinus node abnormalities, including sick sinus syndrome, are probably affected by disturbances in autonomic innervation. Sethi *et al.*[32] found that in 76% of patients their sick sinus syndrome was due to an intrinsic function abnormality of the sino-atrial node, while a disturbance of autonomic regulation was the cause in 24%. Ambrosini and his co-workers[33] studied 134 patients with bradycardia, 12 patients showed clinical evidence of carotid sinus hypersensitivity, 68 patients exhibited sick sinus syndrome and 54 were normal controls. They found that there was little abnormality of sinus node automaticity in patients with carotid sinus hypersensitivity compared with patients with sick sinus syndrome. This suggests that the basis of sinus node dysfunction in these patients is an abnormal carotid sinus.

AUTONOMIC MODULATION OF THE ATRIOVENTRICULAR NODE

There are various antagonistic effects between sympathetic and parasympathetic neuronal activity on the atrioventricular (AV) node. On the other hand there is also an interaction between the two limbs of the autonomic tone acting to regulate the AV node. Salata and his co-workers[34] have shown that dynamic vagal control of heart rate and atrioventricular conduction involves both phase-dependent and phase-independent factors. Sympathetic activity appears to affect only the phase-independent factors in the control of heart rate, whereas it affects both phase-dependent and phase-independent factors in the control of atrioventricular conduction. Butrous *et al.*[35] have demonstrated that atrioventricular delay, as measured by the AH interval, adjusted itself to changes in heart rate, maintaining 1:1 atrioventricular conduction despite rapid changes in heart rate. This may explain some of the atrioventricular nodal abnormalities in patients with sick sinus syndrome. Poor sinus node function may result in a discordant relationship between the autonomic regulation of both nodes and may produce or exaggerate atrioventricular block.

The effects of autonomic blockade on dual atrioventricular nodal pathway patterns were studied in 15 patients by Paparella and his co-workers[36] who showed that the dual AV nodal pathway pattern is mainly related to the intrinsic structure of the AV node, and the autonomic nervous system only affects the refractoriness and conduction velocity in each pathway. These findings suggest that although dual atrioventricular pathways may be the substrate for atrioventricular re-entry tachycardia, the balance achieved between the electrophysiologic parameters of these two pathways, for example by the effects of autonomic tone, may allow the initiation and continuation of these arrhythmias.

AUTONOMIC TONE MODULATION ON THE QT INTERVAL

There is now a wide belief that the pathogenesis of congenital long QT syndrome is based on the presence of an abnormally dominant sympathetic tone to the left side of the heart[37]. This imbalance is probably responsible for the action potential dispersion which creates a substrate for ventricular arrhythmias. Recently Cinca et al.[38] obtained support for this view by studying the electrophysiologic effects of both left and right stellate ganglion blockade, with a 24 hour interval between the two procedures, in patients with supraventricular tachycardia. They found that right but not left stellate ganglion block caused prolongation of the QT interval. In reviewing the heart rate changes over a 3-year period of 61 newly born babies with long QT syndrome, Vincent[39] observed that these babies showed a lower heart rate trend in comparison to age-matched normal babies. He suggested that the difference supported the hypothesis that these patients had lower than normal right sided cardiac sympathetic activity.

AUTONOMIC TONE MODULATION ON ACCESSORY PATHWAY ELECTROPHYSIOLOGY

The role of autonomic tone on the electrophysiologic properties of accessory pathways has not been studied systematically. Until recently there are several clinical and experimental observations suggesting that such a role exists. The effect of adrenergic tone on the accessory pathway has been reported. Wellens et al.[40] showed that isoprenaline shortened the refractory period of the accessory pathway, and its effect was particularly noticeable when accessory pathway refractory periods were long. Both standing and exercise decrease accessory pathway refractoriness. However, most studies have explained that the effect of autonomic tone is more pronounced on the AV node than on an accessory pathway[41]. These observations were also supported by Brugada et al.[42] who found that the effect of isoprenaline on the conduction of circus movement tachycardia in patients with an accessory atrioventricular pathway was predominantly via the atrioventricular node.

The parasympathetic effect on accessory pathway conduction is controversial. There is theoretical and experimental evidence to suggest that parasympathetic neuronal activity improves conduction through the accessory pathway. Averill et al.[43] reported that atropine caused the disappearance of pre-excitation in 18 of 56 patients with Wolff–Parkinson–White syndrome. However, this finding has been explained by others as an improvement of conduction through the atrioventricular node[44,45]. Wolff[46] studied the natural history of a neonate with Wolff–Parkinson–White syndrome, and proposed that resolution of the arrhythmias and the pre-excitation pattern with age occurred because of autonomic tone modulation, i.e. age-related development of adrenergic innervation and the decrease in the cholinergic tone.

Sympathetic and parasympathetic interaction has also been documented as affecting the accessory pathway. Przybylski et al.[47] studied 21 patients who had previously exhibited pre-excitation, but who showed normal ventricular activation at the time of the study. They found that in nine patients pre-excitation could be induced by carotid sinus massage, whilst in another five patients pre-excitation appeared only during isoprenaline infusion combined with carotid sinus massage. In another case pre-excitation could only be repeatedly induced by carotid sinus massage during isoprenaline infusion[48]. Butrous et al.[49] demonstrated the presence of this interaction clinically by showing the parasympathetic neuronal activity improved the anterograde conduction via the accessory pathway in the presence of high sympathetic tone.

CARDIAC ARRHYTHMIAS DURING NIGHT SLEEP

Although sleep may be associated with a reduction in the frequency of ventricular arrhythmias the reverse has also been documented. Rosen berg et al.[50] identified an individual with ventricular ectopics which increased in frequency and complexity during sleep. They found neurological diseases in this individual, and suggested a neurological mediation of these arrhythmias. There has also been a report of aggravation or development of arrhythmias in patients with acute myocardial infarction during sleep[51]. Otsuka and his co-workers[52] found that there are two types of arrhythmias induced by sleep. The first type is affected by a phasic increase in sympathetic nervous tone by rapid eye movement sleep and the second type is related to an increase in vagal tone during the night.

CONCLUSIONS

The above studies have documented the importance of autonomic tone modulation on electrophysiological parameters of the heart and cardiac arrhythmias. Although this subject is far from being completely understood the importance of both the sympathetic and parasympathetic systems and their interaction is essential to the understanding of patients with cardiac arrhythmias.

References

1. Janes, R. D., Brandys, J. C., Hopkins, D. A., Johnstone, D. E., Murphy, D. A. and Armour, J. A. (1986). Anatomy of human extrinsic cardiac nerves and ganglia. *Am. J. Cardiol.*, **57**, 299–309
2. Randall, W. and Armour, J. A. (1977). Gross and microscopic anatomy of the cardiac innervation. In Randall, W. (ed) *Neuronal Regulation of the Heart*. pp. 13–41. (NY: Oxford Univ. Press)
3. Randall, W., Armour, J. A., Geis, W. P. and Lippincott, D. B. (1972). Regional cardiac distribution of sympathetic nerves. *Fed. Proc.* **1**, 1199–203
4. Randall, W. C. and Ardell, J. L. (1985). Selective parasympathectomy of autonomic and conductile tissue of the canine heart. *Am. J. Physiol.*, **248**, H61–H68
5. Brown, O. M. (1976). Cat heart acetylcholine: structural proof and distribution. *Am. J. Physiol.*, **231**, 781–5
6. Takahashi, M., Barber, M. J. and Zipes, D. P. (1985). Efferent vagal innervation of canine ventricle. *Am. J. Physiol.*, **248**, H89–H97
7. Prystowsky, E. N., Jackman, W. M., Rinkenberger, R. L., Hegar, J. and Zipes, D. P.

(1981). Effect of autonomic blockade on ventricular refractoriness and atrio-ventricular nodal conduction in humans. *Circ. Res.*, **49**, 511–18

8. Zipes, D. P., Barber, M. J., Takahashi, M. and Gilmour, R. F. (1983). Influence of the autonomic nervous system on the genesis of cardiac arrhythmia. *Pacing Clin, Electrophysiol.*, **6**, 1210–20

9. Levy, M. N. (1971). Sympathetic–parasympathetic interaction in the heart. *Circ. Res.*, **29**, 437–45

10. Malliani, A., Schwartz, P. J. and Sanchetti, A. (1969). A sympathetic reflex elicited by experimental coronary occlusion. *Am. J. Physiol.*, **217**, 703–9

11. Weiss, J. and Shine, K. I. (1982). [K$^+$] accumulation and electrophysiological alterations during early myocardial ischemia. *Am. J. Physiol.*, **243**, H318–H327

12. Martins, J. B., Miller, M. J. and Leonard, M. T. (1985). Electrophysiologic effects due to regional sympathetic denervation supersensitivity in the dog ventricle. *Circulation*, **72**, 111–41

13. Kilks, B. R., Burgess, M. J. and Abildskov, J. A. (1975). Influence of sympathetic tone on ventricular fibrillation threshold during experimental coronary occlusion. *Am. J. Cardiol.*, **36**, 45–51

14. Gillis, R. A. (1971). Role of the nervous system in the arrhythmia produced by coronary occlusion of the cat. *Am. Heart J.*, **81**, 677–84

15. Gettes, L. S., Symanski, J. D., Flut, W. F., Johnson, T. A. and Graebner, C. (1986). The intracellular and extracellular changes associated with ischaemia – effects of catecholamines in arrhythmogenesis. *Eur. Heart J.* 7 (Suppl A), 77–84

16. Lombardi, F. (1986). Acute myocardial ischaemia, neural reflexes and ventricular arrhythmias. *Eur. Heart J.*, 7 (Suppl A), 91–7

17. Scheridan, D. J., Penkoske, P. A., Sobel, B. E. and Corr, P. B. (1980). Alpha-adrenergic contributions to dysrhythmias during myocardial ischaemia and reperfusion in cats. *J. Clin. Invest.*, **65**, 161–71

18. Corr, P. B., Shayman, J. A., Kramer, J. B. and Kipnis, R. J. (1981). Increased alpha-adrenergic receptors in ischaemic cat myocardium: A potential mediator of electrophysiological derangements. *J. Clin. Invest.*, **67**, 1232–6

19. Yamada, K. A., Saffitz, J. E. and Corr, P. B. (1986). Role of alpha and beta-adrenergic receptor stimulation in the genesis of arrhythmias during myocardial ischaemia. *Eur. Heart J.*, 7 (Suppl A), 85–90

20. Katz, C., Martin, R. D., Landa, B. and Chadda, K. D. (1985). Relationship of psychologic factors to frequent symptomatic ventricular arrhythmias. *Am. J. Med.*, **78**, 589–94

21. Tavazzi, L., Zotti, A. M. and Rondanelli, R. (1986). The role of psychologic stress in the genesis of lethal arrhythmias in patients with coronary artery disease. *Eur. Heart J.* (Suppl A), 99–106

22. Rowey, P. R., Verrier, R. I. and Lown, B. (1982). Decreased vulnerability to ventricular fibrillation by vasodilator-induced baroreceptor sensitisation. *Cardiov. Res.*, **17**, 106–12

23. Schwartz, P. J., La Rovere, M. T., Zaza, A., Pala, M., Mazzoleni, C. and Specchia, G. (1985). Baroreceptive reflexes and cardiac electrical instability in patients with a myocardial infarction. *New Trends in Arrhythmias*, **11**, 289–92

24. Schwartz, P. J. and Stone, H. L. (1985). The analysis and modulation of autonomic reflexes in the prediction and prevention of sudden death. In Zipes, D. and Jalife, J. (eds.) *Cardiac Electrophysiology and Arrhythmias.* pp. 167–76 (NY: Grune & Stratton)

25. Ewing, D. J., Neilson, J. M. M. and Travis, P. (1984). New method for assessing cardiac parasympathetic activity using 24 hour electrocardiograms. *Br. Heart J.*, **52**, 396–402

26. Magid, N. M., Martin, G. J., Kehoe, R. F., Zheutlin, T. A. *et al.* (1985). Diminished heart rate variability in sudden cardiac death. *Circulation*, **72**, (Suppl. III), 241

27. Kilman, B. S., Verrier, R. L. and Lown, B. (1976). Effects of vagus stimulation upon excitability of the canine ventricle. *Am. J. Cardiol.*, **37**, 1041–5

28. Singh, B. N. and Venkatesh, N. (1984). Prevention of myocardial reinfarction and

sudden death in survivors of acute myocardial infarction: role of prophylactic beta adrenoceptor blockade. *Am. Heart. J.*, **107**, 189–200

29. Norwegian Multicentre Study Group (1981). Timolol induced reduction in mortality and reinfarction in patients surviving acute myocardial infarction. *N. Engl. J. Med.*, **304**, 801–7

30. Campbell, R. W. F. and Bourke, J. (1986). Beta blocking agents in post myocardial infarction patients. *Eur. Heart J.*, 7 (Suppl A), 119–21

31. De Marneffe, M., Jacobs, P., Haardt, R. and Englert, M. (1986). Variations of normal sinus node function in relation to age: role of autonomic influence. *Eur. Heart J.*, 7, 662–72

32. Sethi, K. K., Jaishankar, S., Balachander, J., Bahl, V. K. and Gupta, M. P. (1984). Sinus node function after autonomic blockade in normals and in Sick Sinus syndrome. *Int. J. Cardiol.*, 5, 707–19

33. Ambrosini, F. A., Bertoni, T., Pagnoni, F., Pupilella, T. and Lotto, A. (1985). Has carotid sinus compression any relationship with sinus node function correlations with the stimulation tests? *New Trends in Arrhythmias*, 2, 123–6

34. Salata, J. J., Gill, R. M., Gilmour, R. F. and Zipes, D. P. (1986). Effects of sympathetic tone on vagally induced phasic changes in heart rate and atrioventricular node conduction in the anaesthetized dog. *Circ. Res.*, 58, 584–94

35. Butrous, G. S., Cochrane, T. and Camm, A. J. (1987). Rapid autonomic tone regulation of atrioventricular node conduction in man. *Am. Heart J.*, **113**, 934–40

36. Paparella, N., Alboni, P., Pirani, R., Cappato, R., Thomasi, A. M. and Masoni, A. (1986). Effects of autonomic blockade on dual atrioventricular nodal pathways pattern. *J. Electrocardiol.*, 19, 269–74

37. Schwartz, P. J. (1985). Idiopathic long QT syndrome: progress and questions. *Am. Heart. J.*, **109**, 399–410

38. Cinca, J., Evangelista, A., Montoyo, J., Barutell, C., Figueras, J., Valle, V., Rius, J. and Soler-Soler, J. (1985). Electrophysiologic effects of unilateral right and left stellate ganglion block on the human heart. *Am. Heart J.*, **109**, 46–54

39. Vincent, G. M. (1985). The heart rate of Romano–Ward long QT patients. *Circulation*, **72**, 111–44

40. Wellens, H. J. J., Burgada, P., Roy, D., Weiss, J. and Bar, F. W. (1982). Effect of isoproterenol on the anterograde refractory pathway in patients with Wolff–Parkinson–White syndrome. *Am. J. Cardiol.*, **50**, 180–4

41. Butrous, G. S., Nathan, A. W., Bexton, R. S., Hellestrand, K. J. and Camm, A. J. (1984). The effect of posture and exercise on the electrophysiological properties of direct atrioventricular accessory pathway. *J. Am. Coll. Cardiol.*, 3, 612

42. Brugada, P., Facchini, M., and Wellens, H. J. J. (1986). Effects of isoproterenol and amiodarone and the role of exercise in initiation of circus movement tachycardia in the accessory atrioventricular pathway. *Am. J. Cardiol.*, **57**, 146–9

43. Averill, K. H., Fismoer, R. J. and Lamb, L. E. (1960) Electrocardiographic findings in 67375 asymptomatic subjects: IV Wolff–Parkinson–White syndrome. *Am. J. Cardiol.*, 6, 108–29

44. Khair, G. Z., Tristani, F. E. and Bamrah, V. S. (1983). Dynamic QRS variations in Wolff–Parkinson–White syndrome: electrocardiograph and clinical observation. *Am. Heart J.*, **105**, 878–82

45. Duthie, R. J. (1946). Mechanism of the Wolff–Parkinson–White syndrome. *Br. Heart J.* 8, 96–102

46. Wolff, G. S., Han, J. and Curran, J. (1978). Wolff–Parkinson–White syndrome in neonate. *Am. J. Cardiol.*, **41**, 559–63

47. Przybylski, J., Chiale, P. A., Halpern, M. S., Nau, G. J., Elizari, M. V. and Rosenbaum, M. B. (1980). Unmasking of ventricular pre-excitation of vagal stimulation of isoproterenol administration. *Circulation*, **61**, 1030–7

48. Gavrilescu, S. (1976). Manifestation of the Wolff–Parkinson–White syndrome during isoprenaline infusion and carotid sinus massage. *Cardiology*, **61**, 146–9

49. Butrous, G. S., Kaye, G. C., Nathan, A. W., Banim, S. O. and Camm, A. J. (1984). Respiratory modulation of atrioventricular accessory pathway conduction. *Circulation*, **70**, II, 217

50. Rosenberg, M. J., Eugene Uretz, M. S. and Denes, P. (1983). Sleep and ventricular arrhythmias. *Am. Heart J.*, **106**, 703–9
51. Otsuka, K. (1980). Studies of digitalis induced arrhythmias by recordings of 24 hour continuous electrocardiograms. *Fukuoka Igaku Zasshi*, **71**, 631–44
52. Otsuka, K., Vanaga, T., Ichimaru, Y. and Seto, K. (1982). Sleep and night-type arrhythmias. *Jpn Heart J.* **23**, 479–85

5
Haemodynamic consequences of cardiac arrhythmias

G. KAYE and A. J. CAMM

INTRODUCTION

Modern haemodynamic techniques have allowed a greater degree of understanding of the effects of cardiac arrhythmias. The haemodynamic consequences relate to a number of factors which include: the ventricular rate and the regularity of the rhythm, the presence or absence of cardiac disease, the relationship between atrial and ventricular systole, the synchronicity of ventricular contraction, the preservation and level of autonomic tone and disease in other organs[1,2].

FACTORS INFLUENCING HAEMODYNAMIC STATUS DURING TACHYCARDIA

Heart rate

Incremental change in ventricular rate during right atrial pacing produces an initial increase in cardiac output and a linear reduction in stroke volume at rates up to 160 beats per minute (bpm)[3-5]. Ross et al.[6] found a modest decline in the cardiac index at heart rates of 120 bpm or greater, with a substantial fall in stroke volume index at rates of 80–90 bpm. In the normal heart the maximal increase in output occurs with modest increases in heart rate, around 70–90 bpm, and the above variables decline at rates above 160 bpm[7]. In the abnormal heart the fall in output occurs at lower rates.

Ventricular pacing, compared to atrial pacing at similar rates, leads to a reduction in systemic arterial pressure, an increase in atrial pressures and a fall in cardiac output[8]. Gilmore and colleagues[9] showed a significant decrease in stroke work and cardiac output during both left and right ventricular pacing, compared to atrial pacing at similar rates. There was no haemodynamic difference between right and left ventricular pacing.

Change in regularity of rhythm

An important determinant of cardiac output is the diastolic filling time. Greenfield et al.[10] showed a strong correlation bettween peak left ventricular power and stroke work and the two preceding RR intervals. Forward arterial blood flow falls significantly during short RR intervals in both atrial fibrillation and with atrial or ventricular ectopics with short coupling intervals. Braunwald and Frahm[4] have shown a direct relationship between the end-diastolic ventricular muscle length and peak systolic pressure, possibly via Starling's mechanism. Thus long RR intervals may produce enhanced ventricular contraction.

Synchronicity of ventricular contraction

Data concerning the haemodynamic effects of altered ventricular activation and contraction are conflicting. Some studies have shown 100% differences in stroke output during ventricular pacing at different sites emphasizing the importance of alterations in the sequence of contraction[11]. Samet et al[12], using synchronized atrial and ventricular pacing, concluded that atrial transport is a critical feature, and that abnormal ventricular contraction has little import. More recent evidence, however, suggests that disordered left ventricular activation is an important haemodynamic determinant[13]. Pacing from the left ventricular apex has been reported to be haemodynamically better than pacing from other sites, but not consistently so. Ventricular ectopic beats produce a significant reduction in stroke output and peak power, and this may be related to a combination of the coupling interval and altered sequence of contraction[14]. In addition there is a greater reduction in flow with ventricular ectopic beats compared to atrial ectopics at the same coupling interval[15,16].

Ventricular function

In the normal heart, as previously described, increase in heart rate results in an improvement in cardiac performance with an increase in output and ventricular power[7,17]. These values reduce, sometimes dramatically, at rates around 160–180 bpm. In disease states there is often a small increase in cardiac performance with increased rate, but this often reduces at rates of 120–140 bpm[7], much lower in comparison to the normal heart. This may be a primary consequence of reduced resting left ventricular function. Processes that affect both the contraction and relaxation of the ventricular myocardium alter resting function and, during arrhythmias, may be of sufficient import to account solely for any deleterious haemodynamic effects. Ventricular function per se, however, is not an accurate predictor of the haemodynamic outcome of tachyarrhythmias. It is recognized that tachycardias in the presence of severe left ventricular dysfunction may be remarkably stable, whereas similar arrhythmias in an otherwise normal heart may be associated with syncope or the features of shock. In broad terms, however, left ventricular function does to a certain extent influence the haemodynamic effects of arrhythmias, but other separate factors determine the overall outcome. There is no evidence that isolated impairment of right ventricular function determines the haemodynamic outcome of tachycardias.

Of interest is the observation that chronic arrhythmias, either atrial or ventricular, may produce irreversible heart failure in otherwise previously normal hearts[18].

Atrial and ventricular synchronicity

The booster pump effect of the atria in supplementing ventricular filling is well established, and significant alteration in the normal AV relationship is haemodynamically deleterious[19]. Atrial pacing is better than ventricular pacing and the beneficial effects of atrial synchronized pacing during ventricular tachycardia are well known. Conversion of atrial fibrillation to sinus rhythm at comparable ventricular rates produces a significant increase in cardiac output and patient well being[20-22].

The optimal PR interval is 0.1–0.2 seconds and the PR effect increases with heart rate[23]. The importance of the atrial contribution is emphasized in myocardial disease, a well known example being the adverse haemodynamic effect at the onset of atrial fibrillation in patients with mitral stenosis.

Autonomic tone

The adjustment to deleterious haemodynamic events at the onset of tachycardia depends upon the functional integrity of the cardiac and peripheral autonomic nerves and loss of these reflexes, e.g. in diabetes, cardiac transplantation or Chagas' disease, demonstrates their importance in the maintenance of blood pressure and flow to distant organs. The effects of the same arrhythmia in different patients may be related to the status of central and peripheral autonomics. Tachycardias reduce cardiac filling time, stroke volume, systemic arterial and pulse pressure and reduce distension of the carotid and aortic baroreceptors, effectively increasing sympathetic and reducing vagal efferent tone[24].

In man, reflex changes in autonomic tone are usually effective in restoring and maintaining blood pressure and cardiac output during supraventricular tachycardia, on occasion to similar levels prior to the onset of the arrhythmia. Curry[25] defined four phases of the blood pressure response during supraventricular tachycardia: initial profound hypotension, rising blood pressure, an 'overshoot phase' and finally

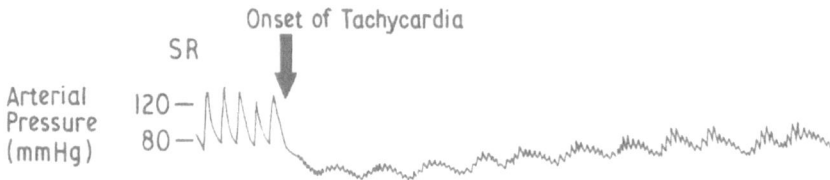

Figure 5.1 Changes in systemic blood pressure at the onset of a paroxysm of supraventricular tachycardia showing an initial hypotensive phase followed rapidly (within 20 seconds) by partial recovery to a mean level below that during sinus rhythm (From ref. 25; reproduced by kind permission of Williams & Wilkins)

stable pressures during established tachycardia (Figure 5.1). These changes occur within 15–30 seconds of the onset. Alterations in tachycardia heart rate are common at arrhythmia initiation, either increasing at first and slowing slightly before becoming stable, or slowing at the onset and then maintaining a constant rate. Curry[25] notes that marked changes in heart rate were seen predominantly in patients with atrioventricular nodal re-entrant tachycardias (AVNRT), rather than during atrioventricular re-entrant tachycardias (AVRT) in association with anomalous atrioventricular (AV) pathways.

Experimental work confirms the relevance of the cardiac autonomics to the stability of the cardiovascular system when under stress. Skinner et al.[26] showed that bilateral vagotomy in dogs blunted the compensatory response to induced atrial fibrillation. Studies in patients with Chagas' disease[27], which in the early stages produces a selective degeneration of the nerve supply to the sino-atrial node, confirm that intact vagal tone is important, but not absolutely essential to reflex cardiac events. Furthermore, the normal changes in heart rate on standing and during tachycardias are initially dependent on parasympathetically mediated events, sympathetic reflexes exerting their maximum effect later. Intrinsic non-autonomic influences may also be present[28-30].

Disease in other organs

The symptomatology of arrhythmias is conditioned, in part, by disease in other systems. Atherosclerosis of the cerebral vessels may produce symptoms not seen in patients with normal vasculature. Syncope at the onset or during tachyarrhythmias is not uncommon even in the presence of normal cerebral vessels, and may reflect temporarily inadequate compensatory mechanisms. Cerebral blood flow is often impaired during arrhythmias and Stokes–Adams attacks are a well described consequence. Cerebral flow is significantly reduced during both ectopic beats and rapid arrhythmias. Ventricular tachycardias tend to cause more cerebral hypotension than atrial arrhythmias at similar rates[31,32].

Coronary artery flow may be reduced by up to 40% during atrial tachyarrhythmias and by up to 60% during ventricular tachycardias. Ectopics produce a variable degree of impairment of flow depending on the coupling interval. The reduction in flow has important patho-physiological consequences. Tachyarrhythmias reduce coronary flow. Ventricular tachyarrhythmias[31] which are often of ischaemic origin, may further aggravate underlying ischaemia possibly potentiating the mechanism of the arrhythmia. ST segment depression during supra-ventricular arrhythmia is well recognized and is thought to be significant, but may be related to marked reduction in coronary flow in the absence of atherosclerosis.

Total renal blood flow significantly falls during rapid arrhythmias of any origin. In dogs, atrial and ventricular premature beats produced similar reduction in flow (8–10%), whereas atrial fibrillation caused a 20% reduction and ventricular tachycardia a 60% reduction at similar ventricular rates[15]. The fall in renal blood flow was maintained for the duration of the arrhythmia and renal vascular resistance markedly increased[33]. Change in mesenteric blood flow during tachyarrhythmias may be variable, and is related to the degree of shunting of blood to more vital areas. The reduction in cerebral, renal and mesenteric flow is corrected within seconds of arrhythmia termination[33]. Severe anaemia modifies the haemodynamic consequences of arrhythmias as does the state of hydration. Tachyarrhythmias occurring in the presence of low plasma or blood volume have a greater deleterious haemodynamic effect than those in the hydrated state, although the ultimate effect will depend on intact neural reflexes and the presence of disease in other organs. These arrhythmias are a common complication of shock and may reflect deranged metabolic state rather than intrinsic myocardial disease. These arrhythmias may be potentially disastrous even though cardiac function is normal and despite the presence of high sympathetic tone.

SPECIFIC ARRHYTHMIAS

Sinus bradycardia

Providing that stroke volume is not limited by significant myocardial or valvular disease severe bradycardias, down to 30 bpm or sometimes less, may be surprisingly well tolerated even in the elderly. Usually, stroke volume increases as the heart rate slows but at very slow rates cardiac output falls and the filling pressures increase[2].

Supraventricular tachycardia

On the basis of cardiac electrophysiology common supraventricular arrhythmias are of the following types:

(1) automatic atrial and re-entrant tachycardias,
(2) atrioventricular re-entrant tachycardia (AVRT),
(3) atrioventricular nodal re-entrant tachycardia (AVNRT).

Patients often tolerate these arrhythmias well although cardiovascular collapse is recognized, especially with rapid rates. Syncope may often occur at the onset of the paroxysm, and dyspnoea, weakness, chest pain and dizziness are common. Polyuria is uncommon but strongly associated with atrial arrhythmias, particularly atrial fibrillation and re-entrant arrhythmias associated with the Wolff–Parkinson–White syndrome[34].

During both atrioventricular nodal re-entrant tachycardia (AVNRT) and atrioventricular re-entrant tachycardia (AVRT) associated with the Wolff–Parkinson–White syndrome there is often a precipitous fall in mean systemic blood pressure at the onset[25,34,35] which may be dramatic, occasionally falling to near zero for a short period. The reduction in pressure is usually corrected within 30 seconds to levels comparable to sinus rhythm. Mean cardiac output falls by up to 40–50% as does stroke volume. Mean pulmonary artery and right atrial pressures rise and the character of the atrial pressure waves changes with superimposition of 'a' and 'v' waves possibly reflecting atrial contraction against a closed tricuspid valve[34]. Goldreyer and colleagues[36] confirmed the presence of large systolic waves in the right atrium during induced supraventricular tachycardias and were unable to differentiate 'a' and 'v' waves. In their series of eight cases pulmonary systolic and diastolic pressures increased, mean brachial artery pressure fell (from a mean of 141 mmHg in sinus rhythm to a mean of 99 mmHg during SVT) and the mean cardiac index decreased by an average of 38%.

During AVNRT the re-entrant circuit occurs within the atrioventricular node and the atria and ventricle contract virtually simultaneously. The atria, therefore, contract against closed AV valves with subsequent marked increase in intra-atrial pressures. During AVRT, however, atrial and ventricular depolarization may be disassociated by as much as 100 ms and, although atrial pressures rise, the increase may not be as marked during AVNRT. 2-D Echocardiography during these arrhythmias[37] demonstrated that atrial end-diastolic volumes did not change significantly, compared to sinus rhythm, whereas there was a significant increase in atrial end-systolic volumes during both arrhythmias possibly reflecting the rise in intra-atrial pressures. Interestingly, atrial end-systolic volume increased more during AVRT than AVNRT, but not significantly.

Pulsus alternans, although usually associated with impaired left ventricular function, may occur during paroxysmal supraventricular arrhythmias in the presence of a normal left ventricle (Figure 5.2). Goldreyer et al.[36] noted pulsus alternans in all of their cases of induced supraventricular tachycardia. It is common at the onset of tachycardia and may wax and wane as the arrhythmia progresses. Its mechanism is obscure, although it has been suggested that it is partially related to alterations in the contractile state of a proportion of the myocardium secondary to failure of electromechanical coupling of some cells resulting in alternate 'weak' contractions. The subsequent stronger

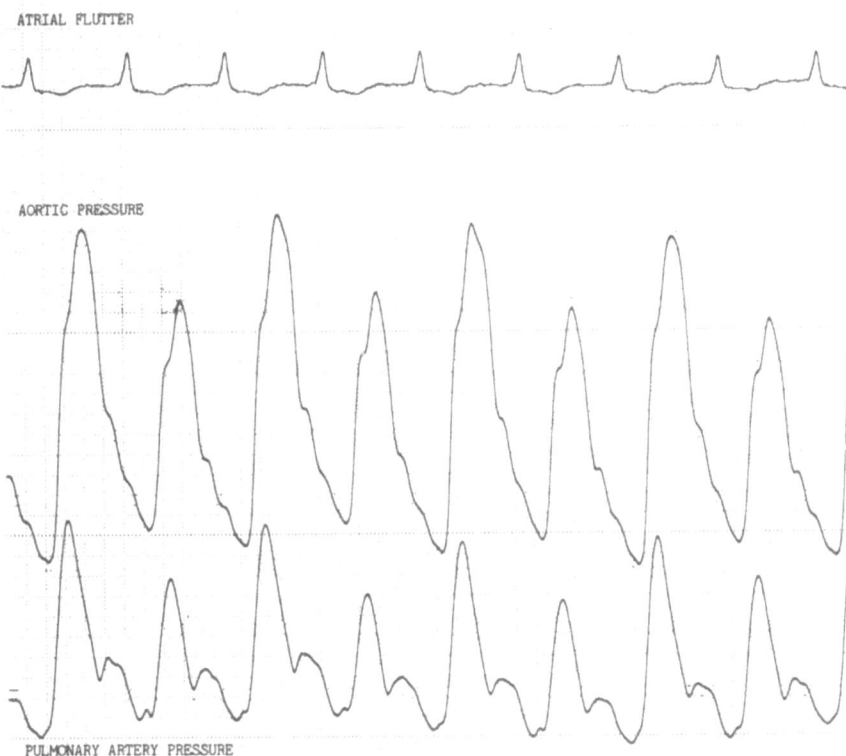

ATRIAL FLUTTER

AORTIC PRESSURE

PULMONARY ARTERY PRESSURE

Figure 5.2 Aortic and pulmonary artery pressures during atrial flutter in a patient with normal left ventricular function clearly showing simultaneous pulsus alternans in both systemic and pulmonary circulations

beat would represent contraction of all cells, some of which would be potentiated[38].

Atrial fibrillation

The loss of synchronized atrial contraction and the irregularity of the ventricular rhythm and rate, particularly with exercise, sufficiently alters the diastolic filling time to produce significant haemodynamic impairment especially in the presence of underlying cardiac disease. Separating the effects of loss of atrial transport, the ventricular rhythm and rate and the underlying cardiac process makes the haemodynamic assessment of this arrhythmia difficult.

During exercise Blumgart[39] noted that the ventricular rate during atrial fibrillation often achieved a higher level and declined more slowly with rest compared with patients with sinus rhythm. This was partially improved with digoxin[40,41]. A small proportion of patients with atrial fibrillation have a normal exercise response, although this is the exception rather than the rule. With the advent of electrical cardioversion[42] haemodynamic changes were more easily studied. McIntosh and Morris[19] noted a 34% increase in cardiac output immediately on conversion of atrial fibrillation to sinus rhythm in 7 of 11 resting patients. Killip et al.[21] found a similar improvement in patients with rheumatic valvular disease, but no difference in patients without demonstrable heart disease. Considering that the heart rate during atrial fibrillation and during sinus rhythm (immediately on conversion) may not be comparable in many of these studies, there is still compelling evidence that atrial fibrillation is haemodynamically less satisfactory. The improvement in output may not be immediate. Oram et al.[43] noted a significant increase 3–16 days after DC cardioversion, there having been no haemodynamic benefit immediately after, which they attributed to an anaesthetic effect. Graettinger et al.[44] noted a significant increase in output 1 h after cardioversion only in patients whose ventricular rate had significantly reduced. Many of the earlier anaesthetic agents were cardiosuppressive, thus accounting for the discrepancies between studies. In many younger patients with otherwise normal hearts and no predisposing factors, so called 'lone atrial fibrillation', there may be little reduction in cardiac output although cardiac efficiency is reduced purely due to the loss of atrial transport. In these cases there is often little haemodynamic detriment although patients feel symptomatically better after cardioversion to sinus rhythm. For some time lone atrial fibrillation has been thought of as benign but recent data from the Framingham Study[45] suggest that there is a significant mortality and morbidity from thromboembolism and this arrhythmia can no longer be considered as wholly innocuous.

The improvement in cardiac function on conversion of atrial fibrillation may be lost as a result of maintenance therapy designed to prevent recurrence. Many such drugs are negatively inotropic although evidence from a small study suggests that quinidine is not. Digoxin, although good at controlling the ventricular rate, is unreliable at preventing initiation of paroxysms.

Factors which initiate atrial fibrillation are controversial but a recent study[46], based on 24 h Holter monitoring, suggests that increased vagal tone is an important determinant. There were significant changes in P wave morphology and lengthening of AV conduction prior to paroxysms of atrial fribrillation, and more episodes occurred during sinus bradycardias associated with sleep.

Atrial flutter

There are few detailed haemodynamic studies. Cardiac output depends on a number of factors including the ventricular rate and the AV relationship. At slow ventricular rates, approximately 100 bpm, cardiac output is usually maintained although McIntosh and Morris[19] noted a reduction in output in one case of atrial flutter with a slow ventricular rate. In their patient, with idiopathic cardiomyopathy, they studied cardiac output during both atrial fibrillation and flutter at ventricular rates similar to sinus rhythm. During atrial flutter output was reduced to $2.5 \, \mathrm{l \, min^{-1} \, m^{-2}}$ (rate 79 bpm) compared to atrial fibrillation $(3.1 \, \mathrm{l \, min^{-1} \, m^{-2}}$ at 79 bpm) and sinus rhythm $(3.2 \, \mathrm{l \, min^{-1} \, m^{-2}}$ at 75 bpm). At high ventricular rates cardiac output depends on atrial synchronicity. Output is reduced during atrial flutter with 2:1 AV block compared to sinus rhythm at comparable ventricular rates. Leguime[47] noted a 35% reduction in output during atrial flutter with 2:1 block compared to sinus rhythm whereas Astrand et al.[48] reported that cardiac output during sinus tachycardia (154 bpm) and atrial flutter with 1:1 conduction (222 bpm) were similar, supporting the view that syn chronized atrial contraction at rapid ventricular rates significantly aids ventricular filling and increasing degrees of AV block impair cardiac efficiency.

Atrial tachycardia

Much of the initial investigation into the haemodynamic consequences of atrial tachycardia was performed during narrow complex arrhythmias which, under current terminology, would be subdivided into re-entrant arrhythmias or otherwise, as previously mentioned. The haemodynamic data have been discussed in the section on re-entrant arrhythmias and, to date, there has been no study specifically to investigate the haemodynamic differences between automatic atrial tachycardia and junctional tachycardia.

Ventricular tachycardia

Haemodynamic investigation of ventricular tachycardia has proven difficult due to its often rapid clinical deterioration, but the advent of electrophysiological and non-invasive techniques has partially overcome this. In general, patients often tolerate atrial arrhythmias better than ventricular arrhythmias at comparable rates. This is not, however, the rule and differentiation of ventricular from atrial tachycardia on the presence or absence of cardiovascular collapse is notoriously unreliable. Ventricular tachyarrhythmias often arise in the setting of cardiac disease, commonly ischaemia, and the level of left ventricular impairment does not always predict the haemodynamic consequences.

Ventricular tachycardias are arbitrarily divided on the basis of rate. Ventricular flutter usually occurs at rates greater than 250 bpm whereas ventricular 'tachycardia' can be as slow as 120 bpm. Both arrhythmias may degenerate to ventricular fibrillation when contraction becomes totally disorganized, cardiac output and systemic pressure fall and filling pressures increase. Theoretical mechanisms for ventricular dysfunction during ventricular tachycardia include:

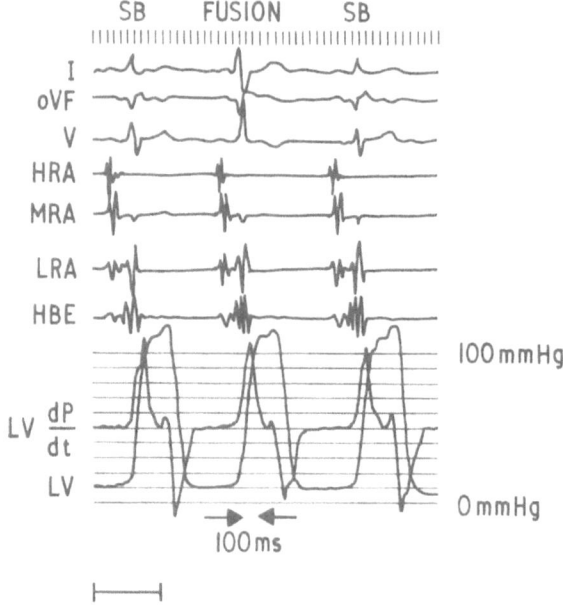

Figure 5.3a, b, c The effect of paced ventricular depolarization on left ventricular function as assessed by left ventricular (LV) pressure and the first derivative of LV pressure (dP/dt). (a) Shows little change in LV pressures with a VPB occurring sufficiently late in diastole to produce a fusion beat, whereas (b) and (c) show progressive reduction in LV pressure and LV dP/dt with increasing prematurity of the paced beat (From reference 49 with permission)

(1) Asynchronous ventricular contraction,
(2) Reduced diastolic relaxation,
(3) Incordinate diastolic relaxation,
(4) Atrioventricular valvular regurgitation,
(5) Ischaemia,
(6) Impaired ventricular contractility, e.g. cardiomyopathies.

The haemodynamic effects of premature beats have been extensively studied and the data extrapolated to tachycardia. The haemodynamic effects of ventricular premature beats (VPBs) depend to a degree on the coupling interval. VPBs occurring late in diastole often have no deleterious effects (Figure 5.3a), whereas those with short coupling intervals produce significant reduction in cardiac output, left ventricular systolic pressure and the first differential of left ventricular pressure, dP/dt (Figure 5.3a, b)[49]. Coupling intervals at 85–97% of the normal RR interval are sufficiently premature to reduce left ventricular stroke volume and stroke work, systemic blood pressure and peak left ventricular systolic pressure with little effect on left ventricular end-diastolic pressure (LVEDP)[50]. Isolated ventricular ectopics cause little change

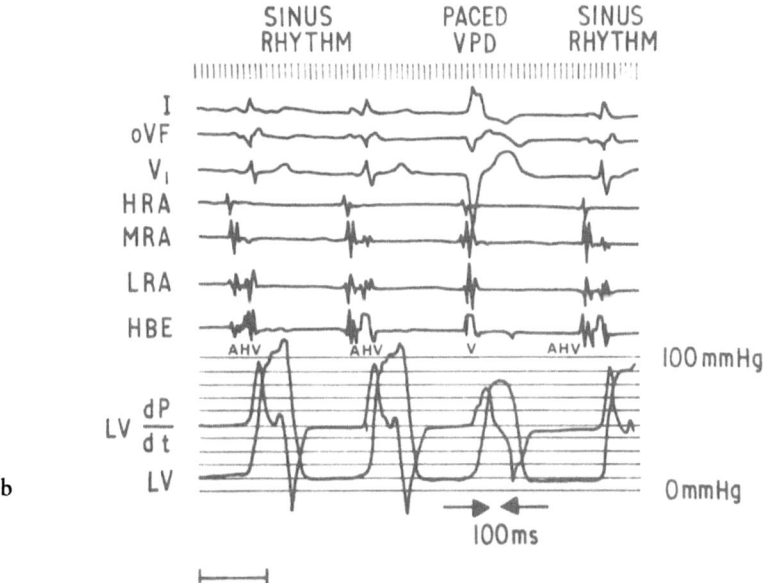

b

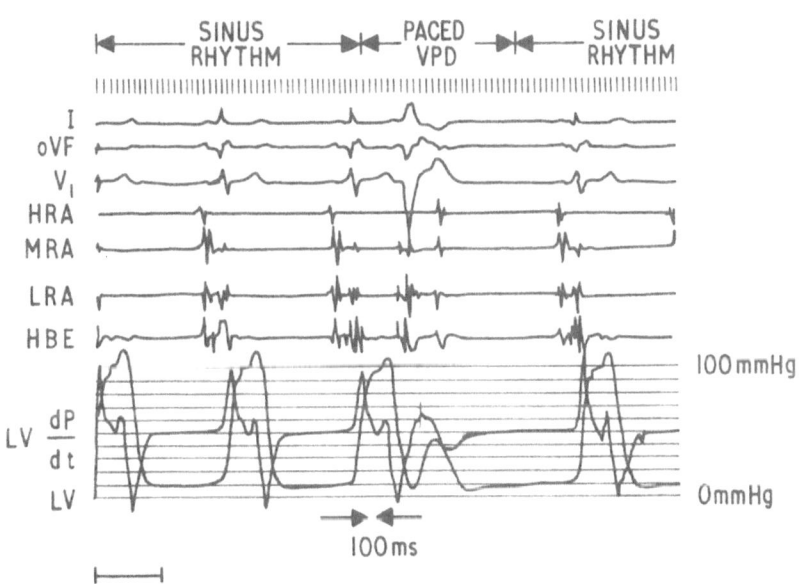

c

in end-diastolic pressures, whereas salvos often produce a significant reduction in peak left ventricular systolic pressure and increase LVEDP. Eber et al.[51] studied the pattern of contraction of VPBs both in experimental animals and in man using contrast ventriculography. Ectopics arising from the left ventricular apex produced a characteristic pattern, which they termed an 'hourglass' appearance, compared to ectopics arising from the left ventricular base, which gave a 'teardrop' pattern. The same ventricular deformation was seen during experimental ventricular tachycardia in dogs and induced tachycardia in man. The results emphasize the importance of ordered ventricular contraction for optimal cardiac function and suggest that apical VPBs are haemodynamically more effective than basal VPBs, supporting an earlier concept[31] that the site of origin of ventricular arrhythmias determines the haemodynamic consequences. Saksena et al.[49] compared the effects of VPBs, ventricular pacing (at an unspecified site) and sustained ventricular tachycardia on left ventricular function in 20 patients and the results are shown in Tables 5.1 and 5.2. There was a decremental change in peak left ventricular systolic pressures with increased pacing rates and a significant reduction in LVEDP. During sustained VT (Table 5.2) a similar reduction occurred as with pacing and VPBs. However, there was a significant increase in LVEDP and little correction of the fall in systolic pressures with time. The reductions of left ventricular systolic pressure during VT and pacing were of a similar order (Figure 5.4). In general, the more rapid the ventricular rate the greater the fall in LV systolic pressure. This contrasts with atrial tachycardias which, although often associated with a precipitous reduction in systemic pressure at the onset, are often corrected to near control levels within a few seconds. This may be related to the recruitment of different neurogenic reflexes during atrial and ventricular arrhythmias. Myocardial relaxation, as assessed by negative dP/dt, is reduced at the onset of tachycardia and during rapid ventricular pacing[49] possibly related to an alteration in ventricular depolarization (Table 5.1). During VT negative dP/dt remains depressed (Table 5.2). Rapid ventricular pacing, however, produces an equivalent degree of left ventricular impairment as does ventricular tachycardia, even though the sequence of ventricular depolarization is different. Data from this study suggest that ventricular end-diastolic volume is an important determinant of left ventricular function during ventricular tachycardia. Similar results were seen by Lima et al.[52] who measured left ventricular pressure and simultaneous 2-D echocardiography during induced ventricular tachycardias in man. Two groups were studied, one with impaired left ventricular function (left ventricular ejection fraction < 40% – group 1) and the other with normal left ventricular function (ejection fraction > 50% – group 2). During VT there was a significant reduction in left ventricular end-diastolic volumes in group 1 but little change in group 2. End-systolic volumes decreased in group 1 and increased in group 2, and there was a similar reduction in peak systolic pressures in both groups, from 123 ± 15 mmHg to 40 ± 10 mmHg in

Table 5.1 Effect of ventricular pacing on left ventricular function. LVEDP = left ventricular end-diastolic pressure, dP/dt = first derivative of left ventricular pressure. p Values show significance compared to sinus rhythm. There is a significant rate related decrease in ventricular function during pacing. (From reference 49 with permission)

	Sinus rhythm	Ventricular pacing (600 ms)	Ventricular pacing (400 ms)
LV Peak systolic BP (mmHg)	123 ± 19	99 ± 22 ($p < 0.01$)	79 ± 16 ($p < 0.01$)
LVEDP (mmHg)	22 ± 9	17 ± 5 ($p > 0.1$)	20 ± 5 ($p > 0.1$)
Peak dP/dt (mmHg/s)	1400 ± 620	890 ± 240 ($p < 0.01$)	805 ± 215 ($p < 0.01$)
Negative dP/dt (mmHg/s)	1220 ± 520	805 ± 210 ($p < 0.01$)	612 ± 150 ($p < 0.01$)

Table 5.2 Left ventricular function during sustained ventricular tachycardia as measured from the first tachycardia beat (VT_1) to the 50th beat (VT_{50}) showing a significant reduction in peak LV systolic pressures, peak dP/dt, negative dP/dt (an index of myocardial relaxation) and a significant increase in LVEDP (From reference 49 with permission)

	Sinus rhythm	VT_1	VT_5	VT_{10}	VT_{20}	VT_{50}
LV peak systolic BP (mmHg)	123 ± 19	77 ± 23 ($p < 0.05$)	61 ± 24 ($p < 0.01$)	62 ± 23 ($p < 0.01$)	58 ± 22 ($p < 0.01$)	57 ± 20 ($p < 0.01$)
LVEDP (mmHg)	22 ± 5	22 ± 9 ($p > 0.2$)	25 ± 13 ($p > 0.2$)	24 ± 12 ($p > 0.2$)	24 ± 11 ($p > 0.2$)	23 ± 9 ($p > 0.2$)
Peak dP/dt (mmHg/s)	$1,400 \pm 620$	810 ± 580 ($p < 0.05$)	580 ± 330 ($p < 0.01$)	575 ± 340 ($p < 0.01$)	550 ± 280 ($p < 0.01$)	580 ± 314 ($p < 0.01$)
Negative dP/dt (mmHg/s)	$1,220 \pm 520$	525 ± 270 ($p < 0.05$)	400 ± 260 ($p < 0.01$)	445 ± 300 ($p < 0.01$)	364 ± 260 ($p < 0.01$)	470 ± 310 ($p < 0.01$)

group 1 and 118 ± 18 mmHg to 38 ± 16 mmHg in group 2. The heart rate during VT in group 2 was lower that that in group 1. In both groups stroke volume fell as a result of reduced ventricular filling with a corresponding increase in LVEDP, and the authors concluded that in group 1 the prime mechanism for these changes was incomplete ventricular relaxation, whereas in group 2, the results suggested that incoordinate contraction and relaxation was the main problem. These conclusions rest on analysis of 2-D echocardiography which has known limitations, and no mention is made of mitral valve function during the arrhythmias, although the authors note that some patients had significant regurgitation during sinus rhythm. Nevertheless, it is an interesting observation and might explain why patients with differing levels

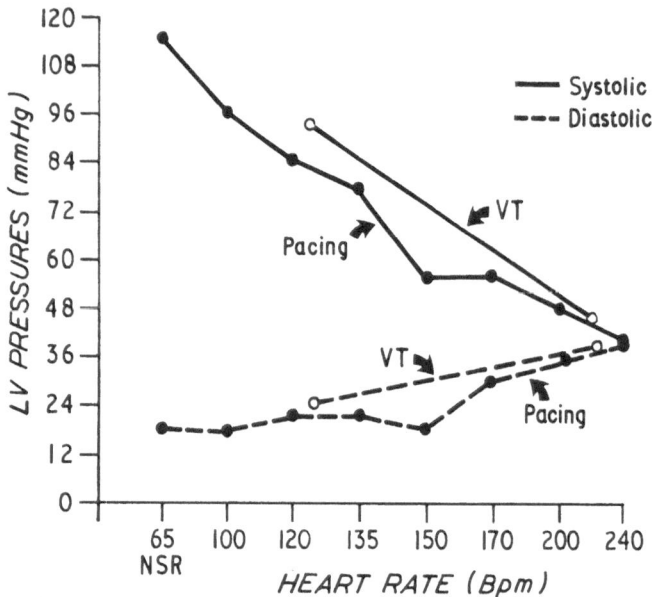

Figure 5.4 The effect of both incremental ventricular pacing and ventricular tachy-cardia (VT) at different rates on left ventricular pressures as compared to a baseline measurement during sinus rhythm (NSR). There is a linear reduction in peak systolic pressure and an increase in diastolic pressure with increasing ventricular rates. The changes in pressures are of a similar order of magnitude comparing ventricular pacing and tachycardia. (From reference 49 with permission)

of resting left ventricular function produce similar hypotension during VT. Mitral regurgitation at the onset of VT has been implicated as an important determinant of left ventricular dysfunction, and this may be related to the fall in left ventricular pressure seen during some arrhythmias. Mitral valve opening may be markedly altered during VT as compared to sinus rhythm[53] and is characterized by intermittent and infrequent opening, particularly during rapid arrhythmias. In Rosenbloom's study[53] the mean VT cycle length was 255 ± 58 ms (230 bpm) in patients with ventricular dysfunction compared to 305 ± 79 ms (197 bpm) in patients with preserved valvular excursion. Ejection fraction, assessed echocardiographically, was significantly reduced particularly in the val vular dysfunction group. This was found to be related to the rapidity of the tachycardia. Slower tachycardias, 420 ms (140 bpm) were associated with little change in ejection fraction. There was surprisingly little change in left ventricular segmental wall motion during VT as compared to sinus rhythm. Those patients with abnormal segmental wall motion in sinus rhythm had a deterioration during the arrhythmia but only two patients of 13 showed new wall motion abnormalities. Torres et al.[54] studied changes in segmental left ventricular function during ventricular pacing in dogs in an attempt to correlate this to the site of pacing. Using 2-D echocardiography in the mid ventricular short axis view in closed chest dogs they were able to predict, with reasonable accuracy, the site of ventricular premature beats and ventricular pacing.

CONCLUSIONS

There are multiple inter-related factors which determine the overall haemodynamic effect of cardiac arrhythmias, some of which are independent of myocardial function. Autonomic reflexes play an important role in haemodynamic changes, and more studies are required to establish their part in the initiation of arrhythmias as well as during sustained tachycardias. The multiplicity of interacting events makes the prediction of myocardial function from changes seen during an arrhythmia unreliable and each patient must be considered separately. Current interest in cardio- and vasoactive peptides may lead to a better understanding of the physiological changes that occur during arrhythmias in patients with both normal and impaired myocardial function.

References

1. Samet, P. (1973). Haemodynamic sequelae of cardiac arrhythmias. *Circulation*, 67, 399–407
2. Sinno, M. Z. and Gunnar, R. M. (1976). Haemodynamic consequences of cardiac dysrhythmias. *Med. Clin. N. Am.*, 60 (1), 70–80
3. Corday, E. and Irving, D. W. (1961). *Disturbances of Heart rate, Rhythm and Conduction.* (Philadelphia: WB Saunders Co.)
4. Braunwald, E. and Frahm, C. J. (1961). Studies on Starling's Law of the Heart. IV. Observations on the haemodynamic function of the left atrium in man. *Circulation*, 24, 633–42
5. Samet, P., Castillo, C., Bernstein, W. H. and Fernandez, P. (1968). Haemodynamic results of right atrial pacing in cardiac subjects. *Dis. Chest.*, 58, 133–7
6. Ross, J., Linhart, J. W. and Braunwald, E. (1965). Effects of changing heart rate in man by electrical stimulation of the right atrium. *Circulation*, 32, 549–58
7. Benchimol, A. and Liggett, M. S. (1966). Cardiac haemodynamics during stimulation of the right atrium, right ventricle and left ventricle in normal and abnormal hearts. *Circulation*, 33, 933–44
8. Samet, P., Bernstein, W. H., Levine, S. and Lopez, A. (1965). Haemodynamic effects of tachycardias produced by atrial and ventricular pacing. *Am. J. Med.*, 38, 905–10
9. Gilmore, J. P., Sarnoff, S. J., Mitchell, J. H. and Linden, R. (1963). Synchronicity of ventricular contraction: Observation comparing haemodynamic effects of atrial and ventricular pacing. *Br. Heart J.*, 25, 299–307
10. Greenfield Jr, J. C., Harley, A., Thompson, H. K., and Wallace, A. G. (1968). Pressure–flow studies in man during atrial fibrillation. *J. Clin. Invest.*, 47, 2411–21
11. Lister, J. W., Klotz, D. H., Jomain, S. L., Stuckey, J. H. and Hoffman, B. F. (1964). Effects of pacemaker site on cardiac output and ventricular activation in dogs with complete heart block. *Am. J. Cardiol.*, 14, 494–503
12. Samet, P., Bernstein, W. H. and Levine, S. (1965). Significance of the atrial contribution to ventricular filling. *Am. J. Cardiol.*, 15, 195–202
13. Askenazi, J., Alexander, J. H., Koenigsberg, D. I., Belic, N. and Lesch, M. (1984). Alteration in left ventricular performance by left bundle branch block stimulated with atrioventricular sequential pacing. *Am. J. Cardiol.*, 53, 99–104
14. Cohn, K. and Kryda, W. (1981). The influence of ectopic beats and tachyarrhythmias on stroke volume and cardiac output. *J. Electrocardiol.*, 14 (3), 207–18

15. Benchimol, A. and Desser, K. (1971). Phasic renal artery blood flow velocity in man during cardiac arrhythmias. *Am. J. Med. Sci.*, **261**, 161–6
16. Benchimol, A., Desser, K., Wang, T. F. and Mori, K. (1976). Influence of pacemaker-induced tachycardia with a A-V block on left ventricular blood velocity in man. *Am. Heart J.*, **91** (2), 178–85
17. Ricci, D. R., Orlick, A. E., Alderman, E. L., Ingels, N. B., Daughters, G. T., Kusnick, C. A., Reitz, B. A. and Stinson, E. B. (1979) Role of tachycardia as an inotropic stimulus in man. *J. Clin. Invest.*, **63**, 695–703
18. Packer, D. L., Bardy, G. H., Worley, S. J., Smith, M. S., Cobb, F. R., Coleman, R. E., Gallagher, J. J. and German, L. D. (1986) Tachycardia-induced cardiomyopathy: a reversible form of left ventricular dysfunction. *Am. J. Cardiol.*, **57**, 563–70
19. McIntosh, H. D. and Morris, J. J. (1966). The haemodynamic consequences of arrhythmias. *Prog. Cardiovasc. Dis.*, **182**, 548–55
20. Morris Jr, J. J., Entman, M. L., North, W. C., Kong, Y. and McIntosh, H. D. (1965). The changes in cardiac output with reversion of atrial fibrillation to sinus rhythm. *Circulation*, **31**, 670–8
21. Killip, T. and Baer, R. A. (1966). Cardiac function before and after electrical reversion from atrial fibrillation to sinus rhythm by praecordial shock. *J. Clin. Invest.*, **45**, 658–71
22. Mitchell, J. H. and Shapiro, W. (1969). Atrial function and the haemodynamic consequences of atrial fibrillation in man. *Am. J. Cardiol.*, **23**, 556–67
23. Brockman, S. K. (1965). Cardiodynamics of complete heart block. *Am. J. Cardiol.*, **16**, 72–83
24. Waxman, M. B., Wald, R. W. and Cameron, D. (1983) Interaction between the autonomic nervous system and tachycardias in man. *Cardiol. Clin.*, **1** (2), 143–84
25. Curry, P. (1979). The haemodynamic and electrophysiological effects of paroxysmal tachycardia. In Narula, O. S. (ed.) *Cardiac Arrhythmias; Electrophysiology, Diagnosis and Management.*, pp. 364–82 (Baltimore, London: Williams & Wilkins)
26. Skinner, S. N., Mitchell, J. H., Wallace, A. G. and Sarnoff, S. J. (1964). Haemodynamic consequences of atrial fibrillation at constant ventricular rates. *Am. J. Med.*, **36**, 343–9
27. Marin Neto, J. A., Gallo Jr, L., Manco, J. C., Rassi, A. and Amorim, D. S. (1980). Mechanisms of tachycardia on standing: Studies in normal individuals and in chronic Chagas' heart patients. *Cardiovasc. Res.*, **14**, 541–50
28. Pathak, C. L. (1959). Alternative mechanisms of cardiac acceleration in Bainbridge's infusion experiments. *Am. J. Physiol.*, **197**, 441–4
29. Nolan, J. P. and Short, F. A. (1966). Chronotropic alteration of cardiac performance in man. *Clin. Res.*, **14**, 241–5
30. Kappagoda, C. T., Linden, R. J. and Sivanathan, N. (1979). The nature of the atrial receptor responsible for a reflex increase in heart rate in the dog. *J. Physiol.*, **291**, 393–412
31. Corday, E., Gold, H., deVera, L. B., Williams, J. H. and Fields, J. (1959). Effect of the cardiac arrhythmias on the coronary circulation. *Ann. Intern. Med.*, **50**, (3), 535–53
32. deVera, L. B., Gold, H. and Corday, E. (1958). Simultaneous comparison of antegrade and collateral coronary blood flows. *Circ. Res.*, **6**, 26–8
33. Irving, D. W. and Corday, E. (1961). Effects of cardiac arrhythmias on the renal and mesenteric circulations. *Am. J. Cardiol.*, **6**, 32–40
34. Wood, P. (1963). Polyuria in paroxysmal tachycardia and paroxysmal atrial flutter and fibrillation. *Br. Heart. J.*, **25**, 273–81
35. Saunders Jr, D. E. and Ord, J. W. (1962). The haemodynamic effects of paroxysmal supraventricular tachycardia in patients with the Wolff–Parkinson–White syndrome. *Am. J. Cardiol.*, **9**, 223–36
36. Goldreyer, B., Kastor, J. A. and Kershbaum, K. L. (1976). The hemodynamic effects of induced supraventricular tachycardia in man. *Circulation*, **54** (5), 783–9
37. Kaye, G. C., Giles, M. and Camm, A. J. (1986). Measurement of left atrial volume during supraventricular tachycardia in man. *Clin. Sci*, **71**, 43P

38. Pace, J. B., Priola, D. V. and Randall, W. C. (1966). Alterations in cardiac synchrony and contractility during induced pulsus alternans. *Physiologist*, **9**, 259 (Abstr)

39. Blumgart, H. L. (1942). The reaction to exercise of the heart affected by auricular fibrillation. *Heart*, **11**, 49–56

40. Knox, J. A. C. (1949). The heart rate with exercise in patients with auricular fibrillation. *Br. Heart J.*, **11**, 119–25

41. Graybiel, A. (1964). Auricular fibrillation in an asymptomatic young man. Effects of exercise, digitalisation, atropinisation and restoration of normal rhythm. *Am. J. Cardiol.*, **14**, 828–36

42. Lown, B., Raghaven, A. and Newman, J. (1962). New method for terminating cardiac arrhythmias. *J. Am. Med. Assoc.*, **182**, 548–55

43. Oram, S., Weingren, L., Davies, J. P. M., Taggert, P. and Kitchen, L. D. (1963). Conversion of atrial fibrillation to sinus rhythm by direct current shock. *Lancet*, **2**, 159–62

44. Graettinger, J. S., Carleton, R. A. and Muenster, J. J. (1964). Circulatory consequence of changes in cardiac rhythm produced by transthoracic direct current shock. *J. Clin. Invest.*, **43**, 2290–302.

45. Brandt, F. N., Abbott, R. D., Kannel, W. B. and Wolf, P. A. (1985). Characteristics and prognosis of lone atrial fibrillation 30 year follow-up. The Framingham Study. *J. Am. Med. Assoc.*, **254**, 3449–53

46. Gabathuler, J. and Adamec, R. (1985). Declenchment de la fibrillation auriculaire paroxystique. *Arch. Mal. Coeur*, **8**, 1255–62

47. Leguime, J. (1941). Circulatory disturbances in pathologic conditions with high heart rates. *Cardiologica*, **5**, 105–10

48. Astrand, I., Cuddy, T. E., Landegren, J., Malmborg, R. O. and Saltin, B. (1963). Hemodynamic responses to exercise during atrial flutter and sinus rhythm. *Acta Med. Scand.*, **173**, 121–7

49. Saksena S., Ciccone, J. M., Craelius, W., Pannnatapoulous, D., Rothbart, S. T. and Werres, R. (1984). Studies on left ventricular function during sustained ventricular tachycardia. *J. Am. Coll. Cardiol.*, **4** (3), 501–8

50. Takada, H., Takeuchi, S., Ando, K. *et al.* (1970). Experimental studies on myocardial contractility and haemodynamics in extrasystoles. *Jpn. Circ. J.*, **34**, 419–30

51. Eber, L. M., Berkovitz, B. V., Matloff, J. M., Gorlin, R. and Cooke, J. M. (1974). Dynamic characterisation of premature ventricular beats and ventricular tachycardias. *Am. J. Cardiol.*, **33**, 378–83

52. Lima, J. A. C., Weiss, J. L., Guzman, P. A., Wiesfeldt, M. L., Reid, P. R. and Traill, T. A. (1983). Incomplete filling and incoordinate contraction as mechanisms of hypotension during ventricular tachycardia in man. *Circulation*, **68** (5), 928–38

53. Rosenbloom, M., Saksena, S., Rogal, G., Nanada, N. C. and Werres, R. (1984). Two dimensional echocardiographic studies in sustained ventricular tachycardia. *Pacing Clin. Electrophysiol.*, **7**, 136–42

54. Torres, M., Corday, E., Meerbaum, S., Sakamaki, T., Peter, T. and Uchiyama, T. (1983). Characterisation of left ventricular mechanical function during arrhythmias by two-dimensional echocardiography. Location of the site of onset of premature ventricular extrasystoles. *J. Am. Coll. Cardiol.*, **1**, (3), 819–29

6
The morphological correlates of atrial and ventricular tachycardias

M. J. DAVIES

It should be emphasized that morphological changes give a crude indication of electrophysiological function in a tachycardia; the greater success of clinicopathological correlation in conduction defects is based on the total destruction of segments of the conduction system, easily recognized by histological examination.

ATRIAL TACHYCARDIA AND FIBRILLATION

Transient atrial arrhythmias can be provoked by a wide range of pathophysiological mechanisms without morphological abnormality, for which thyrotoxicosis is a good example.

Chronic atrial tachyarrhythmias represent re-entry occurring either within a circumscribed area or throughout the atrial myocardium and non-homogeneous conduction is favoured by the age-related changes that occur in the atrial myocardium of otherwise normal hearts. Numerous authors have quantified the fall in numbers of specialized pacing cells in the sinus node, the increase in atrial connective tissue, the rise in atrial volume and the increasing incidence of small deposits of amyloid in the atria with age[1]. Over 70 years of age, on average, only 10% of the sinus node comprises conduction cells, in contrast to the 50% found in younger subjects. In many subjects over 70 years of age the interatrial septal myocardium may contain more connective and adipose tissue than muscle. The degree of loss of muscle is not evenly distributed throughout the atria and appears unrelated to arteriosclerosis or atheroma.

A wide range of pathological processes accelerate and enhance this non-specific loss of atrial myocardial muscle cells; for example, in end-stage rheumatic valve disease the dilated left atrium often contains very little myocardium. In acute ischaemic heart disease atrial fibrillation is directly linked to the incidence of atrial infarction, but in more chronic states simply represents fibrosis which separates islands of surviving

77

atrial muscle. Infiltration of atrial myocardium by amyloid has a similar pathological result. The association of atrial rather than ventricular arrhythmias with amyloidosis reflects a greater and earlier predilection of atrial myocardium to be involved. A single focus of atrial activity relating to a circumscribed pathological lesion is rare; an exception lies in tumour deposits in atrial muscle. The great majority of cardiac secondary deposits are clinically silent, but in those which do become manifest an atrial tachycardia is common.

VENTRICULAR TACHYCARDIA

Ventricular tachycardias can be divided into those that arise within the ventricular myocardium itself and those which are supraventricular in origin dependent either on re-entrant circuits within the conduction system itself or on an anomalous conduction pathway between atria and ventricles.

Tachycardia arising within the ventricular myocardium

Electrophysiological studies suggest that intraventricular arrhythmias arise due to non-homogeneous intramyocardial conduction leading to re-entry. As an acute phenomenon this may reflect foci of viable but damaged myocytes with abnormal transmembrane potentials, as caused by acute myocarditis or found at the margins of an acute myocardial infarction. In chronic situations many conditions can cause ventricular arrhythmias, but common to most is the disruption of the homogeneous mass of myocardial muscle cells into cords and strands by either fibrosis or infiltration by substances such as amyloid. A reasonable hypothesis is that such replacement creates an anastomosing configuration of muscle bundles ideal for a re-entrant phenomenon.

Ischaemic heart disease

Examination of the fibrous scars that result from previous acute infarction shows that the margins are not clearly defined (Figure 6.1). At the lateral border of the scar, clumps and strands of surviving myocardial muscle are embedded in collagen and in the scarred area itself a thin layer of myocardial muscle survives just beneath the endocardium. This sheet of muscle, only a few cells thick, owes its survival to diffusion of oxygen from the left ventricular cavity and contains variable proportions of conduction (Purkinje fibres) and contractile myocardial cells. The subendocardial sheet of muscle is contiguous with more normal myocardium at the margins of the area of infarction.

Given these facts, the morphological substrate for a re-entrant tachycardia must exist in many ischaemic scars, yet the majority of patients with a healed infarct are not troubled by arrhythmias and additional factors must be implicated.

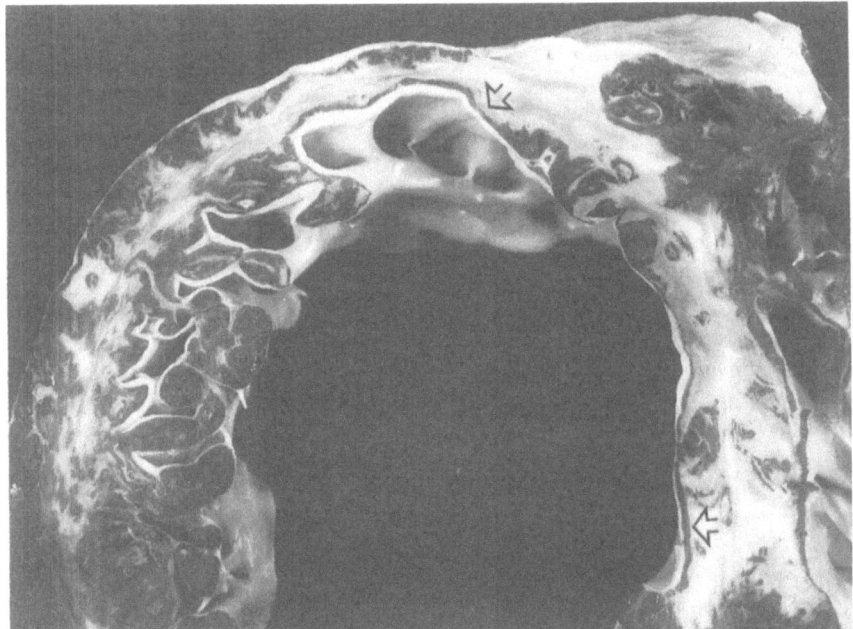

Figure 6.1 Transverse section of ventricular myocardium from a patient with ischaemic heart disease and recurrent ventricular tachycardia. The viable myocardium stains darkly, the collagen is white. In the area of old infarction immediately beneath the thick white endocardium is a thin layer of surviving muscle (arrow). Within the scar are other islands of surviving myocardium

Clinical studies which involve mapping the site of origin of a ventricular arrhythmia followed by curative resection have in part elucidated these problems. Over the area of old infarction potentials are fractionated[2] and the endocardium is activated in advance of the subepicardial surface[3]. Subendocardial resection, particularly at the margins of an aneurysm, is often successful in abolishing the arrhythmia[4], whereas simple aneurysectomy alone may not succeed. It therefore seems established that the source of ventricular tachycardias lies in the surviving subendocardial muscle at the margins of old infarcts, particularly those which are aneurysmal.

Histological examination of the material excised in procedures which abolish ventricular tachycardia[4-7] shows that the endocardium is markedly thickened by elastic tissue and collagen. Beneath the endocardium the tissue is also predominantly collagen, scattered amongst which are islands of myocardial muscle which make up only 10–50% of the tissue mass. Detailed ultrastructural studies confirm that these surviving muscle cells comprise both conduction (Purkinje) and contractile types. The Purkinje cells are predominantly normal in structure, but in contrast many of the contractile muscle cells are structurally abnormal by light

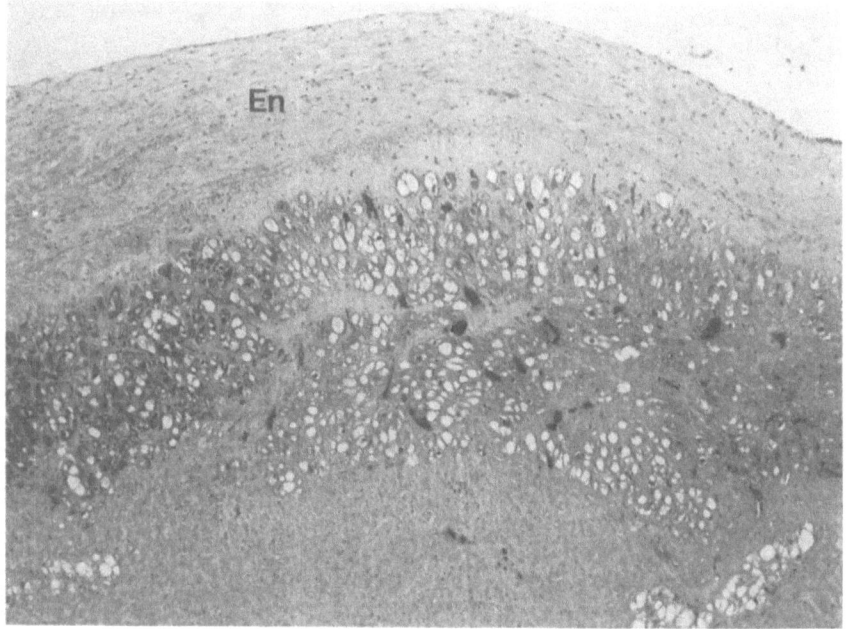

Figure 6.2 Histological appearance of the surviving layer of myocytes just beneath the endocardium in an area of healed infarction. The myocytes are vacuolated due to the reduced number of myofibrils contained with the cell (En, endocardium)

microscopy having undergone what is known as myocytolysis (Figure 6.2), a change thought to reflect chronic hypoxia. The cells appear large and vacuolated due to swelling and myofibrillary loss, but ultrastructural and histochemical studies show the mitochondria and nuclei to be intact and the cell is, therefore, viable. Contractile myocardial muscle cells which have undergone this change come to closely resemble Purkinje cells as seen by light microscopy, but the distinction between the two cell types can still be made based on the ultrastructure of the cell junctions and the presence or absence of transverse tubules[4].

Direct proof of the mechanism by which a sustained ventricular tachycardia is initiated cannot be obtained by these morphological studies but very reasonable hypotheses have been formulated. The particular properties of the surviving subendocardial muscle may lie in a particular geometric arrangement. The area of endocardium over which the circuit is located has been recorded as small (2–3 cm²) up to quite large (10–12 cm²) in size[8]. In theory this area could be studied by reconstructing the microanatomy, but the sheer number of serial sections needed and the fragmented nature of surgical resections precludes such work. The proximity of normal Purkinje cells to damaged but viable contractile cells may be an important factor. Against this is the fact that not all successful resections contain conduction as well as contractile tissue. Progressive endocardial thickening, particularly when associated with marked deposition of elastic tissue, may play a role in both inducing further hypoxia in surviving muscle or by further sub-dividing the subendocardial muscle sheet. In support of this view cases coming to successful surgical ablation have white endocardial thickening over the areas found to be responsible for initiating arrhythmias. Following successful subendocardial resection the endocardium once again is thickened by the formation of elastic and collagen tissue, but the arrhythmia does not recur in the absence of surviving muscle cells[6].

Non-ischaemic arrhythmogenic ventricular disease

Hypertrophic cardiomyopathy is associated with a high incidence of ventricular arrhythmias which predict the risk of sudden death[9,10]. The particular configuration of the muscle cells, arranged in circular whorls around foci of connective tissue, seems an ideal basis for re-entry tachycardia. Other factors potentiating arrhythmia may be focal myocyte damage reported in the literature as 'myocarditis' and anomalous atrioventricular connections[11]. In dilated cardiomyopathy ventricular arrhythmias are common[12], and again diffuse interstitial fibrosis in association with continuing myocyte damage and loss forms the morphological basis. Ventricular arrhythmias are strongly associated with myocardial sarcoidosis when granulomas are present in the myocardium, but arrhythmias also persist in hearts which are scarred, the active process burnt out and granulomas absent. In some cases local aneurysm formation occurs, and the arrhythmias may have a morphological basis similar to that seen in ischaemic disease.

Ventricular arrhythmias also complicate left ventricular hypertrophy due to aortic stenosis or regurgitation and their incidence rises as ventricular function declines[13]. In any hypertrophied ventricle the amount of collagen relative to the number of myocytes rises steadily with the increase in ventricular mass, and in the late stages fibrosis may be the predominant constituent of the myocardium particularly in the subendocardial zone. This degree of hypertrophy is also associated at autopsy with morphological evidence of focal necrosis of myocytes resulting from abnormalities of intramyocardial blood flow. In any ventricle with severe hypertrophy a combination of fibrosis and focal myocyte damage will therefore exist and form a possible basis for arrhythmia. Similar changes affect the right ventricular myocardium in gross hypertrophy, for example in Fallot's tetralogy[14,15].

Right ventricular dysplasia

Right ventricular dysplasia primarily causes dilation of the right ventricle due to replacement of the myocardium by fibrous or adipose tissue. In many cases the principal clinical manifestation is a tachycardia arising

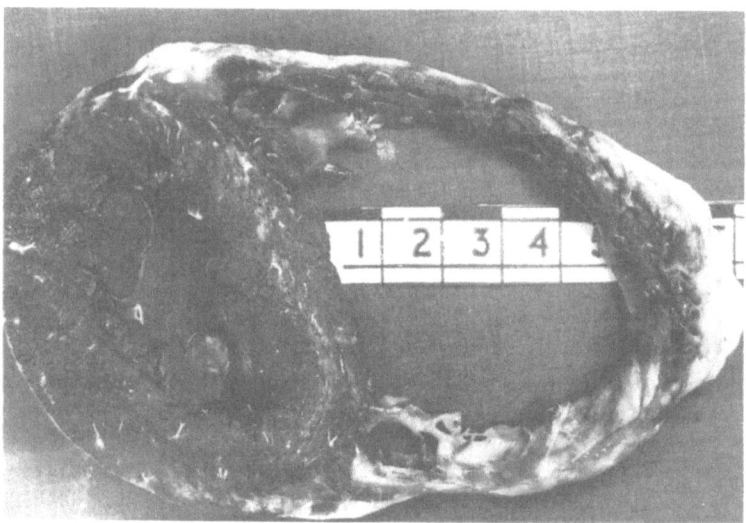

Figure 6.3 Short axis transection across the ventricles in a case of right ventricular dysplasia. The right ventricle is dilated and thin walled. Throughout the right ventricle there is extensive fibrous replacement of the myocardium. The left ventricle is normal in wall thickness and chamber diameter. The subject died suddenly during active sport

in the right ventricle[16]. Review of data in the literature taken in combination with nine autopsy cases seen personally allows the spectrum of the pathological features to be described. The essential macroscopic feature is a dilated right ventricular cavity and a right ventricular wall which is thinned (Figure 6.3). The most common pattern is aneurysmal dilation confined to the anterior wall of the outflow tract (five cases), but the anterior wall may be affected in combination with the lateral and posterior wall (three cases) or rarely the posterior wall is solely affected (one case). The left ventricle is essentially normal in terms of wall thickness, mass and cavity size, but two cases had macroscopic scarring in the subpericardial zone of the posterior wall, three showed an increase in small focal scars and interstitial fibrosis, and in only four cases was the left ventricular myocardium totally normal. The right ventricular myocardium was replaced by fibrous tissue with or without adipose tissue in all cases (Figure 6.4), and in five there was an area of right ventricular wall in which this change was transmural. Infiltration by adipose tissue was not a constant feature, being absent in five cases, whereas islands of myocardial muscle intersected by fibrous tissue were a feature of all cases. Evidence of continuing myocyte damage with a focal inflammatory response in the right ventricle was found in five cases.

The induction of a ventricular tachycardia in these cases must be presumed to be due to the formation of islands and strands of myocardial

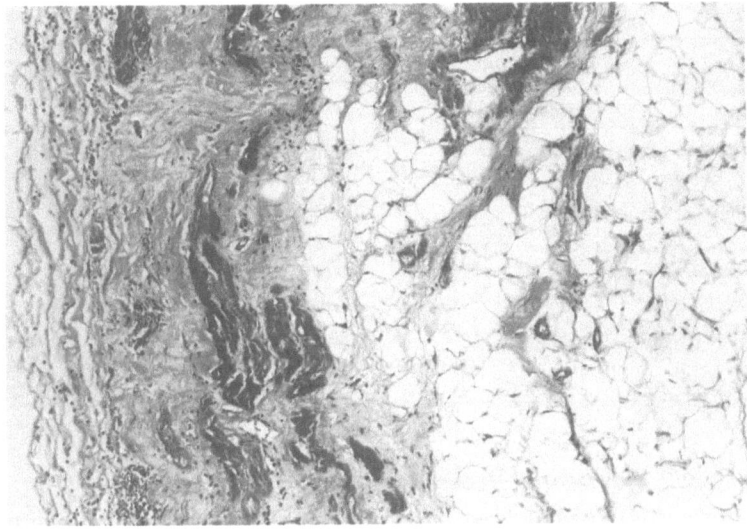

Figure 6.4 Histological section of the right ventricular wall in dysplasia. There are islands of myocardial muscle separated by collagen and adipose tissue

muscle cells separated by fibrous tissue associated with progressive myocyte damage.

The pathogenesis of the disease remains speculatory and it is uncertain if it is acquired or congenital. Familial cases are rare but well described[17]. Adipose tissue is found in the normal right ventricular myocardium, and its presence in ventricular dysplasia could indicate either a progressive myocyte loss or congenital absence of cardiac muscle. Those who believe that the lesion is a congenital lack of right ventricular myocardium use the term right ventricular dysplasia and consider the fat as indicating a failure of the muscle to form. In contrast, those who see the lesion as a progressive cardiomyopathy predominantly affecting the right ventricle cite the presence of extending fibrosis in the right ventricle and minimal left ventricular disease in some cases. There seems no clinical or morphological reason to separate cases with replacement of the right ventricular wall by adipose tissue and fibrosis from those who have fibrosis alone.

Sudden death is a significant risk of the condition, and the hearts seen personally were acquired in a referral practice of unexplained deaths in young subjects in which the local pathologist sought a further opinion. The condition may well be missed unless the features of a dilated right ventricle with focal wall thinning are known to the pathologist. Despite the association with sudden death some cases do survive until old age, the oldest reported being aged 84 at death[16].

Table 6.1

	Idiopathic arrhythmogenic right ventricle	Right ventricular dysplasia	Uhls disease
RV contraction	normal	segmental hypocontraction	generalized hypokinesia
Tricuspid regurgitation	absent	inconstant	gross
Cardiac failure	absent	inconstant	present
RV dilatation	absent	present	gross
Morphology	(a) normal (b) increased interstitial fibrosis	transmural replacement by fat or fibrous tissue	whole right ventricle replaced by fat/fibrous tissue

Ventricular tachycardia in apparently normal hearts

In cases without evidence of a contractile abnormality ventricular tachycardia is regarded as idiopathic or euphemistically as 'innocent'. When these arrhythmias arise in a right ventricle with demonstrable contractile abnormalities the case fits into the spectrum of right ventricular dysplasia; it is in those in which the right ventricle contracts normally that difficulty arises, and biopsy has been claimed to be a valuable adjunct to diagnosis. Four series[18-21] have expressed the view that a right ventricular biopsy is abnormal in over 90% of such cases. However, closer inspection of the 49 cases reported in these series reveals histologic data which are seldom quantified, and to some extent reflect the philosophy of the individual pathologists rather than indicating a specific diagnosis. A proportion of these patients are shown to have an occult acute myocarditis, but if rigid morphological criteria for the diagnosis are adopted it accounts for only seven patients in the 49 overall (14.3%). Twenty-three of the patients (46.9%) showed an increase in interstitial fibrosis of unknown origin, and three showed infiltration by adipose tissue and fibrosis reported as indicating right ventricular dysplasia despite normal ventricular function. The incidence of biopsies which are normal is, therefore, 32.7%. The 23 patients with an isolated increase of fibrosis in the right ventricle had an unquantified and often minimal increase in connective tissue, the significance of which is hard to interpret.

The arrhythmogenic right ventricle – one condition or several?

A spectrum of clinical and pathological changes (Table 6.1) link, on the one hand, patients who have arrhythmias arising in what is a normal ventricle in terms of contractile function and histology to, at the other extreme, patients who are in cardiac failure due to total replacement of the right ventricular muscle by fibrosis, a condition often known as Uhls disease. An individual patient can be placed at a point in this spectrum

Table 6.2

Name	Connections	Eponym
Accessory atrioventricular	right atrium–right ventricle ⎫ left atrium–left ventricle ⎬ parietal atrial septum–posterior IV septum atrial nodal overlay–IV septum	Kent — —
Atriofascicular	atrial septum–penetrating AV bundle	Brechenmacher
Nodoventricular	compact node to IV septum ⎫	Mahaim
Fasciculoventricular	penetrating bundle to IV septum ⎭	
Paranodal	posterior atrial septum–distal AV compact node	James
Intranodal	within compact AV node or between superficial and deep compact node	—

by consideration of all the available clinical and biopsy data. More long-term studies are needed to determine if patients progress from one point to another.

VENTRICULAR TACHYCARDIA DEPENDENT ON CONDUCTION FROM THE ATRIA

In the pre-excitation state the ventricular myocardium is activated earlier than anticipated by a conduction pathway which by-passes the delay normally imposed by the atrioventricular node. Sustained ventricular arrhythmias can result from the establishment of a circuit of activation using the normal conduction pathway as one limb and the anomalous path as the other limb.

A considerable number of accessory conduction pathways are known to be responsible for pre-excitation (Table 6.2). Most are supported by well-documented clinicopathological correlations of one or more cases.

The atrioventricular junction in normal hearts

In normal hearts the atrial and ventricular muscle is separated by the central fibrous body and the fibrous rings of the mitral and tricuspid valves. The normal atrioventricular conduction path (bundle of His) tunnels through the central fibrous body. While usually regarded as solid fibrous structures the valve rings are often deficient, particularly on the right side, but although atrial and ventricular muscle may abut (contiguity) at these sites muscle bundles do not actually run from the atria to ventricles thus establishing continuity of muscle. Similar defects allowing contiguity, but not continuity, are also common in the posterior aspect of the central fibrous body near the coronary sinus.

The atrial muscle close to the base of the insertion of the valve cusps into their rings contains persistent node-like myocardium in up to 25%

of normal hearts[22]. Such cell rests are particularly common in the anterior portion of the tricuspid ring and are almost certainly the structures identified by Kent as accessory pathways. Serial reconstruction however, shows that this ring of nodal tissue in normal hearts does not cross from atria to ventricle and is merely an embryonic remnant.

Within the conduction system itself there is variation in the connections of the atrial muscle to the atrioventricular node. The transition from atrioventricular node to penetrating bundle is normally taken as the point at which the conduction tissue is completely encased by the fibrous body. In some hearts this tunnel remains partially open due to lack of development of the fibrous body, and the potential exists for an unduly late insertion of an atrial input into the bundle of His.

Strands of AV nodal tissue often penetrate into the fibrous body (archipelagos) before the formation of the penetrating bundle proper. These strands form a mass of interweaving bundles isolated within the fibrous body, but very rarely reach the ventricular septum. These islands are prominent in neonatal and infant hearts but disappear with age. While these archipelagos of nodal tissue might form the basis for reentry no formal proof of such function exists, although their role in sudden death has been a matter of speculation[23] both in infants and adults.

Accessory conduction pathways

For the purposes of classification[24,25] accessory pathways can be divided into those which lie in the mitral or tricuspid valve rings (left and right parietal pathways) and those which lie in the septum. Posterior septal paths may activate the myocardium on either side of the midline and may thus be mistaken clinically for parietal pathways.

Parietal pathways

These paths form the bulk of well documented clinicopathological studies. The majority of parietal accessory pathways comprise normal working myocardial cells arranged in a slender bundle joining atria to ventricles. Multiple slender bundles and arborization of the ventricular end over a wide area of ventricular myocardium are common. Isolated examples[24] of accessory paths which arise in the persistent nodal type tissue of the valve rings are described, and in theory can exhibit a delay in conduction in the anomalous path.

On the left side the anomalous bundles run in the epicardial fat skirting but closely applied to the annulus of the mitral valve. On the posterior surface of the left ventricle this site lies close to the left circumflex artery which separates the anomalous path from the coronary

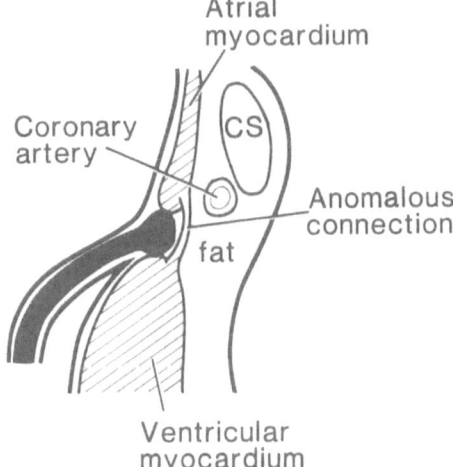

Figure 6.5   Anatomic relations of left-sided parietal pathways

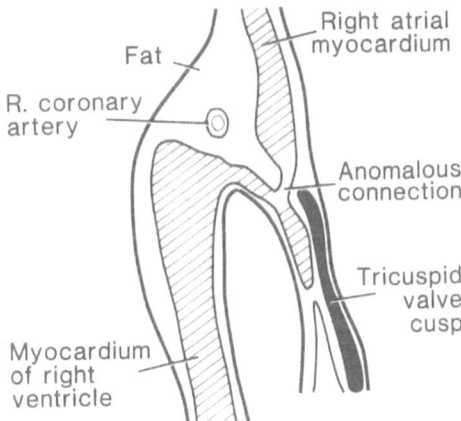

Figure 6.5   Anatomic relations of left-sided parietal pathways

sinus (Figure 6.5). On the right side the annulus is often deficient, being replaced by a pad of fat through which the pathway runs (Figure 6.6).

Septal pathways

In the region of the coronary sinus immediately posterior to the atrio-ventricular node the central fibrous body is almost always deficient, and through this gap muscle strands may connect atria and ventricles. The strands comprise normal atrial muscle.

Connections more anterior in the septum lie close to the atrio-

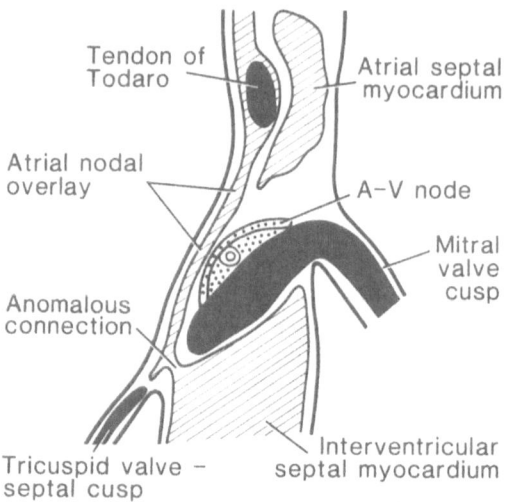

Figure 6.7 Anatomic relations of the atrioventricular node and septal pathways

ventricular node, and some understanding of the microanatomy in this region is necessary for their description.

The compact portion of the atrioventricular node abuts onto the central fibrous body and lies just beneath the endocardium of the right atrium at the apex of the triangle of Koch. The apex of this triangle is made by the insertion of the tendon of Todaro into the base of the septal cusp of the tricuspid valve. The node at this point (Figure 6.7) has a deep portion surrounded by onion skin-like layers of the superficial node, an overlay of transitional cells and finally a layer of ordinary atrial muscle cells. This last layer runs down over the atrial septum into the base of the septal cusp of the tricuspid valve. Since the insertion of the septal cusp of the tricuspid valve is below the apex of the muscular interventricular septum there is an area in which the atrial overlay muscle lies alongside the ventricular septal muscle. The extension of the central fibrous body of the base of the septal cusp is very often deficient in this area allowing contiguity of the atrial and ventricular muscle. If muscle bundles cross through the defect an anomalous pathway is created[11].

Nodoventricular and fasciculoventricular connections

Mahaim described these connections penetrating the fibrous body, and there is no doubt that such strands of muscle are not infrequent in normal hearts particularly at young ages. The connections tend to vanish as the central fibrous body undergoes sclerosis with age. While often used as a theoretical basis for pre-excitation, tachycardia or sudden death proof of their function is often minimal. One documented clinico-pathological case of pre-excitation exists[26], and one case report describes the coincidence of ventricular tachycardia with these pathways with proof of their function in maintaining the arrhythmia[27], but more such detailed electrophysiological pathological studies are needed if the role of these paths is to be confirmed. It may be that nodoventricular and fasciculoventricular connections are simply 'bystanders' in a patient in whom tachycardia originates by re-entry with the AV node itself.

Atriofascicular connections

Such paths theoretically abolish the normal nodal delay leading to a short PR and a normal QRS complex. In incontrovertible cases the connection joins the penetrating bundle within its tunnel in the central fibrous body[28].

Paranodal connections

James[29] described conduction fibres running in the superficial atrial overlay of the node which originated around the Eustachian ridge posteriorly in the atrial septum, and entered the node well anteriorly just before the penetrating bundle commenced. Others[24] have failed to find such connections in normal hearts and their function remains theoretical.

Conditions associated with anomalous pathways

A pre-excitation pattern in the ECG is found in up to 10% of patients with Ebstein's anomaly and up to 50% have episodes of tachycardia[30]. The anomalous pathway is right-sided and when septal probably reflects an abnormal degree of downward displacement of the septal leaflet of the tricuspid valve allowing contact between the atrial overlay fibres and the ventricular septum. The dysplastic cusps in Ebstein's anomaly are often extensively covered by a layer of atrial muscle, and in one reported case this made contact with ventricular muscle in the anterior part of the atrioventricular ring. This is the commonest site for persistence of nodal type ring tissue, and similar contact with the ventricular myocardium occurs in corrected transposition and double inlet left ventricles[31]. In such cases if the conduction system proper is deficient due to the gross defect in septal development atrioventricular conduction may depend solely on the accessory pathway.

There also appears to be an undue association of hypertrophic cardiomyopathy with pre-excitation, and in some families the two are directly linked[32]. The sites of the pathways have been both parietal and septal and usually involve insertion into areas of abnormally arranged ventricular muscle. It is uncertain whether this is a simple persistence of the anomalous connection or whether the abnormal arrangement and growth of the ventricular myocardium establishes connections at a later date in areas where deficiency of the fibrous rings has been present.

An ECG showing a pre-excitation pattern is described as unduly frequent in mitral valve prolapse. One view put forward is that the structural abnormality of the connective tissue of the cusp is also expressed in the annulus allowing a connection of atrial to ventricular to exist or develop, but an alternative explanation to the association is that pre-excitation itself leads to asynchronous contraction inducing prolapse of a structurally normal cusp[33]. In 13 patients with pre-excitation in one study mitral valve prolapse occurred only when conduction via the anomalous pathway was occurring.

There is also an undue association of posterior left parietal pathways with aneurysms of the coronary sinus[34] which has been linked to abnormal persistence of a cuff of atrial muscle associated with the sinus venosus. This muscle may follow abnormal veins entering the aneurysmal sac from the posterior wall of the ventricle.

INTRANODAL RE-ENTRY TACHYCARDIA

AV nodal re-entrant tachycardias are common, and thought to arise in dual conduction pathways close to, or within, the A–V node itself. There is a slow antegrade path and a rapidly conducting retrograde path. Electrophysiological studies suggest both begin and end in nodal tissue[35], and the whole circuit is, therefore, intranodal. Islands of nodal tissue separate from the main node and embedded within the central fibrous body are common particularly in hearts from young subjects; if these form loops connecting with the node an ideal substrate for dual intranodal paths would exist. An alternative view[36] sees one limb of the circuit being made up of atrial myocytes, and thus paranodal in position. Supporting this, surgical dissection of the margins of the node is often successful in abolishing intranodal re-entry. Part of the controversy is semantic and concerned with different definitions of what comprises the node. To the anatomist the node is like half an onion with successive layers. Only the deepest layer has small interweaving myocytes which the electrophysiologist would regard as nodal. The superficial layers are very like atrial myocardium and could form one limb of a re-entry circuit which would be disrupted by dissection around the nodal area. The form of nodal re-entrant tachycardia with a long RP' interval has been postulated to be due to accessory nodal tissue, and residual islands within the central fibrous body are an obvious candidate. However, one autopsy study merely revealed a long and tortuous septal anomalous path made up of normal myocytes[37].

Focal His bundle tachycardia

This is thought to represent an abnormal autonomous focus within the His bundle, and is supported by a single case report showing a focal His bundle lesion with fibrosis at autopsy[38].

TACHYCARDIA WITH A LONG QT INTERVAL

In experimental situations an imbalance of sympathetic stimulation will prolong the QT interval and focus attention on the cardiac ganglia and nerves in human cases. A focal 'neuritis', that is degeneration of axons and an infiltration of the ganglia by lymphocytes, has been described as being present[39]. However, routine examination of the nervous system is difficult, and the immunological and quantitative assessment that would be used by neuropathologists on peripheral nerves has not been carried out. Another study of six cases showed fatty infiltration and mild 'myocarditis' of the node[40]. The morphological basis, if any, of the long QT interval remains to be confirmed. The consensus among many pathologists is that it does not lie in structural abnormalities of the conduction system or of its nerves[41].

References

1. Davies, M. J. (1983). The pathology of atrial arrhythmias. In Davies, M. J., Anderson, R. H. and Becker, A. E. (eds.) *The Conduction System of the Heart.* pp. 203–215. (London: Butterworths)
2. Cox, J. L. (1983). Anatomic-electrophysiologic basis for the surgical treatment of refractory ischaemic ventricular tachycardia. *Ann. Surg.,* **198,** 119–29
3. Josephson, M. E., Horowitz, L. N. and Spielman, S. R. (1980). Comparison of endocardial catheter mapping with intraoperative mapping of ventricular tachycardia. *Circulation,* **61,** 395–404
4. Fenoglio, J. J., Pham, T. D., Harken, A. H., Horowitz, L. N., Josephson, M. E. and Wit, A. L. (1983). Recurrent sustained ventricular-tachycardia: structure and ultrastructure of subendocardial regions in which tachycardia originates. *Circulation,* **68,** 518–33
5. Bolick, D. R., Hackle, D. B. and Reimer, K. A. (1985). Infarct structure in patients with ventricular tachycardia. *Circulation,* **72,** III 346
6. Silver, M. A., Cohen, A. I. and Katz, N. Ml. (1984). Cardiac morphological findings late after partial left ventricular endomyocardial resection for recurrent ventricular tachycardia. *Am. J. Cardiol.,* **54,** 233–5
7. Silver, M. A. (1986). Morphologic substrates of ventricular arrhythmias. *Clin. Prog. Electrophys. Pacing,* **4,** 1–3
8. Horowitz, L. N., Josephson, M. E. and Harken, A. H. (1980). Epicardial and endocardial activation during substained ventricular tachycardia in man. *Circulation,* **61,** 1227–38
9. Bjarnason, I., Hardarson, T. and Jonsson, S. (1982). Cardiac arrhythmias in hypertrophy cardiomyopathy. *Br. Heart J.,* **48,** 198–203
10. McKenna, W. J., England, D., Doi, Y. L., Deanfield, J. E., Oakley, C. and Goodwin, J. (1981). Arrhythmia in hypertrophic cardiomyopathy. Influence on prognosis. *Br. Heart J.,* **46,** 168–72
11. Krikler, D. M., Davies, M. J., Rowland, E., Goodwin, J. F., Evans, R. C. and Shaw, D. B. (1980). Sudden death in hypertrophic cardiomyopathy: associated accessory pathways. *Br. Heart J.,* **43,** 245–51
12. Huang, S. K., Messer, J. V. and Denes, P. (1983). Significance of ventricular tachycardia in idiopathic dilated cardiomyopathy: observations in 35 patients. *Am. J. Cardiol.,* **51,** 507–12
13. Olshausen, K., Amann, E., Hofmann, M., Schwartz, F., Mehmel, H. C. and Kubler, W. (1984). Ventricular arrhythmias before and late after aortic valve replacement. *Am. J. Cardiol.,* **54,** 142–6
14. Karey, R. E. W., Blackman, M. S. and Sondheimer, H. (1982). Incidence and severity

of chronic ventricular dysrhythmia after repair of tetralogy of Fallot. *Am. Heart J.*, **103**, 342–50

15. Deanfield, J. E., McKenna, W. J. and Hallidie-Smith, K. A. (1980). Detection of late arrhythmias and conduction disturbances after correction of tetralogy of Fallot. *Br. Heart J.*, **44**, 248–53

16. Marcus, F. I., Fontaine, G. H., Guiraudon, G., Frank, R., Laurenceau, J. L., Malergue, C. and Grosgogeat, Y. (1982). Right ventricular dysplasia: a report of 24 adult cases. *Circulation*, **65**, 384–92

17. Rakovec, P., Rossi, L., Fontaine, G., Sasel, B., Markez, J. and Voncina, D. (1986). Familial arrhythmogenic right ventricular disease. *Am. J. Cardiol.*, **58**, 377–8

18. Morgera, T., Salvi, A. E., Silvestri, F. and Camerini, F. (1985). Morphological findings in apparently idiopathic ventricular tachycardia. An echocardiographic haemodynamic and histologic study. *Eur. Heart J.*, **6**, 323–34

19. Sugrue, D. D., Holmes, D. R., Gersh, B. J., Edwards, W. D., McLaran, C., Wood, D. L., Osborn, M. J. and Hammill, S. C. (1984). Cardiac histological findings in patients with life threatening ventricular arrhythmias of unknown origin. *J. Am. Coll. Cardiol.*, **4**, 952–7

20. Strain, J. E., Grose, R. M., Factor, S. M. and Fisher, J. D. (1983). Results of endomyocardial biopsy in patients with spontaneous ventricular tachycardia but without apparent structural heart disease. *Circulation*, **68**, 1171–81

21. Hosenpud, J. D., McAnulty, J. H. and Niles, N. R. (1986). Unexpected myocardial disease in patients with life threatening arrhythmias. *Br. Heart J.*, **56**, 55–61

22. Anderson, R. H., Davies, M. J. and Becker, A. E. (1974). Atrioventricular ring specialised tissue in the normal heart. *Eur. J. Cardiol.*, **2**, 219–30

23. Marino, T. A. and Kane, B. M. (1985). Cardiac atrioventricular junctional tissues in hearts from infants who died suddenly. *J. Am. Coll. Cardiol.*, **5**, 1178–84

24. Becker, A. E. (1983). Morphological basis of pre-excitation. In Davies, M. J., Anderson, R. H. and Becker, A. E. (eds.) *The Conduction System of the Heart.* pp. 181–202 (London: Butterworths)

25. Anderson, R. H., Becker, A. E., Brechenmacher, C., Davies, M. J. and Rossi, L. (1975). Ventricular pre-excitation: a proposed nomenclature for its substrates. *Eur. J. Cardiol.*, **3**, 27–36

26. Lev, M., Fox, S. M., Bharati, S., Rosen, K. M., Langendorf, R. and Pick, A. (1975). Mahaim fibres as a basis for a unique variety of pre-excitation. *Am. J. Cardiol.*, **35**, 152

27. Gmenier, R., Ng, C. K., Hammer, I. and Becker, A. E. (1984). Tachycardia caused by an accessory nodo–ventricular tract: a clinico–pathological correlation. *Eur. Heart J.*, **3**, 233–43

28. Brechenmacher, C. (1975). Atrio–His bundle tracts. *Br. Heart J.*, **37**, 853–5

29. James, T. N. (1961). Anatomy of the human A–V node with remarks pertinent to its electrophysiology. *Am. Heart J.*, **62**, 756–71

30. Simcha, A. and Bonham-Carter, R. E. (1971). Ebstein's anomaly: clinical study of 32 patients in childhood. *Br. Heart J.*, **33**, 46–9

31. Anderson, R. H. (1983). Congenitally complete atrioventricular block. In Davies, M. J., Anderson, R. H. and Becker, A. E. (eds.) *The Conduction System of the Heart.* pp. 167–78 (London: Butterworths)

32. Hauser, A. M., Gordon, S. and Timmis, G. C. (1984). Familial hypertrophic cardiomyopathy and pre-excitation. *Am. Heart J.*, **107**, 176–9

33. Drake, C. E., Hodsden, J. E., Sridharan, M. R. and Flowers, N. C. (1985). Evaluation of the association of mitral valve prolapse in patients with WPW type electrocardiogram and its relation to ventricular activation pattern. *Am. Heart J.*, **109**, 83–7

34. Gerlis, L. M., Davies, M. J., Boyle, R., Williams, G. and Scott, H. (1985). Pre-excitation due to accessory sinuoventricular connections associated with coronary sinus aneurysms. A report of two cases. *Br. Heart J.*, **53**, 314–22

35. Miller, J. M., Rosenthal, M. E., Vassallo, J. A. and Josephson, M. E. (1987). Atrioventricular nodel re-entry tachycardia: studies on upper and lower 'common' pathways. *Circulation*, **75**, 930–40

36. Ross, D. L., Johnson, D. C., Denniss, A. R., Cooper, M. J., Richards, D. A. and Uther, D. B. (1985). Curative surgery for atrioventricular junctional ('AV nodal') re-entrant tachycardia. *J. Am. Coll. Cardiol.*, **6**, 1383–92

37. Critelli, G., Gallagher, J. J., Thisene, G., Perticone, F., Coltorti, F. and Rossi, L. (1985). Electrophysiological and histopathologic correlations in a case of permanent form of reciprocating tachycardia. *Eur. Heart J.*, **6**, 130–7

38. Brechenmacher, C., Coumel, P. and James, T. N. (1976). Intractable tachycardia in infancy. *Circulation*, **53**, 377–81

39. James, T. N., Froggatt, P., Atkinson, W. J. *et al.* (1978). Observations on the pathophysiology of the long QY syndromes with special reference to the neuro-pathology of the heart. *Circulation*, **57**, 1221–31

40. Bharati, S., Dreifus, L., Bucheleres, G. *et al.* (1985). The conduction system in patients with a prolonged QT interval. *J. Am. Coll. Cardiol.*, **6**, 1110–20

41. Pellegrino, A., Ho, S. W., Anderson, R. H., Hegerty, A., Godman, M. J. and Michaelsson, M. D. (1986). Prolonged QT interval and the cardiac conduction tissues. *Am. J. Cardiol.*, **58**, 1112–13

7
Diagnosis of cardiac arrhythmias from the surface electrocardiogram

D. W. DAVIES and W. D. TOFF

INTRODUCTION

The resting 12-lead surface electrocardiogram (ECG) is often the first investigation performed in patients with symptoms suggestive of cardiac arrhythmia. During an arrhythmia, the 12-lead ECG alone may disclose the diagnosis, and between attacks it may provide pointers to the likely diagnosis or aetiology of the arrhythmia, such as pre-excitation in the Wolff–Parkinson–White syndrome (Figure 7.1a) suggesting atrio-ventricular re-entry tachycardia (Figure 7.1b), or evidence of myocardial infarction raising the possibility of ventricular tachycardia. In either of these examples, however, atrial fibrillation (Figure 7.1c) might be an alternative cause of symptoms, emphasizing the importance of an ECG during the symptoms in determining the causal arrhythmia.

Misinterpretation of the surface ECG recorded during a cardiac arrhythmia is common[1,2] and may lead to the prescription of inappropriate and potentially life-threatening therapy. This is particularly true for tachyarrhythmias, and it is the purpose of this chapter to indicate how the adoption of a systematic approach to analysis of the surface ECG of cardiac arrhythmias avoids common diagnostic pitfalls, and provides an insight into the aetiology and pathophysiology of the arrhythmias.

BRADYARRHYTIIMIAS

The key to the diagnosis of bradyarrhythmias is the determination of the relationship between atrial and ventricular activity (Figure 7.2). Where the P wave cannot be seen on the surface ECG it can often be disclosed by using oesophageal[3] or intracardiac[4] electrodes. A bradycardia results either from a decrease in the frequency of discharges escaping from the sinus node or from a block in the conduction of the ensuing atrial depolarization to the ventricles.

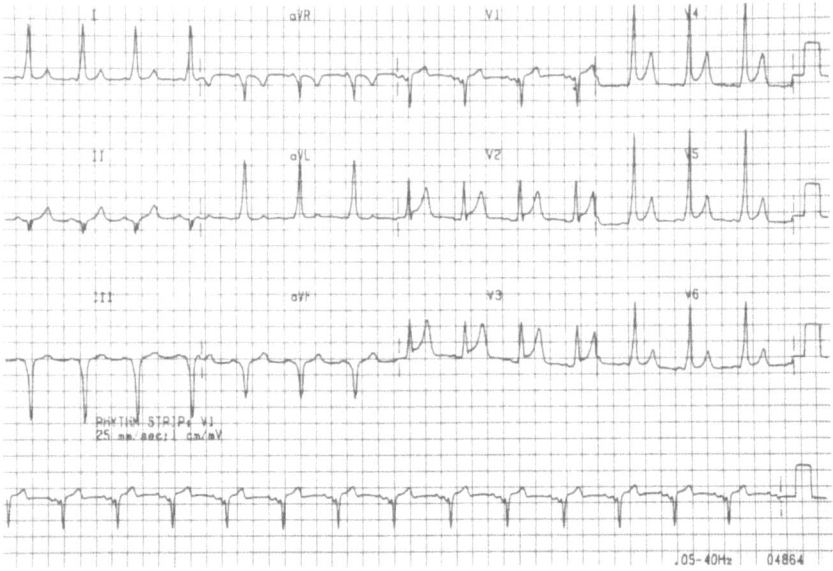

Figure 7.1(a) Twelve-lead ECG showing ventricular pre-excitation by a posteroseptal accessory pathway during sinus rhythm.

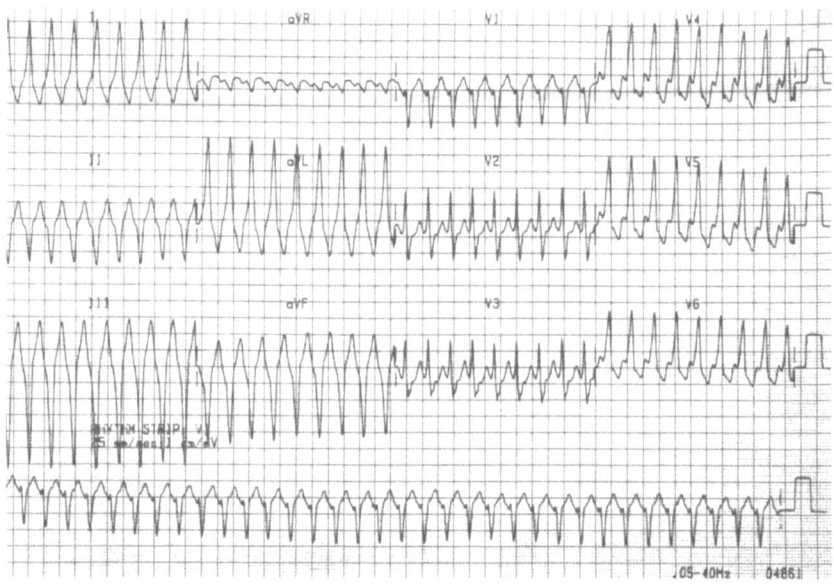

Figure 7.1(b) Twelve-lead ECG from the same patient as Figure 7.1a but during antidromic atrioventricular tachycardia. Note the accentuation of the pre-excitation pattern seen during sinus rhythm as fusion with ventricular depolarization mediated by the His–Purkinje system is lost. The possibility of a pre-excited atrial tachycardia cannot be excluded from this ECG.

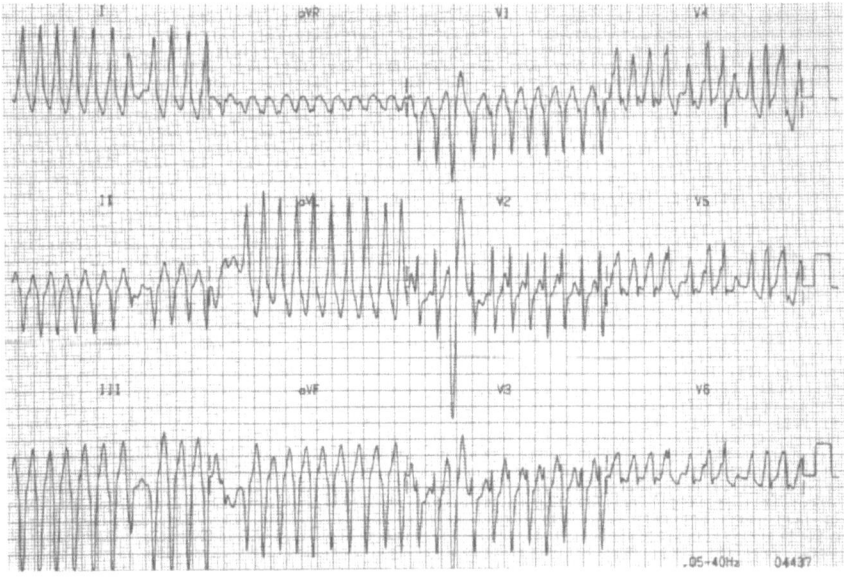

Figure 7.1(c) Twelve-lead ECG from the same patient as in (a) and (b). This shows pre-excited atrial fibrillation. Note the irregular and rapid (up to 300 bpm) ventricular response, similar QRS morphologies to those in (a) and (b) but with variation of QRS width representing varying degrees of fusion between normal and pre-excited ventricular depolarization. This is best seen in leads V4, V5 and V6 in this example.

Sinus bradycardia

Sinus bradycardia may reflect cardiovascular fitness, as in athletes, β-blockade or a disorder such as hypothyroidism. In these conditions the sinus node discharges at a decreased rate, each depolarization being conducted to the surrounding atrial tissue, resulting in P waves of normal morphology, each being followed at a more or less constant interval by a QRS complex.

Sino–atrial dysfunction

Disorders of the sinus node (sino–atrial block or sinus arrest) may result in a bradycardia of a different appearance.

Sino–atrial block

Sino–atrial block is an exit block in the conduction of sinus node depolarization to the surrounding right atrial myocardium. As with atrioventricular block, there are different degrees and analogous terminology is used to describe them[5,6]. First degree sino–atrial block cannot be diagnosed from the surface ECG, as a more or less constant

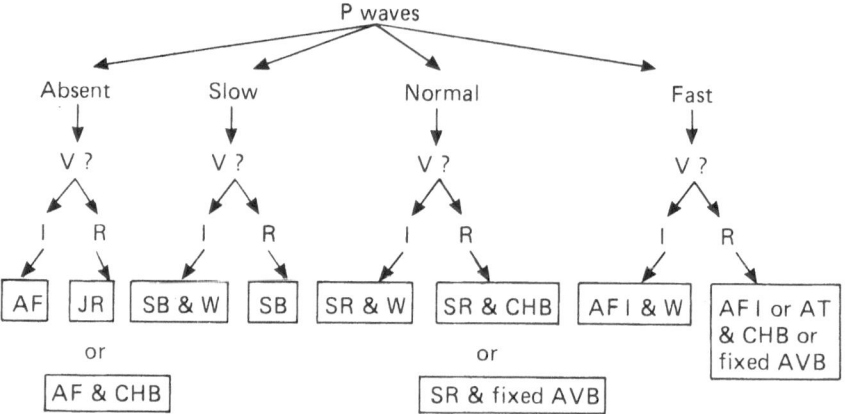

Figure 7.2 Flow diagram of a scheme for differential diagnosis of a bradycardia. Not all the possible diagnoses in this figure are likely (e.g. sinus bradycardia with Wenckebach block), but all are possible. The P waves may be absent during JR because of concealment in the QRST complex. Fixed AVB describes a constant atrioventricular ratio whether the mechanism be Mobitz I (Wenckebach) or Mobitz II AVB as it may be impossible to distinguish between them with certainty.
Abbreviations: AF = atrial fibrillation; AFl = atrial flutter; AT = atrial tachycardia; AVB = atrioventricular block; CHB = complete heart block; I = irregular; JR = junctional rhythm; R = regular; SB = sinus bradycardia; SR = sinus rhythm; V? = ventricular response?; W = Wenckebach AVB

delay is present between the invisible sinus node depolarization and the start of the P wave. Type I second degree sino–atrial block (analogous to Mobitz type I or Wenckebach atrioventricular block) occurs when the sino–atrial conduction time progressively lengthens until one impulse is blocked and a P wave is absent from the surface ECG. As with the R–R interval in Mobitz type I second degree atrioventricular block, the P–P interval progressively shortens until the 'missing' P wave becomes evident as a sudden long pause. This contrasts with sinus arrhythmia in which gradual shortening of the P–P interval is followed by gradual lengthening. The distinction is not always obvious, particularly when the two conditions co-exist, but may be facilitated by the construction of a Schamroth-Dove diagram[7]. Essentially, the length of each P–P interval is plotted against that of the succeeding P–P interval, the first being plotted on a descending Y axis and the second on the X axis. Characteristic distributions about the leading diagonal (which joins points with equal X and Y ordinates) are then observed.

Type II second degree sino–atrial block (block without prior prolongation of sino–atrial conduction time) is characterized by a sudden doubling of the expected P–P interval when block occurs for one cycle. In cases of greater severity, alternate sinus depolarizations may fail to initiate P waves, and it may be impossible to distinguish the resulting appearance from that of sinus bradycardia unless a sudden halving or doubling of the P wave rate is seen at the onset or offset, respectively. Complete, or third degree sino–atrial block causes complete absence of normal P waves. The resultant rhythm depends on the nature of the escape focus.

Sinus arrest

Sino–atrial block may be difficult to distinguish from sinus arrest, in which the sinus node fails to depolarize, but in sinus arrest the pause is not usually a multiple of the expected P–P interval. Both conditions may be mimicked by blocked atrial extrasystoles hidden in the T wave of the preceding QRST complex. Sinus arrest is often associated with a variety of supraventricular tachyarrhythmias in which case the terms 'brady–tachy' or 'sick sinus' syndrome are used[8–11].

Atrioventricular block

Atrioventricular block rarely causes diagnostic difficulty, although it is important to understand the significance of the various types, particularly of second degree block. First degree atrioventricular block is characterized by a prolonged PR interval, each P wave being followed by a QRS complex. When high heart rates occur in association with first degree atrioventricular block, the P wave may be obscured by the preceding T wave. Mobitz type I (Wenckebach) second degree atrioventricular block is characterized by the intermittent failure of a normally timed P wave (i.e. one which is not premature) to be conducted, in association with varying PR intervals[12] (Figure 7.3). This is usually attributed to block occurring in the atrioventricular node, whereas Mobitz type II second degree atrioventricular block (failure of a normally timed P wave to be conducted, without prior variation of the PR interval) is attributed to a more distal, infra-Hisian block. Whilst this is usually the case, the Wenckebach pattern of atrioventricular block can be generated by the His–Purkinje system[13,14] so that its occurrence is not necessarily benign, especially when associated with bundle branch block or in patients with a history of syncope. Complete heart block is diagnosed when the occurrence of P waves at a normal rate bears no relationship to the timing of QRS complexes occurring at a slower rate. During atrial fibrillation, the diagnosis is suggested by a slow and regular QRS rhythm. The diagnosis usually implies infra-Hisian conduction system disease although, when complicating acute inferior myocardial infarction, the usual site of the block is the atrioventricular (AV) node and spontaneous recovery is usual.

The treatment of bradyarrhythmias should be directed to the correction of any remediable cause and the introduction, where appropriate, of cardiac pacing. There is no place in the current therapy of chronic

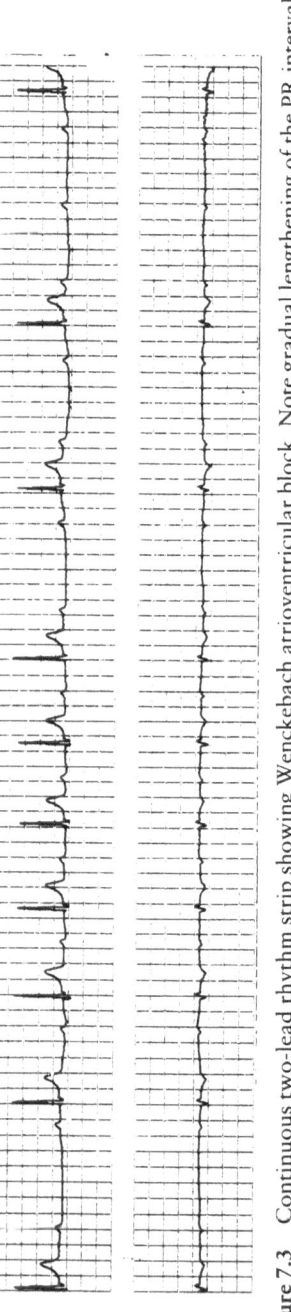

Figure 7.3 Continuous two-lead rhythm strip showing Wenckebach atrioventricular block. Note gradual lengthening of the PR interval before a P wave is not conducted to the ventricles

bradycardias for positively chronotropic drugs such as slow release isoprenaline. Difficulty in management may arise when severe bradycardia is suspected as the cause of unobserved symptoms such as dizziness or syncope. In contrast to the investigation of tachycardias, invasive electrophysiological studies are rarely helpful in deciding therapy. Every effort should be made to document the arrhythmia by ambulatory ECG monitoring although, in some patients, abnormalities such as bifascicular block on the resting ECG may provide sufficient circumstantial evidence to justify pacemaker implantation.

TACHYARRHYTHMIAS

It is in the evaluation of tachyarrhythmias that diagnostic errors are most commonly made. The result of such errors may be the prescription of dangerously inappropriate therapy, the most common mistake being the misdiagnosis of a broad complex tachycardia of ventricular origin as one of supra-ventricular origin with aberrant atrioventricular conduction. Narrow complex tachycardias, however, are also misdiagnosed, usually as a result of an incomplete understanding of the mechanism of the arrhythmia. The surface ECG may offer many helpful clues to correct diagnosis and a systematic approach will ensure that they are not missed (Figure 7.4).

The diagnosis of tachycardias from the surface ECG can be simplified if the arrhythmias are considered according to whether the QRS complexes occur regularly or irregularly and whether they are narrow (< 120 ms) or broad (> 120 ms).

TACHYCARDIA WITH NARROW QRS COMPLEXES

A narrow QRS complex indicates ventricular depolarization via an intact His–Purkinje system. Thus arrhythmias with narrow QRS complexes arise either from the atrium or the atrioventricular junction with anterograde recruitment of the His–Purkinje system. Determination of the cause of a regular narrow complex tachycardia may be impossible from the surface ECG without recourse to vagotonic manoeuvres such as carotid sinus massage or the Valsalva manoeuvre. These may lengthen the PR or RP' interval so that the P waves are separated from the QRS complexes and are thus more easily seen. If P waves can be reliably identified, analysis of their rate, regularity, morphology and relation to the QRS complexes will usually allow a diagnosis to be made.

Sinus tachycardia

Sinus tachycardia is diagnosed from the normal P wave morphology and the clinical setting, e.g. stress, exercise or fever.

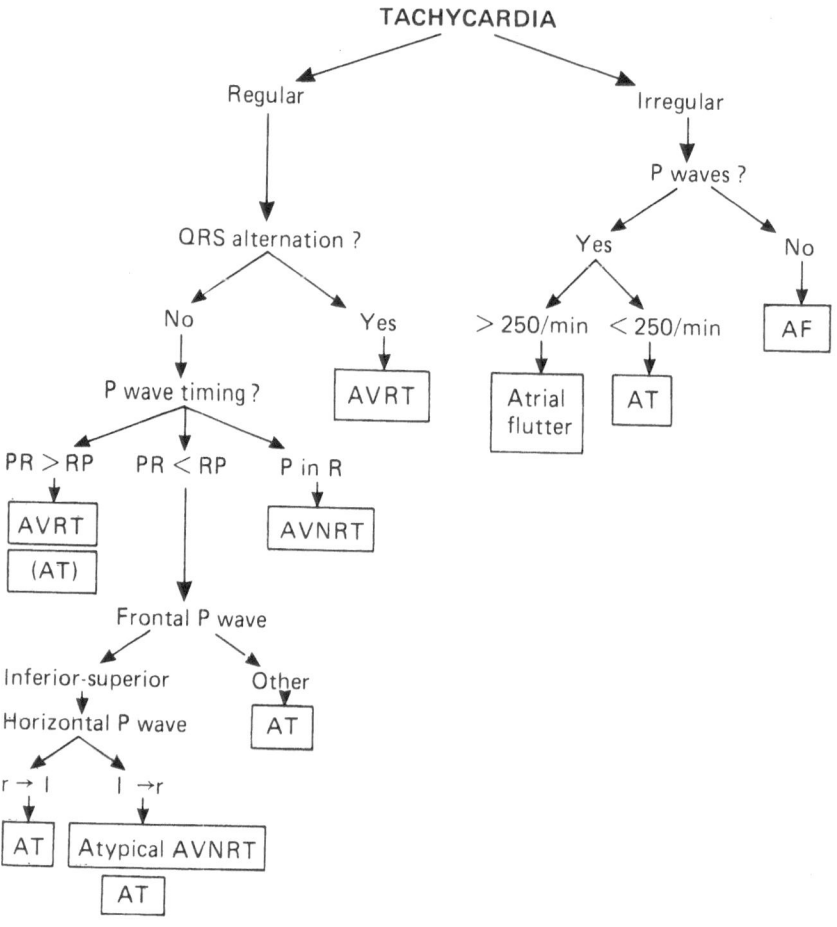

Figure 7.4 Flow diagram for the differential diagnosis of a narrow complex tachycardia. Modified from Bar *et al.*[19] – see text for description. Abbreviations: l = left, r = right. Other abbreviations as in text.

Atrial tachyarrhythmias

Atrial fibrillation

If, during a sustained tachycardia, narrow QRS complexes occur with continuous irregularity, the likeliest cause is atrial fibrillation, in which case discrete P waves will not be seen. Confusion may sometimes arise in chaotic, multiform or multifocal atrial tachycardias (associated with severe respiratory impairment and/or digoxin toxicity) in which irregular and polymorphic P waves precede the QRS complexes, or when Mobitz type I second degree atrioventricular block complicates atrial tachycardia or flutter. In atrial fibrillation the surface ECG reflects the simultaneous activation of multiple areas of the atrium by several small independent areas of re-entry. This results in the characteristic irregular, low amplitude, fibrillatory waves. Conduction to the ventricles is typically irregularly irregular as a result of the frequent but chaotic activation of the AV node which blocks the passage of the majority of impulses, thereby protecting the ventricles from excessive rates. When atrial fibrillation complicates the Wolff–Parkinson–White syndrome (Figure 7.1c), extremely rapid ventricular rates may occur which occasionally lead to ventricular fibrillation. The risks of this occurrence are markedly increased by the administration of drugs that reduce the anterograde refractoriness of the accessory pathway. Thus digoxin, verapamil and lignocaine should never be used to treat atrial fibrillation when the Wolff–Parkinson–White syndrome is suspected.

Atrial flutter

A regular P wave rate of 260–340 per minute implies a diagnosis of atrial flutter, which is usually conducted to the ventricles with variable atrioventricular block, resulting in the classic saw-tooth appearance of the baseline between QRS complexes that characterizes the 'typical' or 'common' variety of atrial flutter. In this form the P waves are predominantly negative in leads II, III and aVF, in contrast to the 'atypical' or 'uncommon' variety in which the P waves are positive in these leads and more discrete, the saw-tooth pattern being absent and the atrial rate lower (250–300/min)[15]. Atrial flutter may also occur at higher rates (340–430/min), and it has been observed that, in contrast to the slower form, to which it sometimes spontaneously converts, the faster form is not readily terminated by rapid pacing in the high right atrium[16]. On the basis of these observations Wells[17] classified the slower form as type I and the faster form as type II. Type I appears to correspond to the classic or common form, although type II is less clearly related to uncommon flutter as the latter usually has rates considerably less than 300 min. At high rates, atrial flutter may be difficult to distinguish from atrial fibrillation, or they may co-exist, leading to the often used term 'flutter-fibrillation'. These classifications based on morphological and rate criteria do not necessarily imply variations in the mechanism of arrhythmogenesis. This is still the subject of debate but there is substantial evidence in favour of a re-entry mechanism[18].

Atrial tachycardia

Atrial tachycardias are diagnosed on the basis of rapidly occurring P waves of altered morphology, although distinction from a junctional re-entry tachycardia (see below) is not always possible without an intracardiac electrophysiology study. Atrial tachycardia is typically slower than atrial flutter (150–250/min), and is characterized by distinct

P waves preceding each QRS complex. The P wave morphology is determined by the site of origin of the tachycardia. It may arise by re-entrant or automatic mechanisms.

The circuits of re-entrant atrial tachycardia are usually entirely within the atrial myocardium, with the exception of the rare sino–atrial re-entrant tachycardia, which is usually clinically insignificant. Intra-atrial re-entry may be accompanied by varying degrees of second degree atrioventricular block, particularly in patients taking AV node depressant drugs. The surface ECG between paroxysms may either be normal or reveal evidence of abnormal atrial activation, such as right or left atrial enlargement. Sino–atrial re-entrant tachycardia, in which the re-entry circuit is thought to be in or around the sinus node, is characterized by a sudden change in atrial rate with little or no change in the P wave morphology, since the atrial activation sequence is unchanged. It may thus be indistinguishable from sinus tachycardia.

Automatic atrial tachycardia is most commonly seen in digoxin toxicity when it is typically conducted to the ventricles with varying degrees of atrioventricular block, reflecting both the enhancement of ectopic automaticity and depression of normal atrioventricular conduction brought about by the drug.

Both atrial flutter and tachycardia may be diagnosed from the surface ECG if the atrioventricular conduction varies, either spontaneously or in response to vagotonic manoeuvres or drugs, so that independent P wave activity is seen (faster than QRS activity) with tachycardia continuing thereafter. This distinguishes the rhythms from junctional re-entry arrhythmias in which such vagal suppression of atrioventricular nodal conduction would usually result in tachycardia slowing or termination.

Junctional tachycardia

Junctional arrhythmias may arise either by re-entry or from enhanced focal automaticity.

Atrioventricular nodal re-entry tachycardia

Atrioventricular nodal re-entry tachycardia (AVNRT) originates from a circuit contained entirely within or immediately adjacent to the atrioventricular node. The relationship of atrial and ventricular depolarization depends on the nature of the re-entry circuit and its site within or immediately around the atrioventricular node. Usually, the circuit consists of a slow anterograde limb and a fast retrograde limb. This arrangement results in almost simultaneous atrial and ventricular depolarization so that the P waves are obscured by the QRS complexes on the surface ECG. Occasionally, an atypical form exists where the fast pathway conducts anterogradely and the slow pathway conducts retrogradely (atypical 'fast–slow' AVNRT). This results in clearly visible inverted P waves in leads II, III and aVF, typically a little over halfway between the QRS complexes. This is one of a number of possible causes of a long RP' tachycardia in which the RP' interval exceeds the PR interval. Other causes are discussed below.

Atrioventricular re-entry tachycardia

In the circuit of orthodromic atrioventricular re-entry tachycardia (AVRT) the AV node is only involved in the anterograde limb, depolarization continuing via the His–Purkinje system (and thus usually with narrow QRS complexes – unless there is bundle branch block) around the ventricles and returning to the atria via an extranodal accessory pathway and thence again to the AV node. The circuit is reversed in the rare antidromic AVRT in which anterograde conduction occurs via the accessory pathway with retrograde conduction through the AV node. The resultant arrhythmia is a regular tachycardia with wide QRS complexes reflecting complete ventricular pre-excitation (Figure 7.1b and see below). In contrast to AVNRT, atrial and ventricular depolarization in AVRT are separated in time by the conduction times of the AV node and the accessory pathway. The location of the P wave within each cycle and its morphology, as assessed by frontal and horizontal axis determination, have accordingly been suggested as useful markers in the differential diagnosis of narrow complex tachycardias[19]. Other features suggested to be of diagnostic value are the presence of an alternation of QRS amplitude[20] (which is thought to be indicative of AVRT, although the mechanism is obscure) and the atrial rate. There is evidence that QRS alternation is more likely at higher heart rates and that when corrected for rate it is, in practice, of little diagnostic value in distinguishing AVRT and AVNRT[21]. Bar *et al.*[19] have nonetheless suggested a clinical diagnostic algorithm using these features. Their algorithm was derived from the retrospective analysis of 187 patients with narrow complex supraventricular tachycardia and a prospective analysis of 57 patients (Figure 7.4). The algorithm relies on the reliable identification of P waves which is often difficult, particularly with rapid tachycardias.

Alternating cycle lengths may be seen with both AVRT and AVNRT (especially after the onset and just prior to termination) and probably represent alternate use, in the same direction, of two or more AV nodal pathways. Prolongation of the cycle length of an initially narrow complex tachycardia by the development of bundle branch block provides extremely useful diagnostic information. This indicates that the tachycardia is AVRT with a lateral accessory pathway on the same side as the bundle branch block. The delayed ventricular depolarization with bundle branch block, results in an equal delay in the tachycardia wavefront reaching the accessory pathway, thus prolonging the tachycardia cycle length. In contrast, contralateral bundle branch block or bundle branch block during AVRT mediated by a septal accessory pathway, do not affect tachycardia cycle length.

An ECG during sinus rhythm without evidence of pre-excitation is unhelpful in distinguishing between AVRT and AVNRT, as accessory pathways which only conduct retrogradely (concealed pathways) are common and may support orthodromic AVRT without producing ventricular pre-excitation during sinus rhythm. Accessory pathways may also not be manifest on the surface ECG because AV nodal conduction to the His–Purkinje system has preceded ventricular depolarization via the accessory pathway. This typically occurs with very lateral left-sided accessory pathways, when the time taken for right and left atrial activation to reach the pathway exceeds the sum of right atrial activation and AV nodal conduction times. Furthermore, AVNRT as well as AVRT, may occur in patients with the Wolff–Parkinson–White syndrome, so that electrophysiological study is usually necessary to differentiate between the two with certainty. It is not possible, however, for atrial and ventricular activity to be independent with AVRT, so the appearance of a 2:1 atrioventricular or ventriculo–atrial ratio during junctional re-entry is diagnostic of AVNRT with its localized circuit within the AV node.

Long RP' tachycardias

The features of an incessant or 'permanent' form of junctional reciprocating tachycardia ('PJRT') with a long RP' interval were clearly described by Coumel et al. in 1967[22]. The anatomical substrate for this form of tachycardia is a retrograde anomalous pathway with a long conduction time and in which anterograde conduction cannot be detected[23]. Electrophysiological studies have usually shown the pathways to be located close to the AV node, although left free wall concealed accessory pathways with long ventriculo–atrial conduction times have also been described[24]. It is rarely possible to distinguish with certainty between PJRT and ectopic atrial tachycardia, so that a formal electrophysiological study is usually required[25,26]. Full electrophysiological evaluation should be considered in patients with long RP' tachycardias as they are frequently incessant, often refractory to medical therapy and in many cases amenable to curative surgery.

Focal His bundle tachycardia

Focal His bundle tachycardia, also known as junctional ectopic tachycardia, is rare, usually occurs in children, and is characterized by narrow, normal QRS complexes during tachycardia, with dissociated P waves. It originates from an abnormal automatic focus in the lower part of the AV node or His bundle either of congenital origin or as a consequence of cardiac surgery.

Accessory pathway localization

Various attempts have been made to define criteria by which accessory pathways may be localized using information derived from the surface electrocardiogram[27-33]. Although most patients in whom accessory pathways come to light are likely to proceed to full electrophysiological evaluation, it is helpful to have knowledge of the pathway's location before proceeding, as this may provide important initial evidence for the existence of multiple pathways. Rosenbaum et al.[27] classified patients with Wolff–Parkinson–White syndrome according to whether the direction of the dominant QRS deflection in the right precordial leads of the surface ECG was upwards (type A) or downwards (type B). Giraud et al.[28] later proposed that the type A configuration resulted from left posterobasal pre-excitation and type B from right lateral pre-excitation. Subsequent studies have made use of both the delta wave polarity and the QRS morphology and axis on the surface ECG to distinguish between different pathway locations[29,30]. The most comprehensive study by Gallagher et al.[29] suggested criteria to separate pathways in up to ten possible locations on the basis of the delta wave polarity during maximum pre-excitation. The latter is not always present at rest,

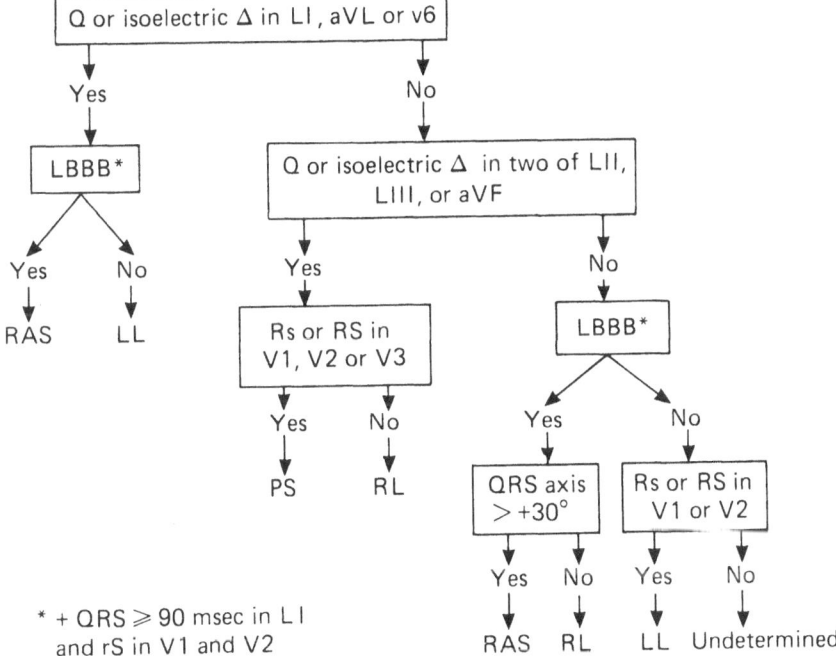

Figure 7.5 Flow diagram for the localization of the site of an accessory pathway according to Milstein et al.[33] Abbreviations: LBBB = left bundle branch block;   LL = left lateral;   PS = posteroseptal;   RAS = right anteroseptal;   RL = right lateral

however, and may only be manifest during rapid atrial pacing. Lemery *et al.*[32] have suggested that the standard surface ECG is limited in its ability to exactly localize accessory pathways. However, Milstein *et al.*[33] have recently proposed a simple algorithm for localizing accessory pathways in the four most common locations (Figure 7.5). In four steps, simple questions are asked regarding the polarity of the delta wave and other features of the QRS morphology, which require only affirmative or negative answers. Using this algorithm, two independent, blinded observers obtained at least a 90% agreement with the results of accessory pathway localization at electrophysiological and/or operative mapping.

TACHYCARDIA WITH WIDE QRS COMPLEXES

Regular wide complex tachycardias clearly present many physicians with diagnostic problems[1,2]. Unfortunately, diagnostic errors in this situation may have serious consequences for the patient[34,35]. There are three ways in which widened QRS complexes may arise:

(1) Depolarization originating in the ventricles;
(2) Conduction of depolarization of either atrial or junctional origin to the ventricles with bundle branch block (either functional or pre-existing);
(3) Conduction of depolarization of either atrial or junctional origin to the ventricles partially or completely by an accessory pathway (i.e. ventricular pre-excitation).

Bundle branch block may complicate a narrow complex tachycardia of any cause, be it regular or irregular. Pre-excitation may also produce wide QRS complexes during all types of junctional tachycardia. Antidromic AVRT is associated with widened QRS complexes and has been discussed earlier. AVNRT is also occasionally accompanied by pre-excited QRS complexes when there is an additional 'bystander' accessory pathway present, independent from the intra-nodal re-entry circuit. Anterograde conduction may then occur in both the accessory pathway and one of the intra-nodal pathways giving a pre-excited QRS appearance almost identical to that seen during sinus rhythm. Nodoventricular (Mahaim) fibres may also cause pre-excited junctional tachycardias. There is debate as to whether they act as one limb of a re-entry circuit (analogous to the accessory pathway in AVRT), or merely as a bystander pathway resulting in pre-excitation of an independent AVNRT, but the QRS pattern of a 'stunted' left bundle branch block morphology is diagnostic.

The correct distinction of ventricular tachycardia from the other wide complex tachycardias is of paramount importance both because of its prognostic implications and the importance of prescribing appropriate therapy. Many workers have addressed this diagnostic problem retrospectively, studying the electrocardiograms of patients in whom subsequent electrophysiological study had conclusively determined the origins of their tachycardias. Most prominent among these investigators have been Wellens and his group[36] and many of the following observations stem from their work. They have established several criteria for distinguishing ventricular tachycardia from supra-ventricular tachycardia with aberrant conduction. Pre-existing bundle branch blocks and pre-excitation can present difficulties in making the distinction solely from the ECG during tachycardia, but where bundle branch block is functional and rate dependent the distinction can almost always be made.

Rate

In distinguishing ventricular tachycardia from supra-ventricular tachycardia with functional bundle branch block, tachycardia rate is unhelpful because although there is a tendency for supra-ventricular tachycardia with aberrancy to be faster than ventricular tachycardia there is too much overlap for this to be diagnostically useful. Similarly, the type of bundle branch block is of little discriminative value.

Atrioventricular dissociation

Although dissociated P waves during tachycardia are diagnostic of ventricular tachycardia, their association may also occur as a result of 1:1 ventriculo–atrial conduction even up to very high rates, and this finding does not exclude ventricular tachycardia. Ventriculo–atrial conduction of some sort occurs in approximately 50% of ventricular tachycardias[36].

Capture beats and fusion beats

Capture beats and fusion beats (which are seen relatively rarely, Figure 7.6) express the conduction of dissociated P waves and are diagnostic of ventricular tachycardia, but again their absence is of no diagnostic significance.

Concordance

Concordance of the V leads (all positive or all negative) is another finding specific to ventricular tachycardia (Figures 7.7a and 7.7b) but its relative rarity in ventricular tachycardia diminishes its value overall.

QRS width

A QRS width exceeding 140 ms was diagnostic of ventricular tachycardia in Wellens' series, although complexes of 140 ms or less were present in 30% of cases of ventricular tachycardia.

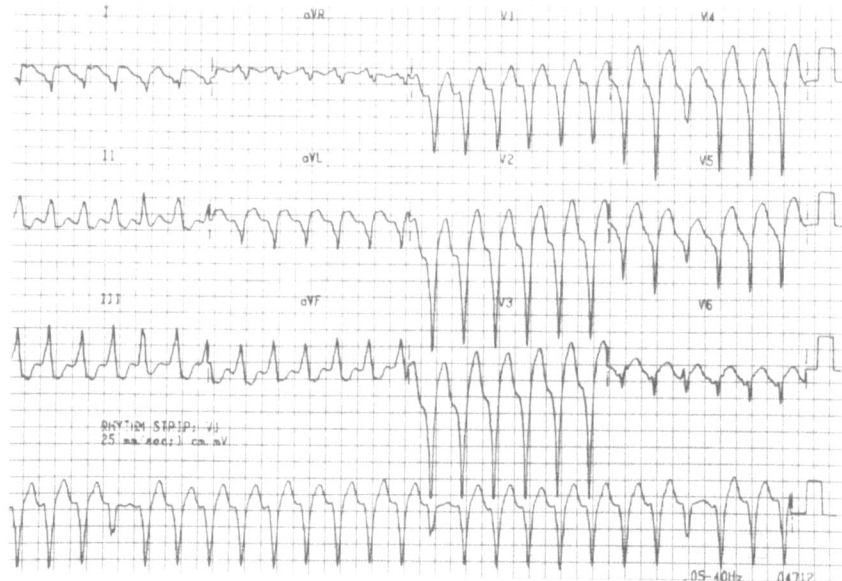

Figure 7.6 Twelve-lead ECG of ventricular tachycardia. This is most easily diagnosed from the fusion beats (3rd beat in V4, 5 and 6, and the 4th, 14th and 22nd beats in the rhythm strip at the bottom. Other features in favour of ventricular tachycardia are the QRS width of 160 ms and a qrS morphology in V6 during a tachycardia with a left bundle branch block appearance

Electrical axis

Left axis deviation is also more common in ventricular tachycardia but by no means universal. A marked shift of axis from the normal range to the left or right at the onset of tachycardia, if this is witnessed, strongly suggests a ventricular origin.

Specific QRS morphologies

Analysis of the QRS morphology in leads V1 and V6 enables distinction of the two arrhythmias in a significant number of cases. Depending on which form of bundle branch block is present, a number of patterns of QRS morphology are diagnostic of ventricular tachycardia. On the other hand, although some patterns are seen more often with aberrancy, none is absolutely diagnostic (Tables 7.1, 7.2 and 7.3).

With a right bundle branch block pattern, monophasic R waves or an RS pattern in V1 are only seen in ventricular tachycardia and a QR pattern is only rarely seen in aberrantly conducted supra-ventricular tachycardia. Obviously triphasic V1 complexes are more common with aberrancy, unless the initial R wave is taller than the subsequent R wave, in which case the diagnosis is ventricular tachycardia. Certain

110

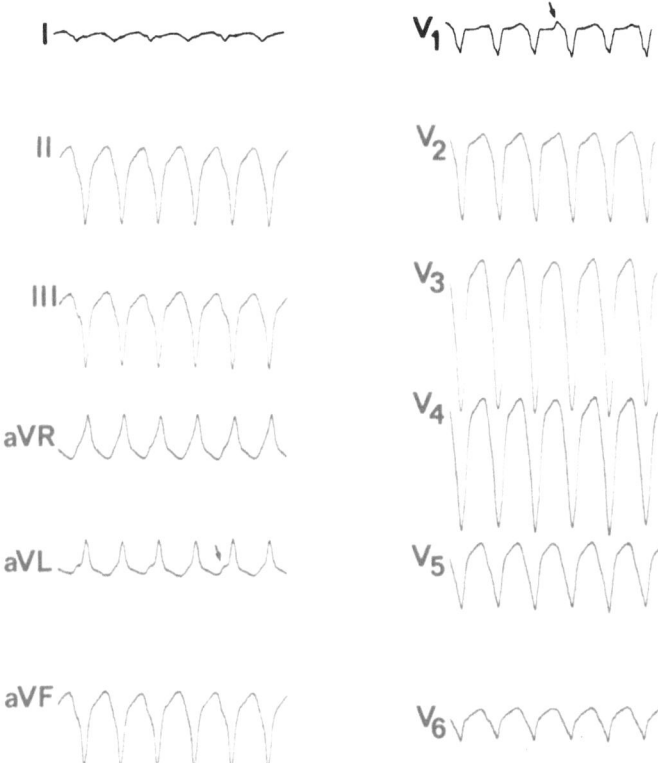

Figure 7.7(a) Twelve-lead ECG of ventricular tachycardia showing negative concordance in the V leads. Note the dissociated P waves (arrowed in leads aVL and V1).

QRS morphologies in V6 during right bundle branch block arrhythmias are also diagnostic of ventricular tachycardia, such as QS, monophasic R and qR. An initial r wave smaller than the subsequent S wave is highly suggestive but not diagnostic of ventricular tachycardia whereas a qRS morphology suggests aberrancy.

With left bundle branch block tachycardias, analysis of the QRS morphology in V1 may provide useful pointers to the diagnosis of ventricular tachycardia. These include a duration of the upstroke of the initial r wave exceeding 30 ms, slurring or notching of the S wave and an interval from the onset of the initial r wave to the trough of the S wave exceeding 70 ms (H. J. J. Wellens, personal communication). In V6, the qR and QS morphologies seem to be specific for ventricular tachycardia.

Pre-existing bundle branch block

Difficulty arises when dealing with pre-existing bundle branch block which can produce complexes wider than 140 ms and can often result

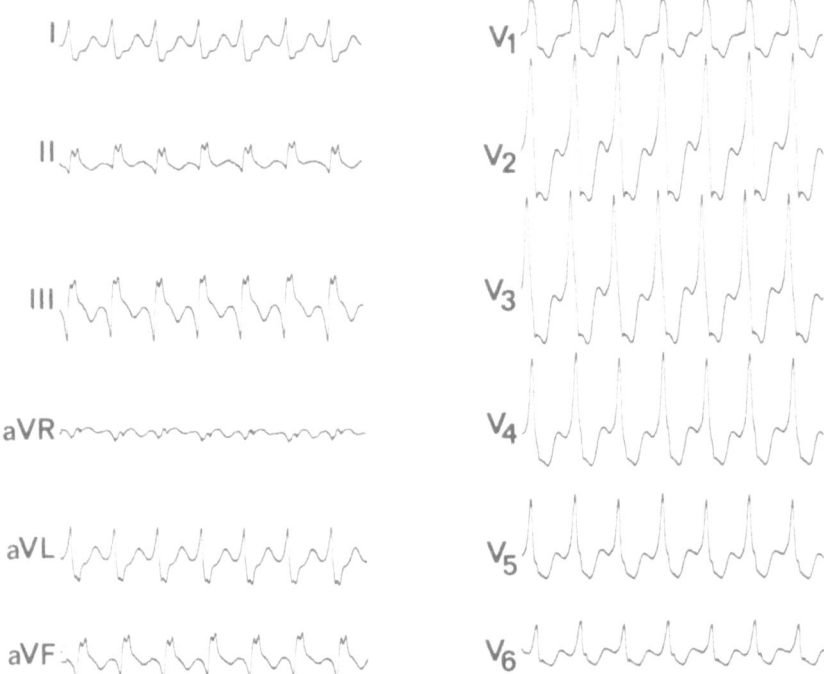

Figure 7.7(b) Twelve-lead ECG of ventricular tachycardia showing positive concordance in the V leads

in significant left axis deviation. However, although this complicates the distinction of the arrhythmias overall, analysis of the ECG during sinus rhythm enables the distinction to be made in individual cases[37]. If the complexes during tachycardia and sinus rhythm are identical then the arrhythmia is of supra-ventricular origin (Figure 7.8) whereas if the QRS complexes are different then the tachycardia is of ventricular origin (Table 7.4).

A pre-excited supra-ventricular tachycardia may on the other hand be impossible to distinguish from ventricular tachycardia because in both instances ventricular depolarization originates in non-specialized myocardium. Thus morphological, axis and width criteria are unhelpful and the diagnosis may have to rely on the discovery of pre-excited sinus rhythm.

Irregular wide-complex tachycardia

The commonest cause of an irregular wide-complex tachycardia is atrial fibrillation conducted with a bundle branch block. Ventricular tachycardia is seldom irregular except in its polymorphic form which is

Table 7.1 Analysis of the morphology of V1 during a tachycardia with a right bundle branch block appearance

V1 morphology	Tachycardia diagnosis	
	SVT with functional RBBB	VT
R	0%	23%
rR	16%	26%
rsR	27.5%	5%
rSR	55%	5%
Rsr	0%	11%
qR	1%	25%
Rs	0%	6%

Abbreviations: RBBB = right bundle branch block; SVT = supra–ventricular tachycardia; V1 = ventricular tachycardia

Table 7.2 Analysis of the morphology of V6 during a tachycardia with a right bundle branch block appearance

V6 morphology	Tachycardia diagnosis	
	SVT with functional RBBB	VT
qRs	64%	5%
RS	30%	23%
rS	6%	41.5%
QS	0%	25%
qR	0%	5%
R	0%	1.5%

Abbreviations: as for Table 7.1

Table 7.3 Analysis of the morphology of V6 during a tachycardia with a left bundle branch block appearance

V6 morphology	Tachycardia diagnosis	
	SVT with functional LBBB	VT
rsR	45%	43%
Rsr	55%	40%
qR	0%	14%
qrS	0%	3%

Abbreviations: LBBB = left bundle branch block; others as in Table 7.1

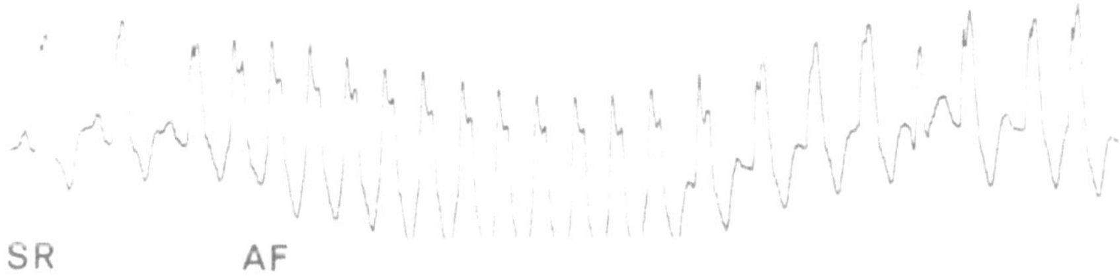

SR   AF

Figure 7.8 Rhythm strip showing the onset of atrial fibrillation in a patient with pre-existing left bundle branch block

113

Table 7.4 Comparison of QRS morphology during tachycardia and sinus rhythm in 25 patients with SVT and 35 patients with VT who had pre-existing bundle branch block (Akhtar, personal communication)

	SVT	*VT*
Identical	23	0
Similar	2	1
Different	0	34

Abbreviations: see Table 7.1

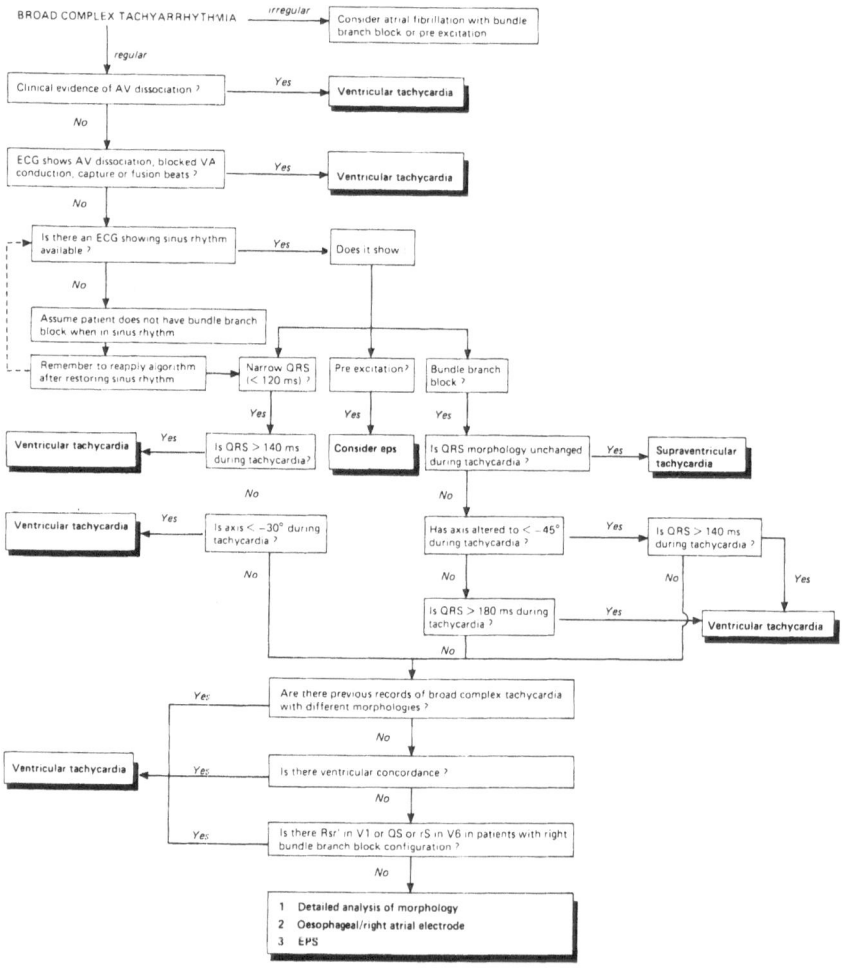

Figure 7.9 Flow diagram for differential diagnosis of a wide complex tachycardia, after Dancy and Ward

rarely sustained. The QRS complexes in the rare bi-directional ventricular tachycardia usually show alternating axis and cycle lengths but are not continuously irregular. Finally, pre-excited atrial fibrillation should be considered. Typically, the width as well as the rate of the QRS complexes varies continuously, with occasional absence of pre-excitation exposing narrow QRS complexes.

Using a combination of the criteria outlined above, Dancy and Ward[38] have suggested an extremely useful algorithm for diagnosing ventricular tachycardia from the surface ECG (Figure 7.9). In cases where the diagnosis of a broad complex tachycardia is in doubt, it should always be assumed to be of ventricular origin and should be treated as such until firm evidence to the contrary is available. This strategy will facilitate the selection of safe and appropriate therapy for those at greatest risk and is unlikely to harm the others. Administration of verapamil in cases of diagnostic uncertainty is a common error and may result in profound haemodynamic deterioration[34,35]. In cases of broad complex tachycardia thought likely, but not certain to be of supraventricular origin, the use of adenosine as a diagnostic and therapeutic agent is presently under investigation and seems likely to be of great value[39]. An intravenous bolus (0.15 mg/kg) terminates or induces atrioventricular block in the vast majority of supra-ventricular tachycardias and is well tolerated and usually ineffective in ventricular tachycardia.

Finally, the clinical history may be of value in cases where the electrocardiographic diagnosis is in doubt. A history of prior myocardial infarction, congestive heart failure or recent angina have strong positive predictive value for ventricular tachycardia[40]. Their specificity, however, is relatively low so their absence (in common with haemodynamic stability at presentation) should never be allowed to weigh against the diagnosis.

CONCLUSIONS

With the adoption of a logical approach to the analysis of the surface ECG during a cardiac arrhythmia, it is rare that the diagnosis will remain in doubt. This approach may be greatly facilitated by the careful application of diagnostic algorithms. Between attacks, the surface ECG should be carefully scrutinized for pointers which may reveal the likely diagnosis and indicate the most fruitful direction for further investigation.

The most important arrhythmia to recognize is ventricular tachycardia, and where the diagnosis is uncertain but this arrhythmia is a possibility, it should be presumptively diagnosed and treated, until such time as an alternative diagnosis can be made with certainty. The chances of successful first line therapy will thereby be improved, and, more importantly, the chances of disastrously inappropriate therapy will be reduced.

References

1. Dancy, M., Camm, A. J. and Ward, D. (1985). Misdiagnosis of chronic recurrent ventricular tachycardia. *Lancet*, 2, 320
2. Nathan, A. W., Elstob, J. E. and Camm, A. J. (1986). The misdiagnosis of ventricular tachycardia – results of a postal survey. *Br. Heart J.*, 55, 513
3. Gallagher, J. J., Smith, W. M., Kasell, J., Grant, A. O. and Benson, D. W. (1980). Use of esophageal leads in the diagnosis of reciprocating supra-ventricular tachycardia. *Pacing Clin. Electrophysiol.*, 3, 336
4. Davies, D. W., Crick, J. C. P., Holt, P. M., Curry, P. V. L. and Sowton, E. (1983). Benefits of long-term recording of the atrial electrogram. *Pacing Clin. Electrophysiol.*, 6 II A, 105
5. Scherf, D. (1969). The mechanism of sinoatrial block. *Am. J. Cardiol.*, 23, 769
6. Robles de Medina, E. O. (ed.). (1978). Definition of terms related to cardiac rhythm. WHO/ISFC Task Force. *Eur. J. Cardiol.*, 8, 127
7. Schamroth, L. and Dove, E. (1966). The Wenckebach Phenomenon in sino–atrial block. *Br. Heart J.*, 28, 350
8. Rasmussen, K. (1971). Chronic sinoatrial block. *Am. Heart J.*, 81, 38
9. Rubenstein, J. J., Schulman, J. L., Yurchak, P. M., and DeSanctis, R. W. (1972). Clinical spectrum of the sick sinus syndrome. *Circulation*, 46, 5
10. Ferrer, M. I. (1973). The sick sinus syndrome. *Circulation*, 47, 635
11. Sigurd, B., Jensen, G., Meibom, J. and Sandoe, E. (1973) Adams–Stokes syndrome caused by sino–atrial block. *Br. Heart J.*, 35, 1002
12. Barold, S. S. and Friedberg, H. D. (1974). Second-degree atrio–ventricular block. A matter of definition. *Am. J. Cardiol.*, 33, 331
13. Zipes, D. P. (1979). Second-degree atrioventricular block. *Circulation*, 60, 465
14. Puech, P. and Wainwright, R. J. (1983). Clinical electrophysiology of atrioventricular block. In Zipes, D. P. (ed.). *Symposium on Arrhymias II, Cardiology Clinics 1* (2). p. 209. (Philadelphia: WB Saunders Co.)
15. Benditt, D. G., Benson, D. W. Jr., Dunnigan, A., Gornick, C. C. and Anderson, R. W. (1984) Atrial flutter, atrial fibrillation and other primary atrial tachycardias. *Med. Clin. N. Am.*, 68, 895
16. Waldo, A. L., MacLean, W. A. H., Karp, R. B., Kouchoukos, N. T. and James, T. N. (1977). Entrainment and interruption of atrial flutter with atrial pacing. Studies in man following open heart surgery. *Circulation*, 56, 737
17. Wells, H. L., MacLean, W. A. H., Hames, T. N. and Waldo, A. L. (1979). Characteristics of atrial flutter; studies in patients after open heart surgery using fixed electrodes. *Circulation,* 60, 665
18. Ward, D. E. and Camm, A. J. (1987). *Clinical Electrophysiology of the Heart*. p. 161. (London; Edward Arnold)
19. Bar, F. W., Brugada, P., Dassen, W. R. M. and Wellens, H. J. J. (1984). Differential diagnosis of tachycardia with narrow QRS complex (shorter than 0.12 second). *Am. J. Cardiol.*, 54, 555
20. Green, M., Heddle, B., Dassen, W. *et al.* (1983). Value of QRS alternation in determining the site of origin of narrow QRS supraventricular tachycardia. *Circulation*, 68, 368
21. Kay, G. N., Pressley, J. C., Packer, D. L., Pritchet, E. L. C., German, L. D. and Gilbert, M. R. (1987). Value of the 12-lead electrocardiogram in discriminating atrioventricular nodal reciprocating tachycardia from circus movement atrioventricular tachycardias utilizing a retrograde accessory pathway. *Am. J. Cardiol.*, 59, 296
22. Coumel, P., Cabrol, C., Fabiato, A., Gourgon, R. and Slama, R. (1967) Tachycardie permanente par rhythme reciproque. I. Preuves du dignostic par stimulation auriculaire et ventriculaire. *Arch. Mal. Coeur*, 60, 1830
23. Gallagher, J. J. and Sealy, W. C. (1978). The permanent form of junctional reciprocating tachycardia: further elucidation of the underlying mechanism. *Eur. Heart J.*, 8, 413

24. Okumura, K., Henthorn, R. W., Epstein, A. E., Plumb, V. J. and Waldo, A. L. (1986) 'Incessant' atrioventricular tachycardia utilizing left lateral bypass pathway with a long retrograde conduction time. *Pacing Clin. Electrophysiol.*, **9**, 33
25. Guarnieri, T., German, L. D. and Gallagher, J. J. (1987). The long R–P' tachycardias. *Pacing Clin. Electrophysiol.*, **10**, 103
26. Castellanos, A., and Myerburg, R. J. (1987). The wide electrophysiologic spectrum of tachycardias having R–P intervals longer than P–R intervals. *Pacing Clin. Electrophysiol.*, **10**, 1382
27. Rosenbaum, F. F., Hecht, H. H., Wilson, F. N. and Johnston, F. D. (1945). The potential variations of the thorax and the esophagus in anomalous atrioventricular excitation (Wolff–Parkinson–White syndrome). *Am. Heart J.*, **29**, 281
28. Giraud, G., Latour, H., Puech, P. and Roujon, J. (1956) Les troubles de rythme du syndrome de Wolff–Parkinson–White. Analyse electrocardiographique endocavitaire. *Arch. Mal. Coeur*, **49**, 101
29. Gallagher, J. J., Pritchett, E. L. C., Sealy, W. C., Kasell, J. and Wallace, A. G. (1978). The preexcitation syndromes. *Prog. Cardiovasc. Dis.*, **20**, 285
30. Willems, J. L., Robles de Medina, E. O., Bernard, R. *et al.* (1985), *J. Am. Coll. Cardiol.*, **5**, 1261
31. Reddy, G. V. and Schamroth, L. (1987). The localisation of bypass tracts in the Wolff–Parkinson–White syndrome from the surface electrocardiogram. *Am. Heart J.*, **113**, 984
32. Lemery, R., Hammill, S. C., Wood, D. L. *et al.* (1987). Value of the resting 12 lead electrocardiogram and vectorcardiogram for locating the accessory pathway in patients with the Wolff–Parkinson–White syndrome. *Br. Heart J.*, **58**, 324
33. Milstein, S., Sharma, A. D., Guiraudon, G. M. and Klein, G. J. (1987). An algorithm for the electrocardiographic localization of accessory pathways in the Wolff–Parkinson–White syndrome. *Pacing Clin. Electrophysiol.*, **10**, 555
34. Stewart, R. B., Bardy, G. H. and Greene, H. L. (1986). Wide complex tachycardia: misdiagnosis and outcome after emergent therapy. *Ann. Int. Med.*, **104**, 766
35. Rankin, A. C., Rae, A. P. and Cobbe, S. M. (1987) Misuse of intravenous verapamil in patients with ventricular tachycardia. *Lancet*, **2**, 472
36. Wellens, H. J. J., Bar, F. W. H. M. and Lie, K. I. (1978). The value of the electrocardiogram in the differential diagnosis of a tachycardia with a widened QRS complex. *Am. J. Med.*, **64**, 27
37. Dongas, J., Lehmann, M. H., Mahmud, R., Denker, S., Soni, J. and Akhtar, M. (1985). Value of preexisting bundle branch block in the electrocardiographic differentiation of supraventricular from ventricular origin of wide QRS tachycardia. *Am. J. Cardiol.*, **55**, 717
38. Dancy, M. and Ward, D. (1985) Diagnosis of ventricular tachycardia: a clinical algorithm. *Br. Med. J.*, **291**, 1036
39. Griffith, M. J., Linker, N. J., Ward, D. E. and Camm, A. J. (1988). Adenosine in the diagnosis of broad complex tachycardia. *Lancet*, **1**, 672
40. Baerman, J. M., Morady, F., DiCarlo L. A., Jr., de Buitleir, M. and Arbor, A. (1987). Differentiation of ventricular tachycardia from supraventricular tachycardia with aberration: Value of the clinical history. *Ann. Emerg. Med.*, **16**, 40

8
Ambulatory electrocardiographic monitoring in the diagnosis of arrhythmias

A. K. BROWN

More than a quarter of a century has elapsed since Holter reported the method of recording long term continuous ambulatory electrocardiograms to which his name is usually attached[1]. Holter monitoring consists of an audiotape to record the ECGs and a rapid scanning device for subsequent analysis. All systems place reliance on a diary of events which is kept by the patient so that symptoms may be correlated with ECG findings on the tape. The patient can also mark the tape to signal specific events. Current recorders permit simultaneous taping of two ECG leads over 24 hours, which facilitates recognition of ventricular ectopic activity. Satisfactory results demand meticulous attention to detail by the technician. The electrodes must be attached perfectly and positioned optimally to provide an ECG which is suitable for arrhythmia analysis. Although the scanning procedures have become more automated recently, visual checking of arrhythmias is still necessary, and analysis of a 24 hour ambulatory ECG tape remains a time consuming and laborious task. Electrocardiograph strips on normal ECG paper are available for analysis of rhythm abnormalities to see if significant arrhythmias coincide with patient-noted events. Charts or histograms may provide graphic evidence of rhythms and their frequency, but it must be emphasized that accuracy depends entirely on the technician's ability to ensure that the beats are recognized correctly by the analyser. The same proviso applies to trend plots showing heart rate against time or ectopic beats against time. Data may also be presented in compressed form so that information for one hour or more is available on a single page. The area involving the abnormal rhythm is enlarged for recognition and interpretation of arrhythmias.

Holter's name should be restricted to the method described by him with its subsequent modifications. Ambulatory or dynamic electrocardiography are wider terms which are used to include all types of ambulatory ECG monitoring including the Holter technique. Real time analysis systems are alternatives which can provide continuous pro-

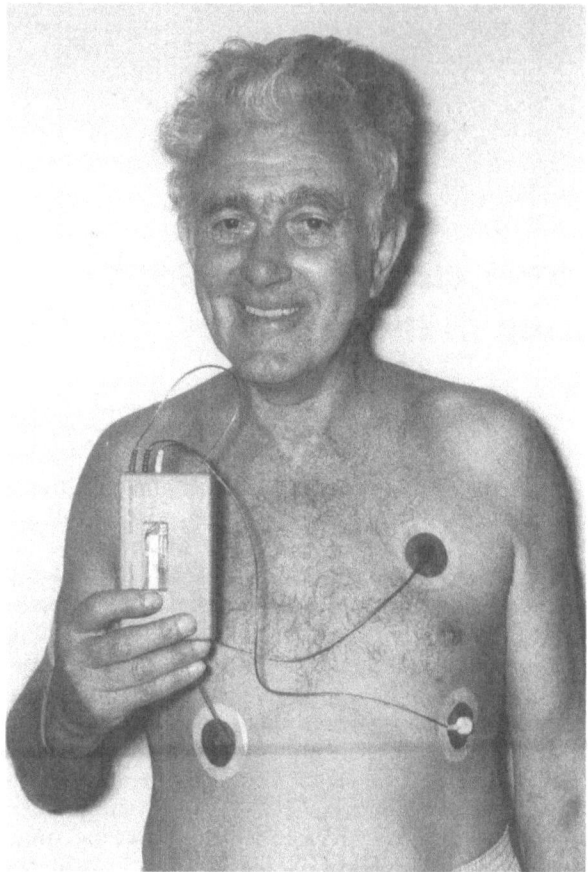

Figure 8.1   Radiotelemetry unit for use on the ward

longed ECG recordings. Immediate ECG analysis is available, and such systems will compete with traditional Holter techniques as accuracy becomes comparable and the storage of data for late retrieval is improved. We use radiotelemetry on the wards (Figure 8.1). Real time records are available and trend charts provide information over 24 hour periods which may be scanned later to retrieve data for analysis (Figure 8.2).

Arrhythmias which occur at infrequent intervals pose a problem for continuous monitoring systems, and various intermittent recorders are described. The Portable Short Electrocardiograph is an inexpensive adaptation of a domestic cassette machine which records an ECG signal by substituting a purpose built printed circuit for the loudspeaker[2]. It may be left with the patient for weeks or months, and playback for analysis of the ECG is affected via a demodulator into a standard ECG

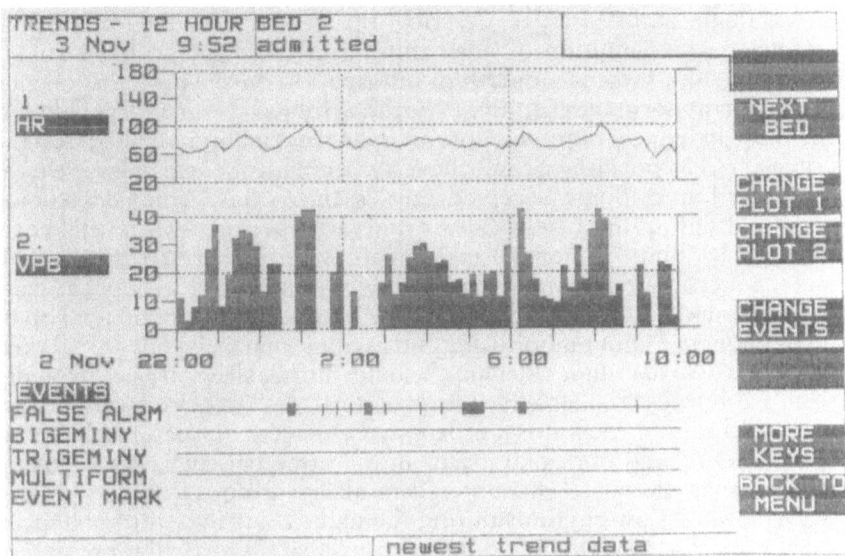

Figure 8.2 Trend plot of telemetry heartrate and ventricular premature beats over 12 hours

machine. Symptoms must last long enough for the patient to apply the electrodes and record the electrocardiograph. A similar restriction applies to transtelephonic monitoring which also has the disadvantage that it requires a dedicated 24 hour hospital based telephone service. Alternatively, battery operated recorders which only record intermittently may be worn for several days. They may record at regular, preselected intervals; may be activated by the patients when symptoms occur, or may be programmed to recognize and record specific arrhythmias such as tachycardia and bradycardia. All intermittent recorders have the problem that there is no way of checking if significant abnormal rhythms have been missed. Both continuous Holter type monitoring and a system for intermittent recording of arrhythmias which occur at long intervals are necessary to provide an adequate ambulatory ECG service.

THE NORMAL AMBULATORY ECG

Before defining a normal recording it is necessary to be able to recognize artifacts which mimic normal rhythms. Artifacts simulating supraventricular or ventricular tachycardia may be caused by poor contact between the skin electrodes, body movements or broken wires; mechanical or electrical faults are prone to cause pauses which may be mistaken for bradycardia and heart block[3].

Although many articles describe the Holter findings in normal people[4-11], the definition of normality in different age groups remains imprecise, and there is a dearth of information on the prognostic value of rhythm abnormalities in these 'healthy' subjects. A major problem is the way in which different groups define normality: the stricter the criteria to select healthy people the fewer significant ventricular arrhythmias are found. Some accepted facts seem to have emerged from a general review of the articles. Heart rate varies between 40 and 180 beats per minute (bpm) in normal individuals, with higher rates in women and smokers. The maximum rate is lower in older age groups, at least partly owing to reduced exercise. Sinus bradycardia (less than 60 bpm) is common on 24 hour monitoring and asymptomatic episodes of marked sinus bradycardia (under 40 bpm), usually during sleep, are occasionally seen. Mobitz I (Wenkebach) and Mobitz II A–V block causing a few dropped beats in 24 hour records may be detected in patients without heart disease, and both may occur in the same patient[12]. Pauses of up to 2 s during sleep are encountered in all age groups and the general occurrence of slow rhythms during the night is attributed to enhanced vagal tone. The majority of adults have atrial and ventricular premature beats on 24 hour tapes and both types of abnormal beat increase with age. Special attention has been paid to ventricular ectopic activity since the early days of coronary care units when the importance of the association between complex ventricular beats and sudden death was recognized. Less than 5% of young adults have frequent and complex ventricular premature beats, and anecdotal experience suggests that this is a benign finding if the subject is otherwise apparently healthy. It is suggested that ventricular PBs are a simple indicator of ageing[13]. In practice Holter recordings are made for clinical reasons, and further investigation is warranted if there are more than 10 ventricular extrasystoles per hour; in those patients with one or more couplets per hour and if bouts of ventricular tachycardia occur. Runs of atrial beats of up to 140 per minute, lasting for 3–10 beats may be found in up to a quarter of cardiac patients, and the phrase 'benign slow atrial tachycardia' has been coined to describe these findings. Bauernfeind and colleagues[14] report apparently healthy people with chronic non-paroxysmal sinus tachycardia. Average waking heart rates are 118–140 bpm with maximum rates of 140–250, and sleeping rates of 70–123. The prognosis of such subjects is unknown. The normal rhythm response to specific activities such as driving, sexual activity, public speaking and various sports are described. Heart rates up to 180 bpm have been recorded after 10 minutes in a sauna[15]. Heart rates rise to levels comparable to moderate physical exertion with most everyday stressful and physical events.

The variety of rhythms which are found on prolonged ECG monitoring in healthy individuals, plus the possibility of technical artifacts, emphasizes the importance of obtaining technically satisfactory recordings. This must be followed by equally careful analysis with regular

Table 8.1 Prolonged ambulatory electrocardiographic monitoring in the investigation of symptoms

Indication	Type of monitoring	Suggested use including time frequency	Comments
Palpitations	Holter or intermittent	repeated 24 h tapes or patient activated or automatic intermittent recordings	empirical drug treatment is rarely justified
Transient cerebral disturbance	Holter or in patient real time system		
(a) Syncope		24 h ECG. Repeated testing often necessary	special care to correlate symptoms with
(b) Other		24 h ECG reserved for known heart disease or negative neurological investigations	arrhythmias particularly in patients with SSS
Chest pain and dyspnoea	Holter or intermittent	repeated 24 h tapes often necessary	alternative investigations, e.g. exercise testing may be appropriate

SSS sick sinus syndrome. NB intermittent includes patient activated devices including transtelephonic and automatic recorders

visual checks to avoid mistaken counting and recognition by the analyser. The correlation of symptoms with ECG abnormalities is essential if inappropriate treatment is to be avoided.

CLINICAL USE OF AMBULATORY ECG MONITORING

The investigation of symptoms (Table 8.1)

Ambulatory arrhythmia detection is widely used for the investigation of palpitations, transient cerebral incidents and for unpredictable bouts of chest pain, chest discomfort and dyspnoea.

Palpitations

Most patients who are distressed or worried by an awareness of erratic heart activity, skipped beats, sensation of the heart stopping or rapid heart rate warrant ambulatory monitoring. Although associated features such as polyuria may give a clue to the abnormal nature of the tachycardia, symptoms may suggest a significant tachyarrhythmia and yet correlate with sinus tachycardia. Potent drugs are consequently avoided, and the value of reassurance in these patients should not be under-estimated[16]. Twenty-four hour tapes are used if symptoms recur on most days, but for episodes occurring at longer intervals we record a single 24 hour ECG and then give the patient a home recorder for up to 3 months.

Transient cerebral disturbance

It is impractical to perform 24 hour ECG monitoring on all patients with transient disturbance of cerebral or brain stem function. Frank blackouts and syncope necessitate prolonged ECG recording, but frequent or major attacks normally require inpatient monitoring rather than ambulatory electrocardiography. Other transient cerebral incidents are less likely to be caused by arrhythmias[17] and 24 hour ambulatory taping is best reserved for patients with known heart disease, or evidence of arrhythmias or unresolved diagnostic problems after full neurological investigation. Many of these patients are elderly and will have abnormalities on prolonged ECG recordings which may be incidental to the symptoms. Repeated 24 hour tapes may be necessary to match symptoms with the cardiac rhythm. It seems reasonable to analyse one 24 hour period fully, but after this, analysis could be deferred until the symptom is reported in order to save technician time.

Unpredictable chest pain, discomfort and dyspnoea

Ischaemia, chest pain and dyspnoea are frequently precipitated by arrhythmias, but most cases present with the acute problem and only require standard electrocardiograms for diagnosis. Unexplained short lasting cardiac pain or dyspnoea may be caused by intermittent arrhythmias, particularly when the main symptom overwhelms the underlying rhythm disturbance. Repeated 24 hour ambulatory ECG monitoring using Holter devices or intermittent recorders for symptoms may be required.

The investigation of cardiac and other disorders (Tables 8.2 and 8.3)

Coronary artery disease

Emphasis has rested on the identification of ventricular ectopic activity (VEA) following acute myocardial infarction. The concept of 'warning arrhythmias' which allow the prediction of life threatening rhythms such as ventricular tachycardia and fibrillation led to the Lown classification of ventricular arrhythmias[18,19]. The consensus of recent opinion is that ventricular fibrillation cannot be predicted by identifying 'warning' arrhythmias during the acute stage of myocardial infarction[20]. The picture is different when prolonged ambulatory ECG monitoring is performed 2–3 weeks after infarction, even though VEA is almost

Table 8.2 Prolonged ambulatory ECG monitoring in acute myocardial infarction (AMI)

Indication	Type of monitoring	Suggested use, time, frequency	Comments
Detection of VEA			
(a) In hospital post CCU	telemetry (real time, trends)	continuous daily	high risk SCD if complex VEA and LV dysfunction. Low predictive value
(b) Subsequent 2–3 weeks	IP telemetry OP Holter	decision of individual physician	complex VEA an independent risk factor. Monitoring to assess drugs
(c) During year after AMI	Holter	decision of individual physician	complex VEA an independent risk factor. Value in management not clear
Sustained VT	IP telemetry	for up to 6 weeks	high mortality when associated with large ant. infarct, CCF ± RBBB. Surgery
After arrest or near arrest	Holter/IP telemetry	prolonged monitoring	consider formal strategy. Exercise testing. 48 h Holter. Trial drugs
Heart block in CCU	Holter	one 24 h tape at least	repeated tapes if symptomatic
Pre-hospital	telemetry	until in CCU	check for paramedics. Probably unnecessary
Rehabilitation programmes	telemetry/Holter	duration of session	for symptomatic patients

VEA ventricular ectopic activity, SCD sudden cardiac death, CCU coronary care unit

Table 8.3   Use of prolonged ECG monitoring in various disorders

Indication	Type of monitoring	Suggested use, time frequency	Comments
HOCM	Holter	all patients 24 h, repeated if symptomatic	asymptomatic VT 8-fold increase mortality
CCF	Holter	decision of individual physician	is it possible to reduce annual death rate by anti-arrhythmic agents?
Mitral valve prolapse	Holter	24 h tape	reserve for symptomatic or abnormalities on resting ECG
Pre-excitation	Holter	24 h tapes	all patients. Repeated in symptomatic
Pacemakers	Holter or intermittent	prolonged monitoring if necessary	detect intermittent faults in pacemaker system. Routine transtelephonic checks. Checking antitachycardia pacemakers
Apnoea	Holter or IP	one or repeated 24 h tapes	investigation of cot deaths, Pickwickian syndrome
Sick sinus syndrome	Holter	repeated 24 h tapes	special care to correlate symptoms with arrhythmias to avoid wrong treatment

invariable. Complex or frequent ventricular ectopic beats (more than 10/h) occur in almost a third of patients, but do provide a risk factor independent of other factors[21]. The need for Holter monitoring to detect VEA in the weeks or months after acute infarction depends on the policy of drug intervention or surgery which is adopted by each unit. A special group in which prolonged ECG monitoring may be useful are those patients with evidence of major AV block or trifascicular block during the acute stage of infarction. Kennedy[12] recommends that those patients who are not permanently paced should be subsequently monitored to see if cardiac conduction returns to normal.

Two different uses for ambulatory monitoring are during the post-coronary care inpatient days and during rehabilitation. We use telemetry to monitor arrhythmias during ward mobilization after discharge from the coronary care unit (CCU). This continuous ECG is observed in the CCU and the same alarms, play back facilities and 24 hour trend data are available as for those patients monitored on the unit. Detection of severe arrhythmias in real time allows rapid treatment, but whether all patients justify this monitoring or whether it can be tailored to use in selected patients at high risk is not yet clear. During formal coronary rehabilitation classes, telemetry or Holter monitoring[22] may be useful on occasion but they are rarely essential. Ambulatory monitoring at home, however, may be valuable in assessing the response to everyday activities and can be a powerful reassuring factor in some cases. It has also been used in a survey of suspected infarction patients selected for home care[23]. To be useful in the management of these patients would require a sophisticated real time telemetric facility. Although telemetry has been proposed for pre-admission care, experience in the United States suggests that the ability to diagnose and treat arrhythmias by paramedical teams is not improved[24].

Sudden cardiac death (SCD)

Ventricular fibrillation is the commonest cause of sudden cardiac death documented by ambulatory monitoring. Bradycardia with asystole is less frequently responsible[25]. In the younger age groups non-coronary heart disease, particularly hypertrophic obstructive cardiomyopathy and the long Q–T syndromes are major causes of SCD, but most sudden deaths overall are caused by ischaemic heart disease, particularly after acute infarction. Extensive myocardial damage, left ventricular dysfunction and complex ventricular ectopic activity identify patients at high risk of SCD following myocardial infarction. Roelandt and Hugenholtz[26] use the concept of mechanical, ischaemic and electrical risk factors in an attempt to predict and prevent SCD in coronary heart disease. Severe mechanical failure requires transplantation or possibly treatment with vasodilators, and ischaemia is helped by reperfusion techniques. The ambulatory ECG has a major role in the investigation of the electrical risk group and in the assessment of the efficacy of treatment. Ventricular arrhythmias are an independent risk factor in the year following acute myocardial infarction[27]. Frequent ventricular extrasystoles (more than 10/h) and complex VEA with couplets and runs of three or more extrasystoles are probably significant. The role of R on T ectopic beats has been controversial. They are rarely found in normal individuals but they are associated with ventricular fibrillation in acute myocardial infarction, congenital long QT syndromes and drug-induced prolongation of QT intervals[28]. The problem of which patient should have ambulatory ECG monitoring; how often and for how long remains a decision for individual physicians. Lown[29,30] bases his strategy on the conviction that sudden cardiac death may be predicted from the detection of complex VEA and the elimination of severe grades of ventricular premature beats will reduce the risk of ventricular fibrillation. He advocates a systematic approach to antiarrhythmic treatment in patients who have suffered 'malignant' ventricular arrhythmias, i.e. ventricular tachycardia or fibrillation with near or actual cardiac arrest. Holter monitoring for 48 hours, combined with treadmill exercise testing, is used to obtain baseline information about ventricular arrhythmias, and both are repeated to assess therapeutic response when taking an antiarrhythmic drug. The aim is to abolish runs of three or more VPBs and R on T ectopics, to reduce couplets by more than 90% and VPBs over 24 hours by more than 50%.

Reviewing the management of ventricular arrhythmias following myocardial infarction, Josephson[31] concludes that rigorous investigation to identify patients at high risk of sudden death is essential if unnecessary, potentially dangerous drugs are to be avoided. Ambulatory monitoring is valuable both for identifying groups of patients at particular risk of SCD and to assess the effectiveness of subsequent treatment. He emphasizes two special groups of patients. In one group, syncope or near syncope draws attention to bouts of non-sustained ventricular tachycardia. When these occur in the second week after infarction, lethal ventricular arrhythmias seem common, and ambulatory monitoring is valuable to see whether the major tachycardias are abolished by treatment. The other group are those patients with spontaneous sustained VT. When this is associated with large anterior infarcts, congestive cardiac failure and possibly right bundle branch block, mortality is high and surgery may be indicated. Prolonged telemetry in hospital for up to 6 weeks is justifiable in these patients. In general, however, predischarge Holter monitoring is a blunt instrument for predicting SCD with a sensitivity under 64% and a positive predictive accuracy of less than 20%. The same problems apply to the recognition of complex and frequent ventricular ectopic beats which are accepted as markers of SCD in the year following acute infarction. Treatment of all these patients with drugs would lead to the majority receiving potentially dangerous agents unnecessarily. Furthermore, it still leaves an approximately equal number of deaths in patients who do not show significant ventricular arrhythmias on prolonged ECG monitoring. Despite the problems ambulatory electrocardiography, supplemented by exercise stress testing and electrophysiological studies, has a role in attempting to identify patients at risk of sudden death.

Cardiomyopathies

In hypertrophic obstructive cardiomyopathy (HOCM), prolonged ambulatory monitoring reveals supraventricular tachycardia or atrial fibrillation in 46–70% of patients, ventricular tachycardia in 7–28% and up to 60% have complex or frequent ventricular ectopic beats[32-34]. Winkle[35] restricts the use of Holter monitoring to symptomatic patients because the prognostic value of recording the arrhythmias is doubtful. However, one series quotes an 8.6% annual mortality in patients with asymptomatic ventricular tachycardia[36]. When coupled with the possibility of reducing sudden death by the suppression of ventricular arrhythmias with amiodarone[37], Holter monitoring seems to be justified in all patients with HOCM.

Two other groups with cardiomyopathy warrant ambulatory monitoring. Ventricular arrhythmias which present late in pregnancy or in the puerperium may indicate peripartal cardiomyopathy[38]. In patients with congestive cardiomyopathy, asymptomatic supraventricular and ventricular arrhythmias and disorders of conduction are frequently found. Holter monitoring is particularly important in demonstrating whether or not symptoms are caused by an arrhythmia.

Congestive cardiac failure

Packer[38] points out that treatment for cardiac failure has improved the lifestyle of patients, but has hardly improved longevity. There is a wide variation in reports of sudden death (4–63%), but it is reasonable to assume that they are due to ventricular tachycardia or fibrillation. Pooling of eight series shows that 87% of patients with CCF have couplets and/or multiform ventricular premature beats, and 54% have non-sustained VT[39]. Evidence that ventricular ectopic activity is an independent risk factor for SCD is lacking. Nevertheless, Holter monitoring is useful in detecting ventricular arrhythmias, in detecting diuretic-induced hypokalaemia and hypomagnesaemia which can be corrected in assessing the effect of withdrawing drugs which may cause arrhythmias, (such as positive inotropes) and in evaluating antiarrhythmic agents.

Valvular heart disease

The cause of sudden death in aortic stenosis is not known, but ambulatory electrocardiograms commonly reveal ventricular ectopic beats. Twenty-four hour recordings in one series showed ventricular tachycardia in 17 of 93 patients with aortic valve disease, and two patients died suddenly[40]. The authors suggest that the arrhythmias are caused by poor left ventricular function. A more specific relationship between arrhythmias and sudden death has been suggested in patients with mitral valve prolapse (MVP). Reports of arrhythmias in patients with MVP are based on hospital referrals, so it is hardly surprising that serious rhythm abnormalities are detected[41]. The indications for ambulatory monitoring remain unclear but patients with ST and T wave changes on standard ECGs warrant prolonged monitoring, because they are more likely to have serious ventricular arrhythmias[42].

Sick sinus syndrome (SSS)

Ambulatory ECG monitoring is the mainstay for the diagnosis of SSS, but strict criteria must be observed if overdiagnosis and overuse of permanent pacing procedures are to be avoided. The recognition of sinus bradycardia and pauses does not necessarily mean SSS. Sinus rates under 50 per minute during the night are common in middle-aged and particularly young adults[43], and sinus pauses are often recorded in young subjects. Marked sinus bradycardia (under 40 b/min) and sinus pauses greater than 2/s are likely to be pathological[44]. Every attempt must be made to establish that symptoms such as syncope or giddiness coincide with ECG findings, and multiple 24 hour recordings may be necessary. Holter monitoring is particularly valuable in the diagnosis and management of the bradycardia–tachycardia syndrome. The use of anti-arrhythmic agents to improve tachycardias may lead to excessive slowing of the heart, and the only drug which is likely to be successful is amiodarone[45].

Pre-excitation

When Wolff–Parkinson–White syndrome or the short PR (Lown–Ganong–Levine) syndrome is diagnosed on standard electrocardiography, routine Holter monitoring is justified as a baseline test. If a patient with a history of palpitations fails to develop them during the 24 hour recording, every attempt should be made to record at the time of symptoms by using patient activated devices. Some patients can be reassured because palpitations are shown to be caused by simple ectopic activity or sinus tachycardia. In those with significant arrhythmias, paroxysmal supraventricular tachycardia can be distinguished from atrial fibrillation or atrial flutter, and appropriate therapy can be prescribed. Routine Holter monitoring in patients complaining of paroxysmal tachycardia with normal standard ECGs may reveal intermittent pre-excitation.

Function of permanent pacemakers

If symptoms of disturbed consciousness recur after implantation of permanent pacemakers, further investigation is necessary to distinguish between pacemaker failure, the 'pacemaker syndrome'[46], intermittent faults in the pacemaker system[47], paroxysmal tachycardia and independent disease such as cerebrovascular insufficiency. Holter monitoring may show intermittent problems owing to faults in the pacemaker system or occasional displacement of the electrode, and bouts of tachycardia will be revealed. Long periods of monitoring are often required and ward based telemetry or home based automatic event recorders may be preferable to routine Holter techniques. Antitachycardia pacemakers also require frequent ambulatory ECG monitoring[35]. Patient activated systems with implanted radiofrequency pacemakers are checked usually by transtelephonic event recorders, and automatic antitachycardia pacemakers are monitored by frequent ambulatory electrocardiograms.

Apnoea

Prolonged ECG monitoring in infants is used in the investigation of sudden 'cot' death. Bradycardia associated with apnoea is found in some subjects with a high risk of sudden death[48]. The relationship is not proved, however, since most healthy infants investigated by ambulatory monitoring show periods of sinus bradycardia and may have junctional escape rhythms, sinus pauses and sinoatrial block[49]. In adults the sleep apnoea syndrome is usually recognized in obese patients with the 'Pickwickian syndrome', although it often affects non-obese patients. Holter monitoring commonly shows arrhythmias including supraventricular and ventricular tachycardias, sinus bradycardia and pauses and atrioventricular block. Serial Holter recordings help to monitor effectiveness of treatment such as weight reduction, nocturnal oxygen supplementation or tracheotomy.

Other uses

Ambulatory electrocardiography is useful in many disorders which are primarily non-cardiac but in which heart problems can be important. Thus diabetics with severe autonomic neuropathy may have functional denervation of the heart. Holter monitoring with trend plotting of R–R intervals against time shows the characteristic loss of beat–beat changes in cycle length[50,51]. Conclusions from three recent articles are used to illustrate the value of ambulatory ECGs in patients with noncardiac disease. Heart rate changes in hyperthyroidism are shown to result from a direct action of T_4 on the heart rather than by the potentiation of catecholamines[52]. Sarcoid heart disease most commonly presents with complete heart block, and should always be considered as a cause in the young patient with CHB. Incomplete heart block, supraventricular and ventricular arrhythmias are also frequent features of sarcoid heart disease[53]. A significantly increased tendency to atrioventricular block and atrial tachycardia is present in patients with ankylosing spondylitis who are HLA B27 positive[54].

Detailed discussion of the large volume of literature concerning the use of ambulatory ECG monitoring in the investigation of antiarrhythmic drugs is beyond the scope of this article. However, several aspects seem worth a mention. Attention is mainly confined to the management of ventricular arrhythmias. Suppression of ventricular premature beats provides a useful method for evaluating the antiarrhythmic properties of a drug, and plasma concentrations can be correlated with antiarrhythmic activity. Hour to hour and day to day variability in VEA[55,56] require dramatic reduction in numbers of ventricular premature beats to distinguish drug effect from spontaneous variability. Using Holter monitoring, the aim of successful treatment should be to reduce VPBs by 75–90% and to abolish runs of ventricular tachycardia[57]. Considerable debate continues on whether suppression of ventricular premature beats is relevant to the prevention of ventricular tachycardia and ventricular fibrillation. Comparisons of the efficacy of antiarrhythmic agents using Holter monitoring and electrophysiological testing show discordance between the results achieved by the two tests[58]. Efficacy is easier to achieve by Holter electrocardiography, but the clinical importance of this has not been confirmed by long term studies. Myerberg and associates[59] have demonstrated that different drug levels are needed to suppress VPBs than to prevent ventricular tachycardia and fibrillation. Accepting this reservation, there are obvious practical attractions to the use of ambulatory electrocardiography in assessing drug therapy in District General hospitals without ready access to electrophysiological studies. The ability of antiarrhythmic agents to provoke or aggravate arrhythmias is increasingly recognized. The problem is to differentiate between inadequate drug dosage, variability or progression of the underlying rhythm disturbance, and a true pro-arrhythmic effect. Simple withdrawal of the drug, plasma levels and electrophysiological tests may help, but the role of ambulatory elec-trocardiography is not clearly established. In the systematic approach to the detection of proarrhythmic effects of drugs advocated by Velebit et al.[60] criteria for the diagnosis of drug induced aggravation of arrhyth-mia are suggested. These include a fourfold increase in the hourly number of VPBs, a tenfold increase in couplets or VT compared to the control period and the first occurrence of VT lasting for one minute or longer. These authors investigated nine drugs and concluded that aggravation of ventricular arrhythmias was caused by all of them. Ambulatory ECG findings are reported for all current antiarrhythmic agents, and the technique is used frequently in comparisons between drugs[61]. Amiodarone exemplifies some of the uses and the snags in using ambulatory monitoring to investigate antiarrhythmic drugs. There is a long delay between the start of treatment and a satisfactory clinical effect and plasma level when routine oral therapy is used. This makes it difficult to judge when prolonged ECG recordings should be made, and after amiodarone is stopped several weeks or longer may be necess-ary before a post drug recording is valid. Subjects treated with ami-odarone may have a satisfactory clinical result with poor Holter findings and vice versa[62,63]. Of 107 patients treated with amiodarone for sustained ventricular tachyarrhythmias 25% had too few VPBs on 24 hour Holter monitoring for statistical analysis, and serial recordings in the remain-ing patients were unable to predict recurrence of arrhythmia[63]. One useful feature is the ability to see if the drug itself or the metabolite, desethylamiodarone, is the active antarrhythmic agent. Using i.v. amio-darone, the antiarrhythmic effect occurs within hours of starting an infusion when serum levels of amiodarone are within the range regarded as effective for oral therapy, whereas desethylamiodarone levels are low[64].

CONCLUSIONS

The widespread use of ambulatory electrocardiographic monitoring makes it difficult to look back and appreciate the benefits which have resulted from the introduction of the technique. It enabled the definition of 'normal' cardiac rhythm in different age groups, and has totally altered the approach to the management of symptomatic arrhythmias. The empirical use of drugs in patients with palpitations is no longer justified, and identification of an abnormal rhythm may be followed by repeat monitoring to assess the efficacy of drug therapy. The sick sinus syndrome and the associated bradycardia–tachycardia syndrome provide a particular example of the important role of ambulatory monitoring in the definition of a condition, diagnosis of individual patients and occasionally in subsequent testing to evaluate treatment. It is also an example of the general need to take special care to match symptoms with the ECG findings to avoid inappropriate treatment. Many patients benefit from the reassurance which can be offered when symptoms are shown to coincide with benign rhythms such as sinus tachycardia.

The use of ambulatory monitoring to investigate asymptomatic individuals remains controversial. It is widely used to detect ventricular ectopic activity particularly after acute infarction, but the predictive value of VEA to identify patients at risk from malignant ventricular rhythms is debatable. Treatment which reduces ventricular premature beats may be unsuccessful in preventing ventricular tachycardia or fibrillation, so the wisdom of relying on a reduction in counts of VEA to show the efficacy of drugs in the prevention of sudden cardiac death is dubious. Similar reservations apply to the use of prolonged ECG monitoring in the evaluation and comparison of antiarrhythmic agents.

Indiscriminate use of ambulatory ECG monitoring runs the risk of reducing the clinical value of the technique. Thus it is important to maintain a good recording technique and to use visual checks of automatic analysis devices. Interpretation must take into account the natural variation found in normal subjects, and symptoms should be correlated with abnormalities whenever possible. Nevertheless, technical improvement in the equipment and new indications for the use of ambulatory electrocardiograms are certain to ensure the continued and increased use of the technique.

References

1. Holter, N. J. (1961). New method for heart studies. *Science*, **134**, 1214–20
2. Brown, A. K., Anderson, V., Burch, J. and Nelson, P. (1982). Home recording of arrhythmias by patients using a portable electrocardiograph. *J.R. Coll Physicians Lond*, **16**, 175–7

3. Kraznow, A. Z. and Bloomfield, D. K. (1976) Artifacts in portable electrocardiographic monitoring. *Am. Heart J.*, **91**, 349–57
4. Hinkle, L. E., Carver, S. T. and Stevens, M. (1969). The frequency of asymptomatic disturbances of cardiac rhythm and conduction in middle aged men. *Am. J. Cardiol.*, **24**, 629–50
5. Clarke, J. M., Shelton, J. R., Hamer, J., Taylor, S. and Venning, G. R. (1976). The rhythm of the normal human heart. *Lancet*, **2**, 508–12
6. Brodsky, M., Win, D., Denes, P., Kanakis, C. and Rosen, K. H. (1977). Arrhythmias documented by 24 hour continuous electrocardiographic monitoring in 50 male medical students without apparent heart disease. *Am. J. Cardiol.*, **39**, 390–5
7. Clee, M. D., Smith, N., McNeil, G. P. and Wright, D. S. (1979). Dysrhythmias in apparently healthy elderly subjects. *Age and Ageing*, **8**, 173–6
8. Romhilt, D. W., Chaffin, C., Choi, S. C. and Irby, E. C. (1984). Arrhythmias on ambulatory electrocardiographic monitoring in women without apparent heart disease. *Am. J. Cardiol.*, **54**, 582–6
9. Rasmussen, V., Jensen, G., Schnohr, P. and Hansen, J. F. (1985). Premature ventricular beats in healthy adult subjects 20 to 79 years of age. *Eur. Heart J.*, **6**, 335–41
10. Orth-Gomer, K., Hogstedt, C., Bodin, L. and Soderholm, B. (1986). Frequency of extrasystoles in healthy male employees. *Br. Heart J.*, **55**, 259–64
11. Ingerslev, J. and Bjerregaard, P. (1986). Prevalence and prognostic significance of cardiac arrhythmias detected by ambulatory electrocardiography in subjects 85 years of age. *Eur. Heart J.*, **7**, 570–5
12. Kennedy, H. L. (1981). *Ambulatory Electrocardiography Including Holter Recording Technology.* (Philadelphia: Lea and Febiger)
13. Petch, M. C. (1985). Lessons from ambulatory monitoring. *Br. Med. J.*, **291**, 617–18
14. Bauernfeind, R. A., Amat Y Leon, F., Dhingra, R. C., Kehoe, R., Wyndham, C. and Rosen, K. M. (1979). Chronic nonparoxysmal sinus tachycardia in otherwise healthy persons. *Am. Intern. Med.*, **91**, 702–10
15. Taggart, P., Parkinson, P. and Carruthers, M. (1972). Cardiac responses to thermal, physical and emotional stress. *Br. Med. J.*, **3**, 71–6
16. Brown, A. K. and Anderson, V. (1980). The contribution of 24 hour ambulatory E.C.G. monitoring in a general medical unit. *J.R. Coll. Physicians Lond.*, **14**, 7–12
17. Luxon, L. M., Crowther, A., Harrison, M. J. G. and Coltart, J. (1980). Controlled study of 24 hour ambulatory electrocardiographic monitoring in patients with transient neurological symptoms. *J. Neurol., Neurosurg. Psychiatry*, **43**, 37–41
18. Lown, B., Fakhro, A. M., Hood, W. B. and Thorn, G. W. (1967). The coronary care unit. New perspectives and directions. *J. Am. Med. Assoc.*, **199**, 188–98
19. Lown, B. and Wolf, M. (1971). Approaches to sudden death from coronary heart disease. *Circulation*, **44**, 130–42
20. Campbell, R. W. F. (1985). DCG in the investigation of ventricular arrhythmias. In Campbell, R. W. F. and Murray, A. S. (eds.) *Dynamic Electrocardiography.* pp. 88–95. (Edinburgh: Churchill Livingstone)
21. Cowan, C. and Campbell, R. W. F. (1986), Antiarrhythmic therapy in post myocardial infarction patients.. *Eur. Heart J.*, **7**, (Supplement A), 145–7
22. Fletcher, G. F. and Cantwell, J. D. L. (1977). Continuous ambulatory E.C.G. monitoring. Use in cardiac exercise programs. *Chest*, **71**, 27–32
23. Brown, A. K., Anderson, V. and Davies, L. (1985). A survey of patients selected by general practitioners for home care of suspected myocardial infarction: Arrhythmia detection using Holter monitoring. *Eur. Heart J.*, **6**, 13–20
24. Cayten, C. G., Oler, J., Walker, K., Murphy, J., Morganroth, J. and Staroscik, R. (1985). The effect of telemetry on urban prehospital cardiac care. *Ann. Emerg. Med.*, **14**, 976–81
25. Roelandt, J., Klootwijk, P., Lubsen, J. and Janse, M. J. (1984). Sudden death during longterm ambulatory monitoring. *Eur. Heart J.*, **5**, 7–20
26. Roelandt, J. and Hugenholtz, P. G. (1986). Sudden death: prediction and prevention. *Eur. Heart J.*, **7**, (Supplement A), 169–80

27. Kulbertus, H. E. (1986). Ventricular arrhythmias, left ventricular function and mortality after acute myocardial infarction. *Eur. Heart J.*, 7, (Supplement A), 123–6
28. Leading article. (1986). R on T ventricular ectopic beats. *Lancet*, 2, 902–3
29. Lown, B. (1982). Management of patients at high risk of sudden death. *Am. Heart J.*, 103, 689–95
30. Lown, B. (1983). Abolishing advanced grades of ventricular premature beats protects patients with recurring malignant ventricular arrhythmias. *Int. J. Cardiol.*, 4, 345–50
31. Josephson, M. E. (1986). Treatment of ventricular arrhythmias after myocardial infarction. *Circulation*, 74, 653–8
32. Ingham, R. E., Rosen, R. M., Goodman, D. J. and Harrison, D. C. (1975). Circulatory electrocardiographic monitoring in idiopathic hypertrophic subaortic stenosis. *Circulation*, 51, II–93
33. Savage, D. D., Seides, S. F., Maron, B. J., Myers, D. J. and Epstein, S. E. (1979). Prevalence of arrhythmias during 24 hour monitoring and exercise testing in patients with obstructive and non-obstructive hypertrophic cardiomyopathy. *Circulation*, 59, 866–75
34. McKenna, W. J., Chetty, S., Oakley, C. M. and Goodwin, J. F. (1980). Arrhythmia in hypertrophic cardiomyopathy: Exercise and 48 hour ambulatory electrocardiographic assessment with and without beta adrenergic blocking therapy. *Am. J. Cardiol.*, 45, 1–5
35. Winkle, R. A. (1981). Current status of ambulatory electrocardiography. *Am. Heart J.*, 102, 757–70
36. McKenna, W. J., Harrison, L., Perez, G., Krikler, D. M., Oakley, C. M. and Goodwin, J. F. (1981). Arrhythmia in hypertrophic cardiomyopathy. II. Comparison of amiodarone and verapamil in treatment. *Br. Heart J.*, 46, 173–8
37. Perloff, J. K. (1984). Pregnancy and cardiovascular disease. In Braunwald, E. (ed.) *Heart Disease.* pp. 1763–81 (Philadelphia: W. B. Saunders)
38. Packer, M. (1985). Sudden unexpected death in patients with congestive cardiac failure: a second frontier. *Circulation*, 72, 681–5
39. Francis, G. S. (1986). Development of arrhythmias in the patient with congestive cardiac failure: Pathophysiology, prevalence and prognosis. *Am. J. Cardiol.*, 57, 3B–7B
40. Oshausen, K. V., Schwarz, F., Apfelbach, J., Rohrig, N., Kramer, B. and Kubler, W. (1983). Determinants of the incidence and severity of ventricular arrhythmias in aortic valve disease. *Am. J. Cardiol.*, 51, 1103–9
41. Winkle, R. A., Lopes, M. G., Fitzgerald, J. W., Goodman, D. J., Schroeder, J. S. and Harrison, D. C. (1975). Arrhythmias in patients with mitral valve prolapse. *Circulation*, 52, 73–81
42. Campbell, R. W. F., Godman, M. G., Fiddler, G. I., Marquis, R. B. and Julian, D. G. (1976). Ventricular arrhythmias in syndrome of balloon deformity of mitral valve. Definition of possible high risk group. *Br. Heart J.*, 38, 1053–7
43. Ferrer, I. (1978). Sleep and the cardiovascular system. *Chest*, 73, 125–6
44. Shaw, D. B. (1985). D.C.G. in the investigation of bradyarrhythmias. In Campbell, R. W. F. and Murray, A. (eds.) *Dynamic Electrocardiography.* pp. 58–73 (Edinburgh: Churchill Livingstone)
45. Brown, A. K., Primhak, R. A. and Newton, P. (1978). Use of amiodarone in bradycardia–tachycardia syndrome. *Br. Heart J.*, 40, 1149–52
46. Kenny, R. A. and Sutton, R. (1986). Pacemaker syndrome. *Br. Med. J.*, 293, 902–3
47. Bleifer, S. B., Bleifer, D. J., Hansmann, D. R., Sheppard, J. J. and Karpman, H. L. (1974). Diagnosis of occult arrhythmias by Holter electrocardiography. *Prog. Cardiovasc. Dis.*, 16, 569–99
48. Guilleminault, C., Arigane, R., Sougnet, M. and Dement, W. C. (1976). Abnormal polygraphic recordings in 'near miss' sudden infant deaths. *Lancet*, 1, 1326–7
49. Southall, D. P., Richards, J., Mitchell, P., Brown, D. J., Johnston, P. G. B. and Shinebourne, E. A. (1980). Study of cardiac rhythm in healthy newborn infants. *Br. Heart J.*, 43, 14–20

50. Murray, A., Ewing, D. J., Campbell, I. W., Neilson, J. M. M. and Clarke, B. F. (1975). R.R. interval variations in young male diabetics. *Br. Heart J.*, 37, 882–5
51. Bennett, T., Riggott, P. A., Hosking, D. J. and Hampton, J. R. (1976). Twenty four hour monitoring of heart rate and activity in patients with diabetes mellitus. A comparison with clinical investigations. *Br. Med. J.*, 1, 1250–1
52. Northcote, R. J., MacFarlane, P., Kesson, C. M. and Ballantyne, D. (1986). Continuous 24 hour electrocardiography in thyrotoxicosis before and after treatment. *Am. Heart J.*, 112, 339–43
53. Fleming, H. A. (1986). Sarcoid heart disease. *Br. Med. J.*, 292, 1095–6
54. Thomsen, N. H., Horsley-Petersen, K. and Beyer, J. M. (1986). Ambulatory 24 hour continuous electrocardiographic monitoring in 54 patients with ankylosing spondylitis. *Eur. Heart J.*, 7, 240–6
55. Winkle, R. A. (1978). Antiarrhythmic drug effect mimicked by spontaneous variability of ventricular ectopy. *Circulation*, 57, 1116–21
56. Morganroth, J., Michelson, E. L., Horowitz, L. N., Josephson, M. E., Pearlman, A. S. and Dunkman, W. B. (1978). Monitoring to assess ventricular ectopic frequency. *Circulation*, 58, 408–14
57. Somberg, J. C., Miura, D. and Keefe, D. L. (1986). The treatment of ventricular rhythm disturbances. *Am. Heart J.*, 111, 1162–76
58. Soo, G. K., Seiden, S. W., Matos, J. A., Waspe, L. E. and Fisher, J. D. (1985). Discordance between ambulatory monitoring and programmed stimulation in assessing efficacy of Class 1A antiarrhythmic agents in patients with ventricular tachycardia. *J. Am. Coll. Cardiol.*, 6, 539–44
59. Myerberg, R., Kesler, K., Kiem, L., Pefkaros, K., Conde, C. and Cooper, D. (1981). Relationship between plasma levels of procaineamide, suppression of premature ventricular complexes and prevention of ventricular tachycardia. *Circulation*, 64, 280–90
60. Velebit, V., Podrid, P., Lown, B., Cohen, B. H. and Graboys, T. B. (1982). Aggravation and provocation of ventricular arrhythmias by antiarrhythmic drugs. *Circulation*, 65, 886–94
61. Campbell, R. W. F. (1985). D.C.G. in the investigation of antiarrhythmic therapy. In Campbell, R. W. F. and Murray, A. (eds.), *Dynamic Electrocardiography*. pp. 117–28 (Edinburgh: Churchill Livingstone)
62. Waxman, H. L., Groh, W. C., Marchlinski, F. E., Buxton, A. E., Sadowski, L., Horowitz, L. N., Josephson, M. E. and Kastor, J. A. (1982). Amiodarone for control of sustained ventricular tachyarrhythmia: clinical and electrophysiological effects in 51 patients. *Am. J. Cardiol.*, 50, 1066–74
63. Sokoloff, N. M., Spielman, S. R., Greenspan, A. M., Rae, A. P., Brady, P. M., Kay, H. R. and Horowitz, L. N. (1986). *J. Am. Coll. Cardiol.*, 7, 838–41
64. Brown, A. K., Holt, D. W. and Anderson, V. (1986). A practical regimen for intravenous amiodarone. *Br. J. Clin. Pract.*, 40, (Suppl 44)

9
The role of electrophysiological study in the diagnosis of arrhythmias

E. ROWLAND

INTRODUCTION

Invasive electrophysiological testing has become the definitive investigation in the majority of arrhythmias, and clinical electrophysiology has grown from the ability to record electrical activity directly from the heart as a branch of cardiology. Earliest recordings identified local atrial and ventricular electrograms, but it was the subsequent recording of His bundle activity followed by the introduction of programmed stimulation that led the way towards a sophisticated investigation procedure having diagnostic, mechanistic, therapeutic and prognostic implications.

Invasive electrophysiological study has not replaced, but is an adjunct to, surface electrocardiographic interpretation. Surface recordings are limited in their inability to register the complex pattern of depolarization of the AV conduction system. However, this shortcoming did not prevent early pioneers in electrocardiography from applying their knowledge of the physiological behaviour of the components of AV conduction in making complex deductions on the mechanisms of most arrhythmias. Electrophysiological study has often achieved little more than confirm these deductions, but the test has found a role in clinical practice for providing accurate diagnoses where surface ECG patterns cannot be precise. For example, atrial activity may be difficult to discern on the surface ECG either because of low amplitude or because of rapid QRS complexes, and the precise identification by intracardiac studies may be crucial for an accurate diagnosis.

Simple recordings made during an established arrhythmia play a small part in the role of invasive study. The use of programmed stimulation allowed the diagnostic role to be extended into the study of paroxysmal arrhythmias, the study of detailed local electrophysiological behaviour thereby allowing mechanisms of arrhythmia to be identified and confirmed. Again many of these principles had been proposed before the era of invasive electrophysiological study, adding further weight to the doctrine that surface electrocardiography and invasive electrophysiology are complementary techniques in the approach to the treatment of patients with arrhythmia. Providing this philosophy is appreciated, unnecessary invasive studies on patients will be avoided and the maximum benefit obtained when they are necessary.

ELECTROPHYSIOLOGICAL TECHNIQUE

Equipment

As with other catheterization procedures electrophysiological studies require a high level of patient safety, and in view of the time these studies may take to perform a greater degree of patient comfort than with routine angiographic procedures is necessary. Good quality fluoroscopy facilities are essential, preferably with video tape and freeze-frame facilities, but the capability of undertaking angiography is also desirable. Biplane facilities are recommended if detailed endocardial mapping is to be performed. Full resuscitation facilities including a reserve defibrillator are essential, and in those cases in whom rapid ventricular arrhythmias are likely to occur the use of adhesive defibrillator pads for the duration of the study is recommended. At least three standard ECG leads should be continuously monitored during the study to ensure that axis change and bundle branch block patterns can be accurately detected. Facilities for recording a 12 lead ECG must be available. A minimum suitable combination would be leads I, AVF and VI, but the addition of a lateral chest lead is preferable. Most centres elect to monitor the electrocardiographic signals on a high quality multichannel oscilloscope capable of displaying the high frequency components of the intracardiac electrograms faithfully. Close and detailed analysis of the traces usually requires hard copy, and either an ink jet, UV or photographic recorder are suitable, these being the only recorders capable of displaying signals with a frequency response up to 1 kHz. Detailed analysis of activation patterns may require paper speeds of 200 mm/s.

The catheters used for electrophysiological study are generally constructed from woven Dacron, having small (surface area 12–17 mm²) ring and tip electrodes arranged in pairs. Modern technological improvements allow 6F multipolar catheters to be constructed so that at least two, and often considerably more, bipolar electrograms can be obtained from each catheter. With three or four catheters routinely being used it is not unusual for eight bipolar electrograms to be available for analysis. The precise arrangement used will depend upon the nature and purpose of the study and the degree of detail required in both clinical and research terms. The number of channels displayed at any one time will be limited by the number of amplifiers and the number of channels on the recorder. Providing that the display need not be simultaneous even a relatively modest system can make use of multipolar catheters. However, it cannot be recommended that electrophysiological studies are undertaken with a system of less than three surface ECG channels and four intracardiac channels. The amplifiers used for intracardiac signals require filtering of those signal components outside the range 40–500 Hz, and with continuously variable gain capable of recording signals of $50\,\mu V$ without any significant mains voltage interference. Each channel should be electrically isolated, and should be capable of providing a front end calibration signal. At present the use of low frequency endocardial recordings or unipolar intracardiac signals has little place in routine electrophysiological investigation. Bipolar recordings are generally used, the electrodes being 5 or 10 mm apart. This spacing offers sufficiently discrete local electrograms for accurate timing without compromising electrical separation. 5 mm spacing is recommended for a more accurate mapping of activation sequences.

A stimulator is essential if information beyond simple recording of spontaneous rhythms is to be obtained. It should be capable of delivering up to three premature stimuli synchronized to either paced or spontaneous rhythm, as well as rapid continuous pacing over a wide range of heart rates. The device must be capable of delivering constant current stimuli, and should preferably have two output channels so that synchronous atrial and ventricular pacing can be performed. Ideally the onset of all pacing sequences should be capable of being synchronized to spontaneous rhythm.

Patient selection

Electrophysiological studies are time consuming, expensive and not without potential complications. They should not be undertaken lightly, and the goals of the study should be clarified beforehand. Every effort should be made to document spontaneous arrhythmias prior to the investigation, especially when the nature of the arrhythmia is not clear from the history, examination and preliminary investigations.

There are few contraindications to electrophysiological study. Obviously radiation poses a risk to women of childbearing age. Unstable angina and drug toxicity are two other contraindications. It is probably unwise to undertake studies in those with severely depressed left ventricular function.

Vascular complications are infrequent providing careful attention to catheterization technique is taken. With femoral vein access, phlebitis and/or thromboembolus occur in 0.5–1.0% of studies, and heparinization, which should be routine when arterial catheters are used, should be considered in those thought to be at high risk from venous thrombosis.

Catheterization technique

Electrophysiological studies in general require only venous access. A number of entry sites can be used but the femoral vein is the most convenient. Multiple (usually no more than three) catheters can be inserted via the right femoral vein, a catheter introduced from this site offers the optimal route for obtaining the His bundle electrogram. Left atrial and left ventricular activity can be recorded with a catheter in the coronary sinus, a site that can more easily be obtained by a catheter introduced through either subclavian vein.

The precise arrangement of electrodes used depends on the nature and goals of the study. Most studies require a His bundle electrogram and a tripolar catheter that allows both proximal and distal His bundle activity to be recorded is recommended. Where atrial stimulation and recording are required a quadripolar catheter is invaluable, one bipole for pacing and the other bipole for sensing. This latter bipole ensures local atrial capture which cannot always be verified by observing surface ECG P waves. The right atrial appendage offers a stable site for reliable stimulation without the likelihood of producing phrenic nerve stimulation. However, this site is several centimetres from the sinus node and a position close to the SVC/RA junction is essential if direct sinus node recordings are required. A bipolar catheter often suffices for ventricular stimulation, as the QRS complexes can be used to ensure ventricular capture. The apex of the right ventricle and the right ventricular outflow tract are the most frequently used sites for ventricular stimulation, although the right ventricular inflow tract may be useful in the study of some patients with ventricular tachycardia.

Conduction intervals and principles of stimulation

Electrophysiological investigation rests on two principles – (1) the intracardiac recording of patterns of activation and (2) the response of the various components of the electrical system of the heart to programmed stimulation. In the former domain conduction intervals as well as the pattern of impulse propagation are examined. By recording the His bundle electrogram AV conduction can be divided into the discrete components involved in propagating an impulse from the sinus node to the ventricles (Table 9.1). The PA interval measures conduction across the right atrium but is of little clinical value. The AH interval indicates AV nodal conduction time, and the HV interval the time for conduction through the His–Purkinje system. It is important for purposes of standardization to ensure that a proximal His bundle potential is being recorded, obtained by ensuring that the low right atrial signal is of larger amplitude than the His bundle electrogram. Normal values have been obtained for conduction times through these discrete areas (Table 9.1)[1].

When ventricular depolarization is normal, conduction throughout the fascicular components of the AV conduction system must be equal. When there is bundle branch block the HV interval reflects conduction time through the unblocked fascicle(s) with the shortest conduction

Table 9.1 Normal values for intracardiac conduction intervals and regional refractory periods in the adult

Interval		Duration (ms)
PA	Right atrial conduction time	25–55
AH	AV nodal conduction time	60–110
HV	His–Purkinje conduction time	30–55
AERP	Atrial effective refractory period	180–270
AVNERP	AV nodal effective refractory period	220–400
AVNFRP	AV nodal functional refractory period	320–480
VERP	Ventricular effective refractory period	180–260

time – complete or partial disruption of the interrupted fascicle(s) cannot be discriminated. It may, however, be feasible to identify proximal and distal right bundle branch block based on the interval between the His bundle electrogram and the time of activation of the right ventricular apex[2].

Further observations on the pattern of normal activation are descriptive, based on, for example, the spread of anterograde activation across the left atrium after depolarization of the low right atrium, and activation of the upper ventricular septum and right ventricular outflow tract after activation of the right ventricular apex. The pattern of retrograde atrial depolarization resulting from conduction over the normal AV node–His bundle axis can also be observed. Low right atrial activity precedes coronary sinus depolarization, which is then followed by high right atrial depolarization simultaneously with the onset of spread of activation across the left atrium.

It is important to distinguish the conduction of electrical impulses from the principles of refractoriness that characterize the response of cardiac tissue to premature stimulation. Although a variety of abnormalities can be identified on the basis of abnormal impulse conduction much of the interpretation during electrophysiological study rests on the identification of abnormal responses to premature stimulation. The response of myocardial tissues to stimulation is expressed in terms of refractoriness, various measurements having been defined. They can be measured directly in tissues which can be stimulated directly. Alternatively, the values can be measured indirectly by examining the ability of areas that cannot be stimulated directly (e.g. the AV node) to propagate impulses generated at a proximal site. Tissue characterization in electrophysiological terms can also be seen in values that have combined refractoriness and conduction behaviour. Normal myocardial tissue responds differently to AV nodal tissue. Atrial and ventricular myocardium essentially demonstrate the 'all or nothing' phenomenon in which premature stimuli are conducted at the same velocity irrespective of the prematurity of the stimulus. In fact there is a small degree of delay with stimuli very close to the effective refractory period. AV nodal tissue by contrast demonstrates decremental conduction, i.e. reduced conduction velocity (increased conduction time) with increasingly premature stimuli over a wide range of intervals.

The distinctive components of refractoriness and conduction in electrophysiological behaviour are important concepts if the mechanisms of arrhythmia, particularly with regard to the influence of programmed stimulation, are to be understood. Similarly the conceptual differences between the mechanisms of re-entry and focal automaticity need to be appreciated. While the former can usually be initiated and terminated by premature stimulation, automatic rhythms cannot although they demonstrate overdrive suppression.

SINUS NODE FUNCTION

Although surface ECG recordings provide the mainstay of diagnosing sinus node disease electrophysiological study may occasionally be of value. Two measurements of sinus node function have been established, sinus node recovery time and directly or indirectly measured sinoatrial conduction time.

Sinus node recovery time (SNRT)

Cardiac cells demonstrating intrinsic automaticity will be transiently suppressed at the end of a period of overdrive pacing. This phenomenon of overdrive suppression is measurable as the interval between the last externally paced beat and the first spontaneous or return beat from the automatic area[3]. When testing sinus node function, atrial pacing close to the sinus node is performed for at least 30 seconds at a rate just above the intrinsic sinus rate. The interval between the last stimulus and the first atrial depolarization originating at the high right atrium is taken as the sinus node recovery time. What does this value represent and what are its determinants? The last stimulated atrial depolarization is conducted across the sino–atrial junction and depolarizes the sinus node. Following sinus repolarization and spontaneous diastolic depolarization the sinus node discharges and an impulse is conducted back across the sino–atrial junction to depolarize the atria. Therefore, besides incorporating sino–atrial conduction time this value is related to the rate and duration of pacing, as well as the underlying intrinsic sinus rate. There are a number of explanations for the variability of the measurement, including the integrity of conduction from the atria into the sinus node as well as a pacemaker shift within the node. In practical terms it is important to repeat the tests a number of times and to examine the effect of a range of paced rates. Correction for underlying intrinsic sinus rate can be achieved by subtracting the SNRT from the sinus cycle length thereby obtaining the *corrected* SNRT. Values in excess of 525 ms are abnormal (Figure 9.1). Failure of the last paced beat to be conducted

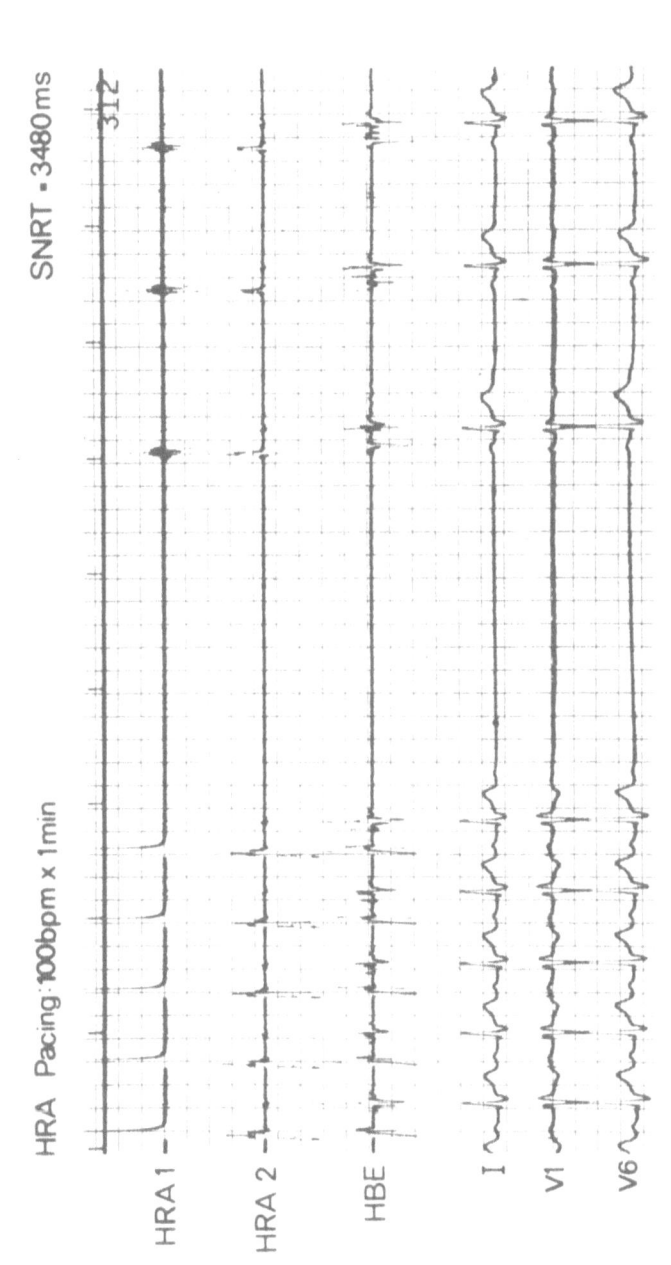

Figure 9.1 Prolonged sinus node recovery time (SNRT) in a patient with sino–atrial disease following right atrial pacing at 100 bpm for 1 minute. (HRA 1 and 2 = High right atrial electrograms, HBE = His bundle electrogram; surface ECG leads I, V1 and V6; paper speed 25 mm/s)

into the sinus node may result in a false negative SNRT; this may, however, result in a prolonged pause after the first return beat[4]. Such secondary pauses may also indicate significant sinus node disease and a nomogram has been established to allow identification of abnormal pauses[4].

Sino-atrial conduction time (SACT)

Although sinus node dysfunction may result from an inability of the sinus pacemaker cells to generate impulses (disordered automaticity), the perinodal structures may be diseased and prevent conduction of impulses between the sinus node and the atrium. Various methods have, therefore, been devised for measuring sino–atrial conduction time. Two methods measure SACT indirectly by examining the influence of premature stimulation on the atrial response. In the first method the influence of stimuli of increasing prematurity is measured[5]. Atrial premature beats are delivered after every eighth sinus beat, and the interval between the last sensed beat and the atrial premature beat compared to the time between the atrial premature stimulus and the next spontaneous sinus beat. These measurements can be normalized by dividing each by the spontaneous sinus cycle length.

The second method uses short (eight beat) episodes of atrial pacing at a rate that just exceeds the intrinsic sinus rate (this rate is assumed not to disturb sinus node automaticity), and measures the interval between the last paced beat and the first return sinus beat[6]. SACT is the recovery interval minus the mean sinus cycle length. In both techniques SACT measures the combined time an impulse takes to travel into the sinus node and then back to the atrium. The individual unidirectional components cannot be identified from each other.

The ability to record sino–atrial activity has provided the first direct measurement of SACT[7]. With an electrode positioned at the high right atrial/SVC junction low frequency signals preceding atrial activity are thought to represent sinus node depolarization.

There is little agreement between the various methods for assessing sinus node function. This may reflect measurement by the tests of different facets of sino–atrial behaviour and various modifications have been suggested in an attempt either to increase the accuracy of the measurements or to increase the sensitivity of the tests. The recent introduction of a more mathematically derived approach to measurements of sinus node automaticity and sino–atrial conduction[8] may allow these separate facets to be identified more accurately, but further experience in a wide variety of patients with sinus node dysfunction will be necessary before it becomes a routine method of assessment. Whether the use of pharmacological adjuncts (e.g. verapamil or disopyramide) which suppress sinus node activity, thereby provoking latent dysfunction will increase the diagnostic sensitivity of these tests remains to be seen.

Clinical electrophysiological testing of patients with suspected sinus node dysfunction lacks the sensitivity and predictive accuracy to make it a reliable test in all patients. However, these tests have good specificity and, therefore, have a role in diagnosis when other tests are normal but where there remains a high index of suspicion that there is underlying sinus node disease.

AV CONDUCTION

Despite the inability of surface ECG recordings to reveal the individual function of the specific components of the AV conduction system, the anatomical location of conduction system disorders can usually be deduced from standard electrocardiographic criteria. Electrophysiological testing, therefore, has a useful but limited role in the assessment of patients with AV conduction disturbances. Its value centres not on making the diagnosis of the degree and type of AV block but on diagnosing the anatomical level of the conduction disturbance, and from this allowing prognostic comments to be made concerning the likelihood of progression to higher grade block, for which pacemaker implantation might be indicated.

In the symptomatic individual every effort should be made to obtain ECG documentation during symptomatic episodes rather than relying on electrophysiological testing. When symptoms can be correlated with bradycardia knowledge of the location of AV conduction block is irrelevant. Where the symptoms are consistent with intermittent high grade AV block and there is resting AV conduction disturbance it was previously felt that precise electrophysiological diagnosis was important. The rationale for this approach had been the apparently good prognosis for second degree type I AV block[9], and, therefore, that confirmation by intracardiac study of the proximal nature of the block might remove the need for pacing in the asymptomatic patient. Recent work[10] has, however, suggested that the prognosis is poor in both forms of second degree block and in both it can be improved by pacing. Interestingly, the prognosis was uninfluenced by the additional presence of bundle branch block. If this study is confirmed the place of intracardiac study would seem to be limited to those with symptomatic first degree AV block in whom ambulatory monitoring cannot reveal higher degrees of AV block (Figure 9.2).

Intraventricular block

The majority of studies have examined the role of electrophysiological investigation in patients with fascicular conduction disturbances. The HV interval indicates conduction time in the unblocked fascicle. These studies have concentrated on bifascicular block and on examining the integrity of the remaining fascicle. A number of prospective studies used measurement of the HV interval in patients with bifascicular block to predict those at risk of complete heart block and sudden death[11-13].

145

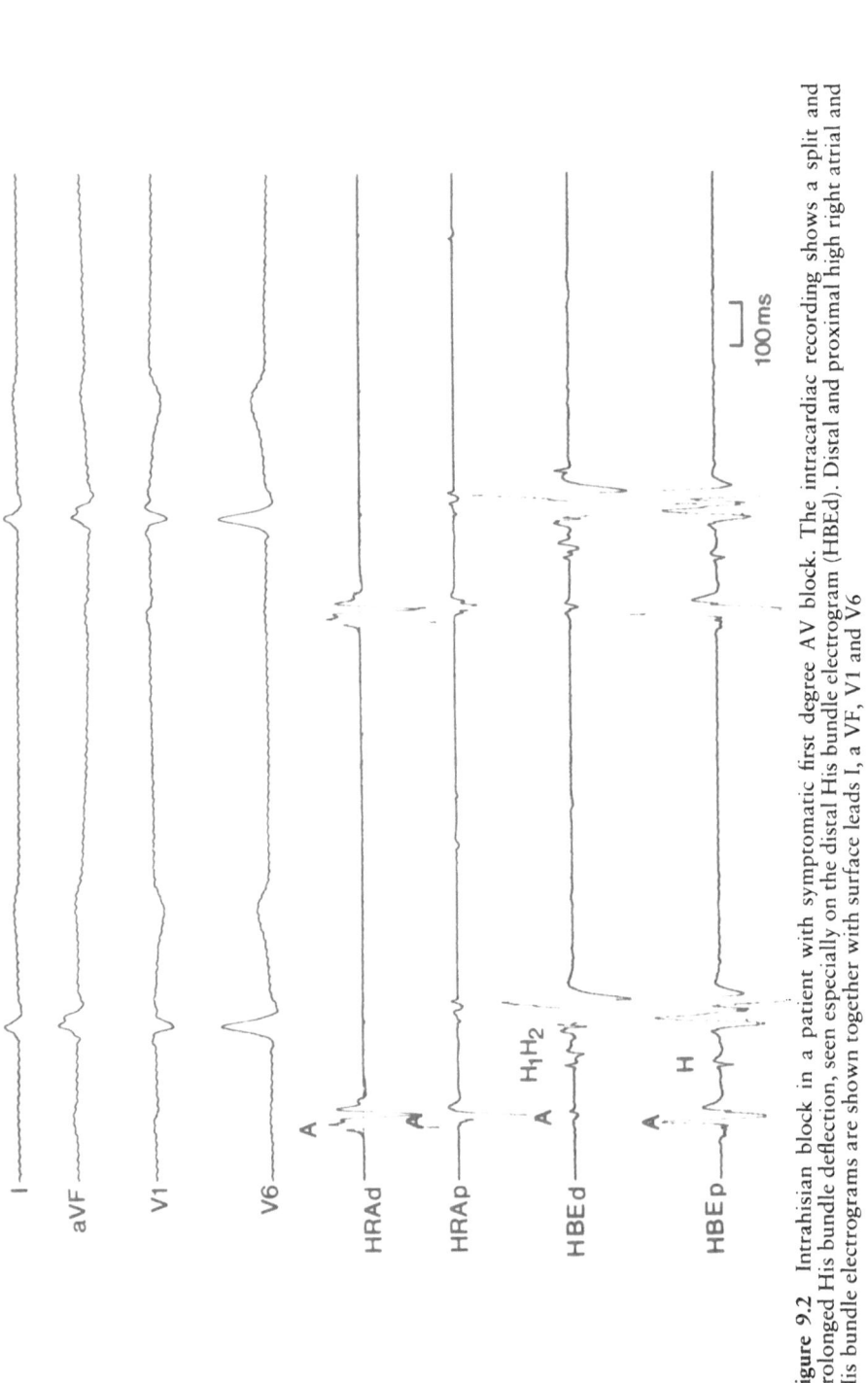

Figure 9.2 Intrahisian block in a patient with symptomatic first degree AV block. The intracardiac recording shows a split and prolonged His bundle deflection, seen especially on the distal His bundle electrogram (HBEd). Distal and proximal high right atrial and His bundle electrograms are shown together with surface leads I, a VF, V1 and V6

Arguably the most important contribution made by these studies has been to demonstrate that the prognosis is determined principally by the nature of the underlying cardiac disease rather than the extent of conduction system disease, and that in many cases sudden death is due to ventricular arrhythmia or myocardial infarction and less frequently to the development of complete heart block. Additionally, in almost half the patients examined there was disease at the level of the AV node and not in the remaining intact fascicle. These studies conflict in their conclusion as to the value of the HV interval as an independent predictor of mortality. Furthermore, the rate of progression to complete heart block in the asymptomatic patient with bifascicular block is low, in the region of 1% per year. This overall value can, however, be broken down more precisely by knowledge of the HV interval. When there is a modest prolongation of the HV interval (55–70 ms) the incidence of progression to second degree AV block or complete heart block is approximately 1% per year. More marked prolongation of the HV interval (70–100 ms) is associated with a 4% per year incidence of high grade AV block, and this incidence increases to 8% when the HV interval exceeds 100 ms. There is, however, no evidence that pacing improves the prognosis, although it may be helpful in the management of symptoms. Therefore, electrophysiological study seems advisable only in those with symptoms, when non-invasive studies have been negative, not solely to clarify abnormal conduction in the remaining fascicle but also to establish, with ventricular stimulation, whether there is inducible sustained ventricular tachycardia[14].

SUPRAVENTRICULAR ARRHYTHMIAS

Atrial flutter and fibrillation

Intracardiac electrophysiological study has little or no part to play in the diagnosis of these arrhythmias. The diagnosis should always be evident on surface electrocardiographic recordings save for the rare case of atrial paralysis in which there may be insufficient atrial muscle to produce a surface deflection, and an invasive study may demonstrate islands of atrial activity amongst a generally inexcitable atrium (Figure 9.3).

Paroxysmal supraventricular tachycardia

As with the other arrhythmias referred to in this chapter diagnosis of the precise mechanism of supraventricular tachycardia can usually be obtained from surface ECG recordings[15]. However, it was electrophysiological studies which provided the precise diagnosis and allowed surface recordings to be interpreted with more precision than had hitherto been possible[16]. Thus intracardiac electrophysiological study remains the 'gold standard' for diagnosing the precise mechanism

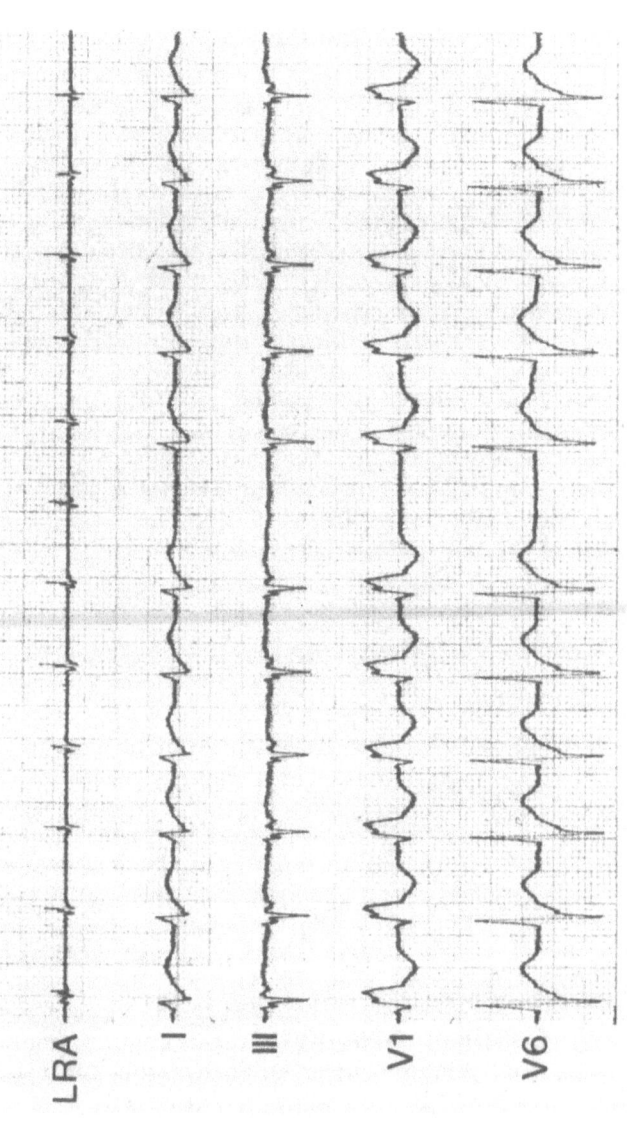

Figure 9.3   Low right atrial (LRA) electrogram in a patient with atrial paralysis. Persistent tachycardia with pauses but without evidence of atrial activity on the surface ECG was documented. Intracardiac study revealed the ectopic atrial rhythm. Low right atrial (LRA) electrogram together with leads I, III, V1 and V6. (paper speed 25 mm/s)

of tachycardia, thereby allowing antiarrhythmic treatment possibilities to be clarified. For example, the absence of pre-excitation on the resting ECG does not exclude the presence of an accessory AV pathway that may be surgically amenable. The majority of cases of paroxysmal supraventricular tachycardia are associated with re-entry either within the AV node or in association with an accessory pathway. Less frequently re-entry may occur in the region of the sinus node or there may be re-entry or focal activity within atrial myocardium.

An approach to treating patients with paroxysmal supraventricular tachycardia can be based on whether it is associated with a normal QRS complex during sinus rhythm or whether there is associated pre-excitation.

PSVT with normal QRS in sinus rhythm

Where the surface ECG does not suggest a mechanism of tachycardia electrophysiological studies are initially directed towards determining whether there is retrograde conduction and its physiological behaviour if present. Re-entry tachycardia associated with either an AV nodal circuit or in association with an accessory AV pathway requires retrograde conduction from ventricle to atrium, and for the pathway to be capable of maintaining 1 : 1 VA conduction at least to the rate of the tachycardia. Where there is poor retrograde conduction (i.e. retrograde block at rates well below the rate of documented tachycardia) an accessory AV pathway can almost certainly be excluded but AV nodal tachycardia cannot. The retrograde pathway involved in AV nodal re-entry is often richly innervated by the autonomic nervous system, and profound changes in retrograde behaviour may occur with sympathetic stimulation. The physiological behaviour of the retrograde pathway in response to incremental pacing or premature stimulation provides the first mechanism for differentiating AV nodal pathways from accessory AV pathways[17]. A retrogradely conducting AV nodal pathway usually demonstrates decremental properties and will activate the low septal right atrium before other atrial sites. Conversely, an accessory AV pathway shows fixed retrograde conduction time and may, depending upon its position, activate other atrial sites before the low right atrium. It may be difficult to separate out these two possibilities when the accessory AV pathway is septal, as some AV nodal pathways conduct retrogradely without demonstrating decremental properties. Additionally, where there is retrograde conduction over a single AV nodal pathway as well as a left lateral accessory pathway retrograde conduction may preferentially occur at slow pacing rates over the AV nodal pathway, because of the proximity to the site of ventricular pacing when this is right ventricular. Therefore, it is always important to examine a wide range of rates and premature intervals in order to achieve decremental conduction in the AV nodal pathway and to allow the consistent conduction over the accessory pathway to predominate.

Atrial stimulation (either incremental pacing or atrial premature stimuli) may reveal dual AV nodal pathways with increasing rate or increasing prematurity, the AH interval remaining fixed or prolonged until at a critical interval or cycle length this faster conducting pathway becomes refractory. The AH interval suddenly lengthens as a second nodal pathway conducts the atrial impulse. Providing conduction over this second pathway is sufficiently slow the propagating impulse may be able to use the faster pathway in a retrograde direction to re-enter the atrium (to produce an echo beat), and if the slower pathway has them recovered excitability AV nodal re-entry tachycardia may ensue (Figure 9.4). Dual AH pathways and echo beats are both suggestive of a substrate for sustained AV nodal re-entry tachycardia, but are probably also present in a percentage of subjects who never experience PSVT. Therefore, manipulation of AV nodal conduction either with catechol-amines or drugs, such as verapamil, which slow AV nodal conduction may be necessary to provoke sustained supraventricular tachycardia.

Either ventricular or atrial pacing may induce sustained supra-ventricular tachycardia and allow the pattern of retrograde conduction to be studied in detail. The diagnosis of the precise mechanism of tachycardia depends upon the timing, location and physiological response of the retrogradely conducting pathway. Sustained tachycardia, therefore, represents the optimal situation for its study. Where low septal right atrial activation precedes the onset of the ventricular component of the His bundle electrogram the diagnosis of AV nodal re-entry is not in doubt (Figure 9.5). Where septal atrial activation occurs coincident with septal ventricular activation both AV nodal re-entry and a septal accessory AV pathway are diagnostic possibilities. Discrimination may rely upon determining whether the His bundle is part of the re-entry circuit or whether it is a common final pathway for ventricular acti-vation[18]. Ventricular premature stimuli delivered just after anterograde His bundle activation will only advance retrograde atrial activation when there is an accessory AV pathway (Figure 9.6). Similarly, in re-entry circuits involving an accessory AV pathway the bundle branch ipsilateral to the accessory pathway will be involved in the tachycardia circuit. Therefore, the influence of bundle branch block on the timing of retrograde atrial activation should be carefully observed[19]. Bundle branch block may occur spontaneously, but may also be induced by manipulation of the His bundle catheter against the septum.

Less frequently there may be AV re-entry associated with a posterior septal accessory AV pathway which conducts slowly, shows decremental retrograde conduction and is associated with incessant tachycardia having a long RP' pattern. It may sometimes require electrophysiological study to distinguish this from an atrial tachycardia arising in the septum or coronary sinus[20].

Sinus node re-entry tachycardia is uncommon, but may be difficult to differentiate on ECG criteria from an atrial tachycardia arising from the high right atrium.

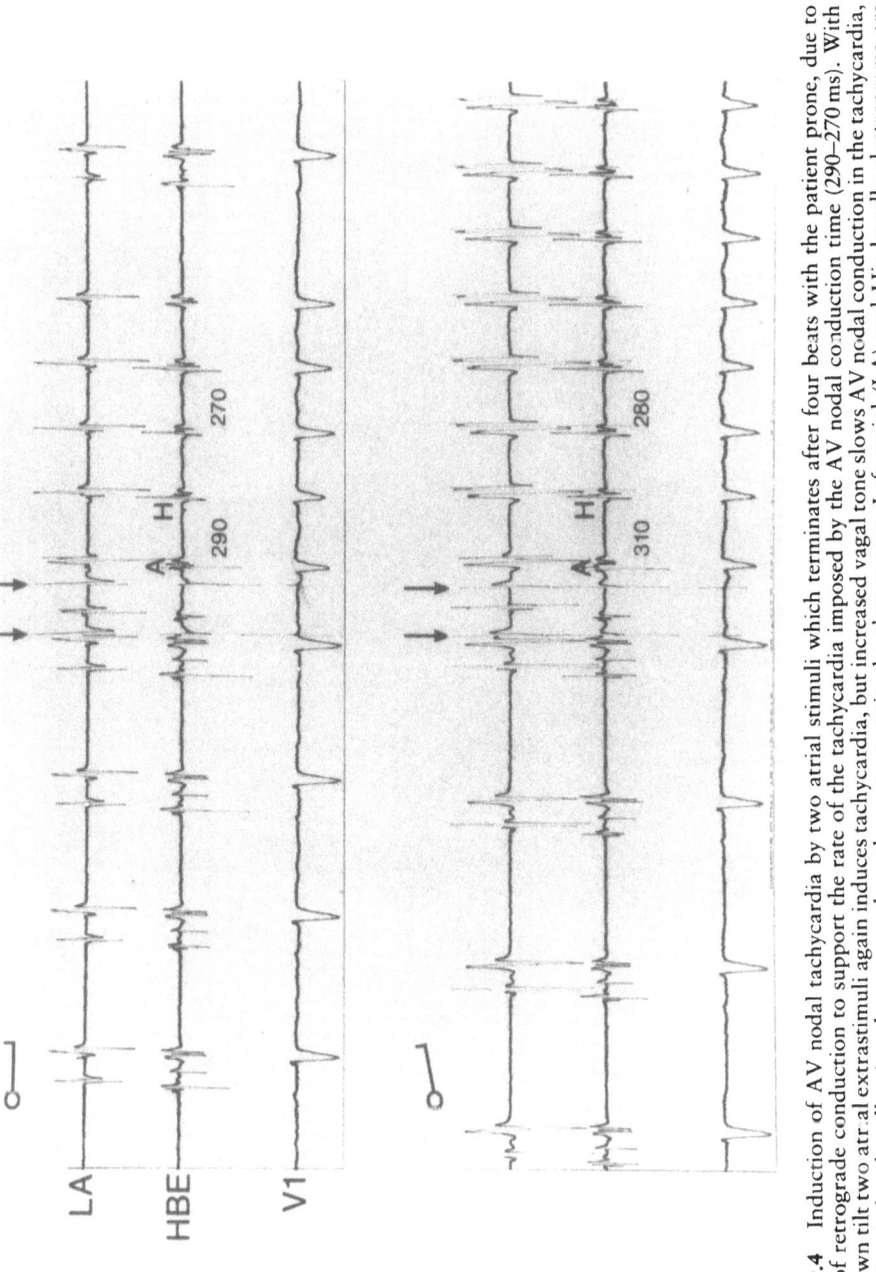

Figure 9.4 Induction of AV nodal tachycardia by two atrial stimuli which terminates after four beats with the patient prone, due to failure of retrograde conduction to support the rate of the tachycardia imposed by the AV nodal conduction time (290–270 ms). With head-down tilt two atrial extrastimuli again induces tachycardia, but increased vagal tone slows AV nodal conduction in the tachycardia, (310–280 ms) thereby allowing the retrograde pathway to sustain the slower rate. Left atrial (LA) and His bundle electrograms are shown together with lead V1

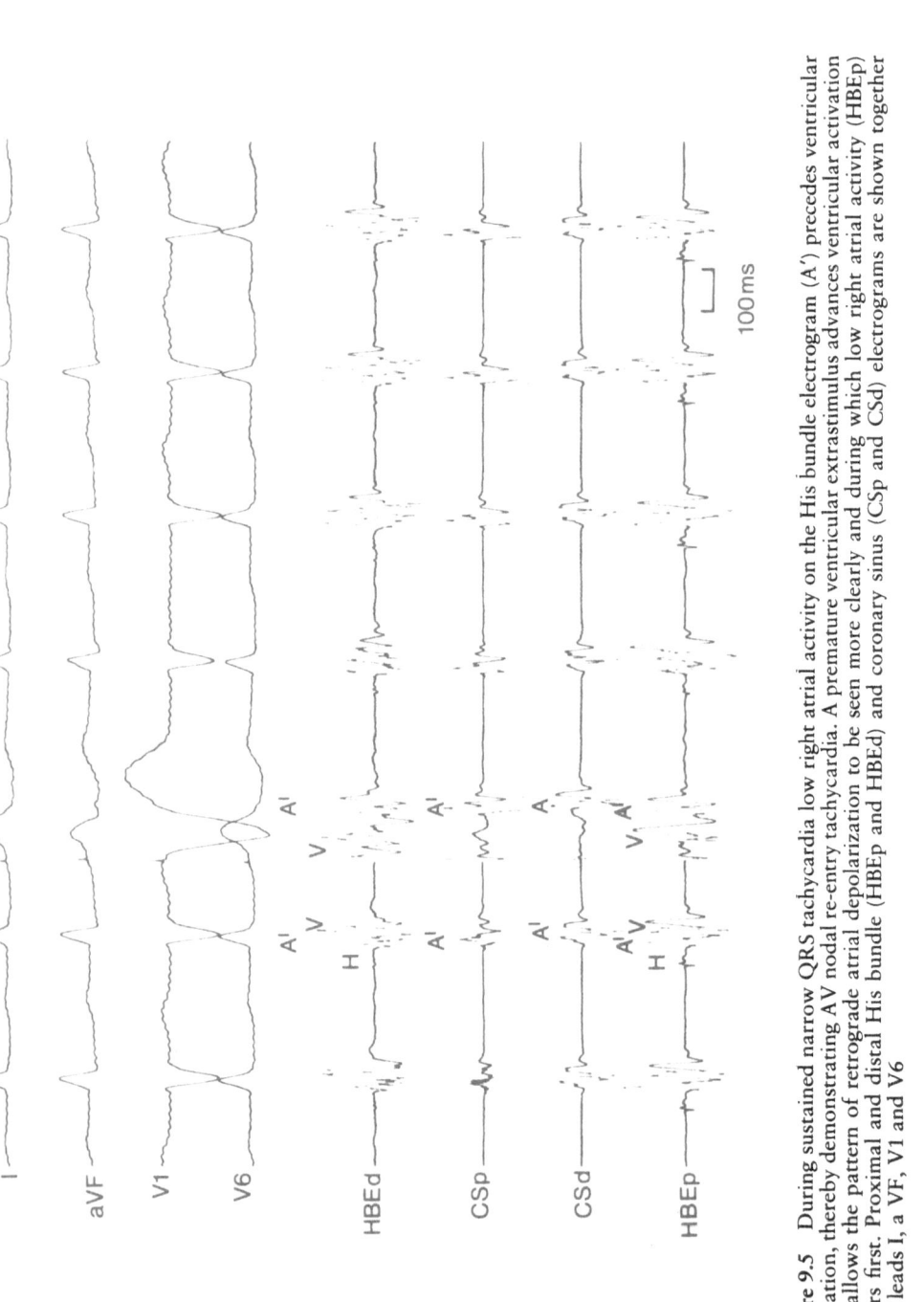

Figure 9.5 During sustained narrow QRS tachycardia low right atrial activity on the His bundle electrogram (A') precedes ventricular activation, thereby demonstrating AV nodal re-entry tachycardia. A premature ventricular extrastimulus advances ventricular activation and allows the pattern of retrograde atrial depolarization to be seen more clearly and during which low right atrial activity (HBEp) occurs first. Proximal and distal His bundle (HBEp and HBEd) and coronary sinus (CSp and CSd) electrograms are shown together with leads I, a VF, V1 and V6

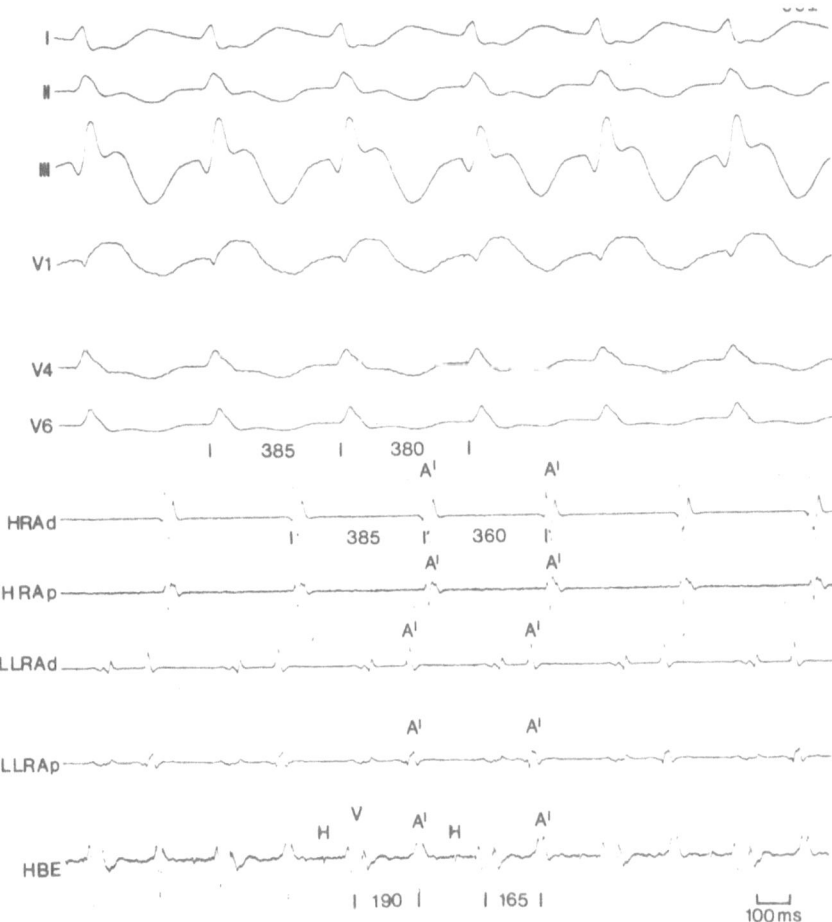

Figure 9.6 During re-entry tachycardia, in a patient with Ebstein's anomaly, associated with a right-sided accessory AV pathway, a late ventricular premature stimulus is delivered with a coupling interval of 380 ms, and causes a minimal degree of fusion (4th QRS complex). The cycle length of the tachycardia is 385 ms, and right bundle branch block is established – the retrograde VA interval measured on the His bundle electrogram (HBE) is 190 ms. The stimulus is delivered while the His bundle is refractory, but it results in paradoxically early atrial depolarization (360 ms) due to the shortened retrograde conduction time (165 ms). Distal and proximal high right atrial (HR A) and low lateral right atrial (LLRA) electrograms are shown with leads I, II, III, V1, V4 and V6

PSVT in the presence of ventricular pre-excitation in sinus rhythm

When the mechanism of tachycardia is suggested by the presence of pre-excitation on the resting electrocardiogram, electrophysiological diagnosis is usually directed towards confirming the participation of an accessory AV pathway in the mechanism of tachycardia and clarifying the anterograde functional properties of the accessory pathway. The investigator should bear in mind that multiple mechanisms of tachycardia may be present in patients with pre-excitation. Similar techniques as outlined in the previous section are used to localize and characterize the retrograde pathway during supraventricular tachycardia.

Atrial fibrillation is more prevalent in patients with the Wolff–Parkinson–White syndrome than in the general population, and more so in those with PSVT. The primary purpose of the study must, therefore, be to establish whether the patient would be at risk should atrial fibrillation occur spontaneously, unless this arrhythmia has been previously documented. The consequence of atrial fibrillation can be assessed by electrophysiological study (Figure 9.7). Measurement of the effective refractory period of the accessory pathway and highest rate of 1:1 conduction over the accessory pathway have been shown to correlate with the ventricular rate during atrial fibrillation. Induction of atrial fibrillation, however, remains the definitive test but it may not always be sustained. Assessment of anterograde behaviour requires stimulation at a site as close to the accessory pathway as possible to avoid possible errors due to intra-atrial block or functional properties before the stimulus reaches the accessory pathway (Figure 9.8).

Narrow QRS tachycardia with AV dissociation

In unusual cases a narrow QRS complex tachycardia may occur with AV dissociation, and the diagnosis is often impossible to make without recourse to intracardiac study. The tachycardia may be due to AV nodal re-entry without atrial involvement, or of His bundle origin either alone or in association with a nodoventricular or fasciculoventricular pathway. Ectopic tachycardia arising from the His bundle has become well recognized in infants and young children, particularly after corrective surgery for congenital heart defects, and especially when this involves the ventricular septum. The diagnosis may be difficult to make when there is 1:1 retrograde conduction, and electrophysiological study may be of value in ruling out other mechanisms of tachycardia. Despite the difficulty often encountered in treating His bundle tachycardia, it is an important diagnosis to make as it may be life-threatening. A similar mechanism of tachycardia may occur in adults, usually irregular and catecholamine-sensitive.

Wide QRS tachycardia

The ECG features that help to differentiate the possible diagnoses in the presence of a wide QRS tachycardia have received considerable attention, and it has been shown that invasive study should rarely be required in order to establish the diagnosis. However, the distinction between VT, SVT with aberration, SVT with anterograde conduction over an

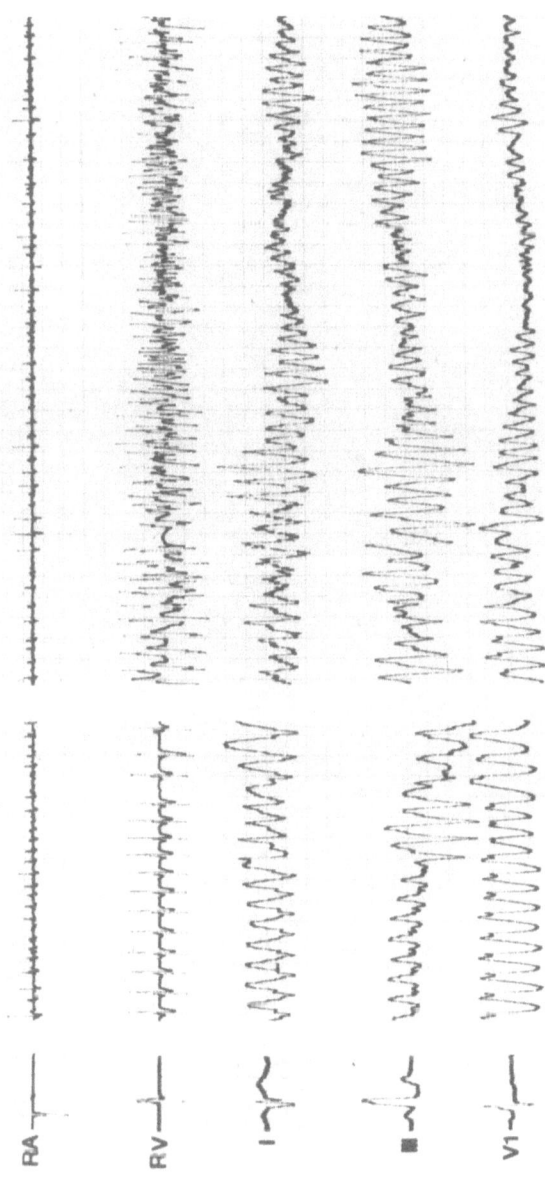

Figure 9.7 Induction of atrial fibrillation during electrophysiological study in a patient with the WPW syndrome is associated with an extremely rapid ventricular response and eventual degeneration into ventricular fibrillation. The left hand panel shows sinus rhythm, the middle panel shows the ventricular response soon after induction of AF, and the right hand panel shows the consequent ventricular fibrillation which ensued after approximately 2 minutes (paper speed 25 mm/s)

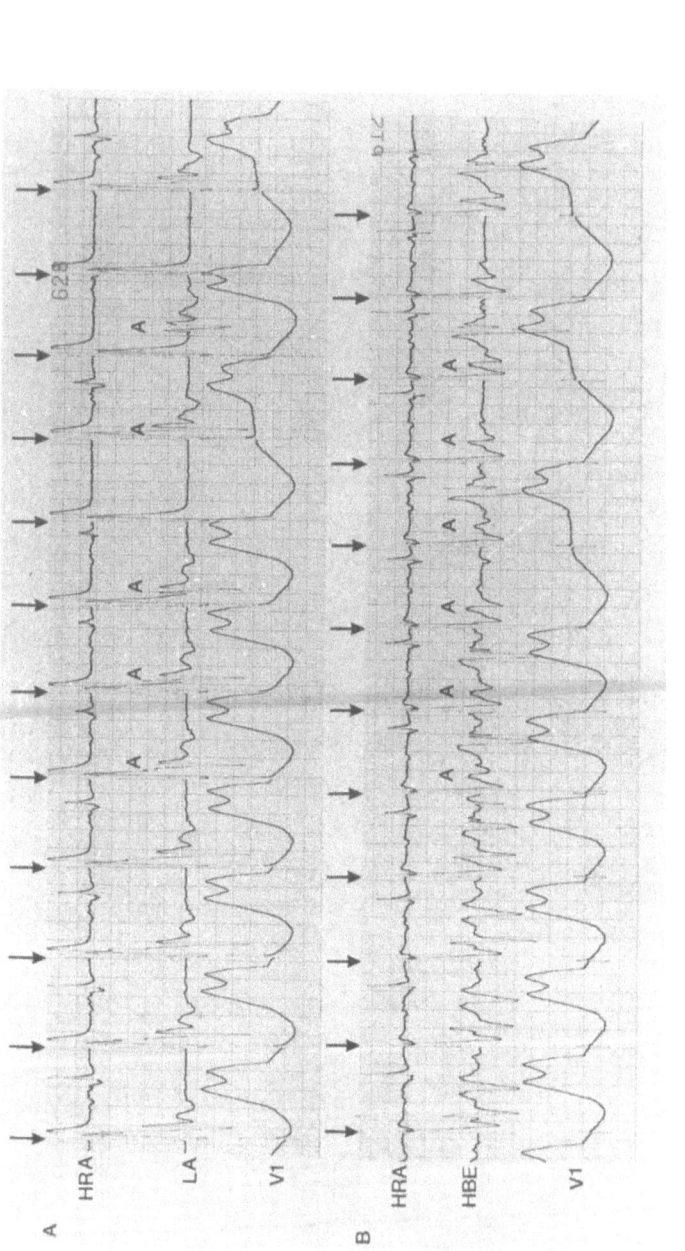

Figure 9.8 Incremental atrial pacing from right atrium (A) and coronary sinus (B) in a patient with the WPW syndrome. Right atrial pacing is associated with second degree intra-atrial block following the eighth stimulus with the result that AV conduction is interrupted. With coronary sinus pacing 1 : 1 intra-atrial conduction is maintained and there is true second degree AV block of the accessory pathway. High right atrial (HRA), left atrial (LA) and His bundle (HBE) electrograms are shown with lead V1 (paper speed 100 mm/s)

accessory AV pathway[21] or tachycardia in association with Mahaim conduction[22] may be impossible when there is 1 : 1 AV association. There are cases in which more than one mechanism coexists (Figure 9.9). The diagnosis of antedromic re-entry tachycardia rests upon the demonstration of an accessory AV pathway used anterogradely, and either AV nodal retrograde conduction or another accessory AV pathway used as the retrograde limb. The essential features of Mahaim conduction are decremental anterograde conduction in association with left bundle aberration and shortening HV interval. The Mahaim pathway may be incorporated in the circuit or may be a 'bystander' in the presence of AV nodal or AV re-entry tachycardia.

Ventricular tachycardia

Ventricular tachycardia may occur in a variety of forms that may have mechanistic, prognostic and therapeutic implications. VT can be sustained or non-sustained, monomorphic (uniform) or polymorphic (multiform). Non-sustained VT is generally defined as lasting more than three beats, but terminating spontaneously within 30 seconds. Sustained VT lasts 30 seconds or more or requires immediate termination by pacing or electrical cardioversion. Monoform VT has a consistent QRS morphology while that of multiform VT is constantly changing, the interval between the changes being usually no more than a few seconds.

The diagnosis of ventricular tachycardia can be made in most patients from ambulatory or 12 lead ECG recordings during a spontaneous attack. Rarely, there may be difficulty in differentiating SVT with aberration from VT. A more frequent indication for invasive study exists when ventricular tachycardia is suspected but spontaneous arrhythmia cannot be documented, and this situation is particularly encountered in patients with syncope of unknown cause. Intracardiac study has, therefore, been predominantly used to guide antiarrhythmic therapy, although it has also provided supportive evidence for some of the mechanisms of VT. Reproducible initiation of VT with single or double extrastimuli is in favour of re-entry and excludes an automatic mechanism, while rapid pacing is the most effective method for induction of triggered activity. Re-entry is also usually characterized by an inverse relationship between the coupling interval of the extrastimulus that initiates tachycardia and the interval from the extrastimulus and the first beat of tachycardia. Re-entry requires conduction delay, and this may be manifest as fractionated electrograms. However, demonstration that such delay is crucial to the mechanism of tachycardia is often difficult, as multiple areas of slow conduction may be present, some of them unrelated to the tachycardia.

The diagnostic role of electrophysiological study depends upon its ability to induce clinically relevant ventricular arrhythmia, predominantly provided by ventricular stimulation. Rarely atrial stimulation may induce a form of ventricular tachycardia characterized by a

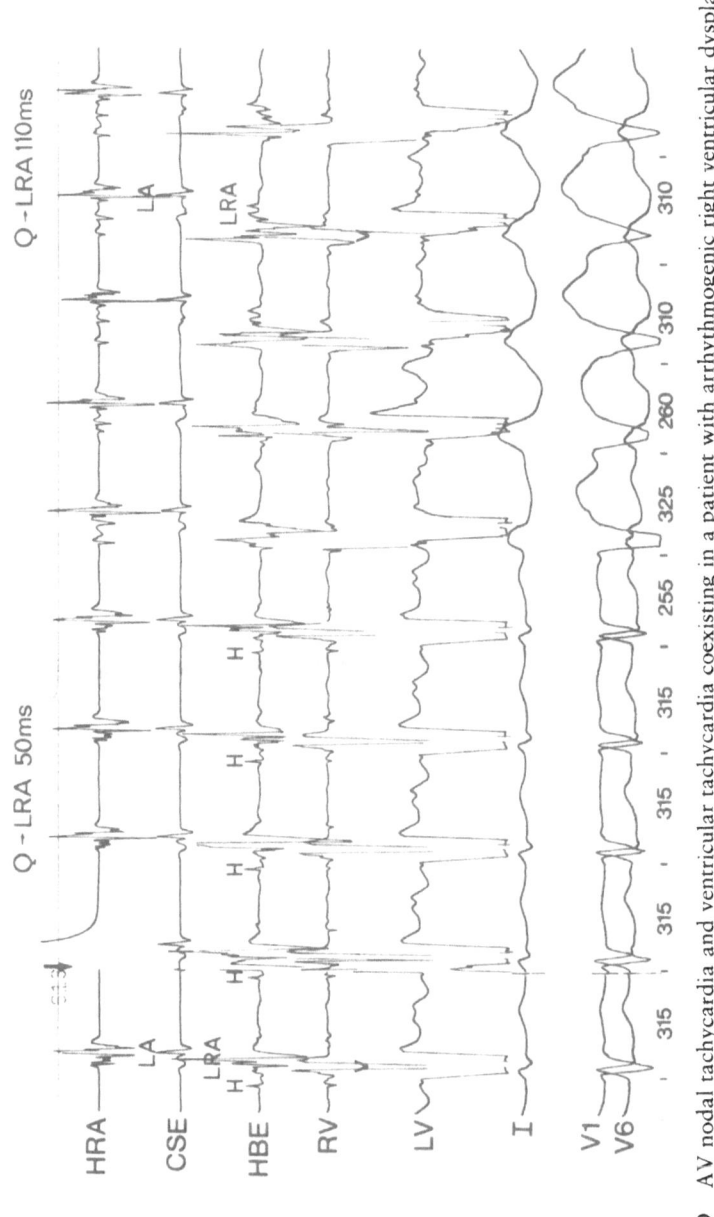

Figure 9.9 AV nodal tachycardia and ventricular tachycardia coexisting in a patient with arrhythmogenic right ventricular dysplasia. During sustained AV nodal tachycardia (cycle length 315 ms) a wide QRS tachycardia occurs spontaneously. High right atrial (HRA), coronary sinus (CSE), His bundle (HBE), right ventricular (RV) and left ventricular (LV) electrograms are shown together with leads I, V1 and V6. There was no evidence of Mahaim conduction

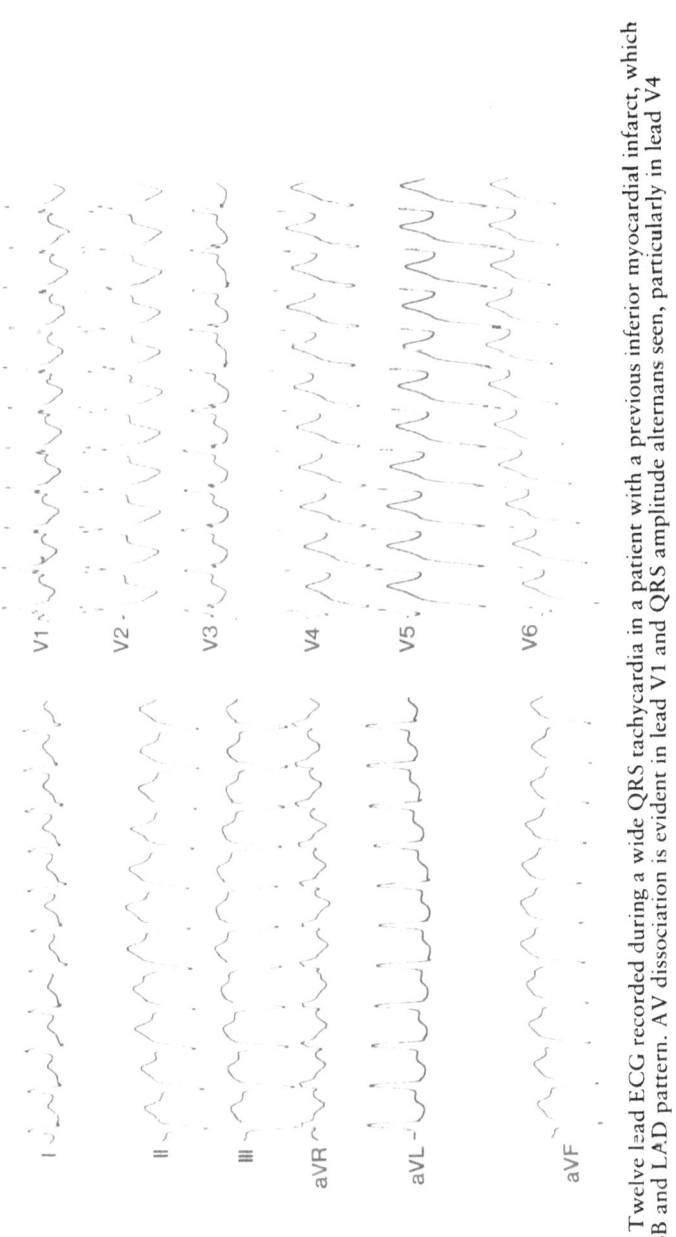

Figure 9.10 Twelve lead ECG recorded during a wide QRS tachycardia in a patient with a previous inferior myocardial infarct, which shows a RBBB and LAD pattern. AV dissociation is evident in lead V1 and QRS amplitude alternans seen, particularly in lead V4

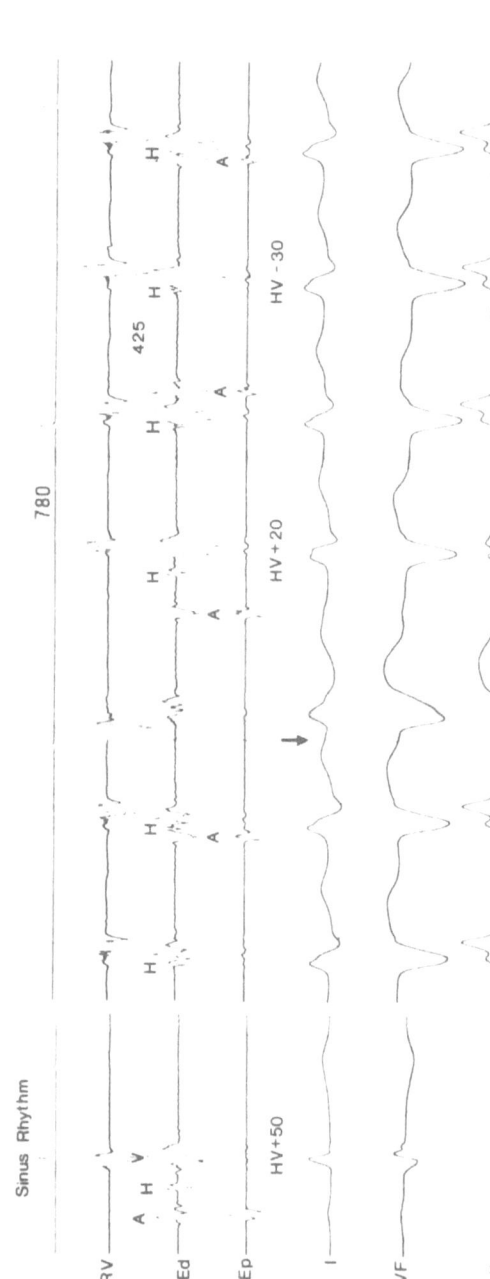

Figure 9.11 Intracardiac recordings from the same patient as in Figure 9.10. Normal intracardiac conduction intervals during sinus rhythm are shown in the left hand panel. During sustained tachycardia His bundle depolarization is evident preceding each septal ventricular deflection on the distal His bundle electrogram (HBEd), but with a negative HV interval (−30 ms). AV dissociation is evident during the tachycardia. Following a ventricular extrastimulus a fortuitous sinus discharge during the compensatory pause is conducted with fusion and with an intermediate HV interval. Distal and proximal His bundle electrograms (HBEd and HBEp) and right ventricular electrograms (RV) are shown with leads I, aVF and V1 (paper speed 100 mm/s)

QRS morphology which has a right bundle branch block and left axis deviation configuration. This so-called fascicular tachycardia may involve the left posterior fascicle, and may be the result of triggered automaticity (Figures 9.10 and 9.11).

A variety of ventricular stimulation protocols have been developed, but as yet there is no agreement on what constitutes the ideal protocol. This subject has been reviewed recently[23] and a few generalizations can be given. The sensitivity of the induction protocol is increased if more extrastimuli are used, if stimuli are delivered after a train of ventricular paced beats rather than in spontaneous rhythm and if more than one drive rate is used. Moreover, there is an increased yield if there is an abrupt change in rate during the drive, if several sites are stimulated and if stimulus intensity is increased. Using a protocol that includes three extrastimuli at two right ventricular sites and multiple drive cycle lengths VT will remain non-inducible in less that 5% of those with spontaneous VT. When more than two extrastimuli are used increased sensitivity is balanced by decreased specificity, as non-specific arrhythmias are induced which may be difficult to interpret when no spontaneous arrhythmia has been documented. Therefore, in those with syncope of unknown origin it seems appropriate to limit stimulation to two extrastimuli. It would also seem that using two stimuli at multiple sites before introducing a third extrastimulus reduces the incidence of non-specific responses.

Never the less, it can be stated that sustained monomorphic ventricular tachycardia is of clinical significance however it is induced. The induction of either non-sustained or polymorphic ventricular tachycardia or ventricular fibrillation must be interpreted in the light of the aggressiveness of the protocol used.

References

1. Josephson, M. E. and Seides, S. F. (1979). *Clinical Cardiac Electrophysiology. Techniques and Interpretations.* p. 28. Philadelphia: Lea and Febiger.
2. Sung, R. J., Tamer, D. M., Garcia, O. L. *et al.* (1976). Analysis of surgically induced right bundle branch block pattern using intracardiac recording techniques. *Circulation,* **54,** 422–6
3. Mandell, W., Hayakawa, H., Danzig, R. and Marcus, H. S. (1971). Evaluation of sinoatrial function in man by overdrive suppression. *Circulation,* **44,** 59–65
4. Benditt, D. G., Strauss, H. C., Scheinmann, M. M. *et al.* (1976). Analysis of secondary pauses following termination of rapid atrial pacing in man. *Circulation,* **54,** 436–40
5. Strauss, H. C., Saroff, A. L., Bigger, J. T. and Giardina, E. G. V. (1973). Premature atrial stimulation as a key to the understanding of sinoatrial conduction in man. *Circulation,* **58,** 86
6. Narula, O. S. *et al.* (1978). A new method for measurement of sinoatrial conduction time. *Circulation,* **58,** 706
7. Reiffel, J. A. *et al.* (1980). The human sinus node electrogram. A transvenous catheter technique and a comparison of directly measured and indirectly estimated sinoatrial conduction time in adults. *Circulation,* **62,** 1324

8. Heddle, W. F., Jones, M. E. and Tonkin, A. M. (1985). Sinus node sequences after atrial stimulation: similarities of effects of different methods. *Br. Heart J.*, **54**, 568–76

9. Strasberg, B., Amat-y-Leon, F., Dhingra, R. C. *et al.* (1981). Natural history of chronic second degree atrioventricular nodal block. *Circulation*, **63**, 1043–9

10. Shaw, D. B., Kekwick, C. A., Veale, D., Gowers, J. and Whistance, T. (1985). Survival in second degree atrioventricular block. *Br. Heart J.*, **53**, 587–93

11. Scheinman, M. M., Peters, R. W., Morady, F. *et al.* (1983). Electrophysiologic studies in patients with bundle branch block. *Pacing Clin. Electrophysiol.*, **6**, 1157

12. McAnulty, J. H., Rahimtoola, S. H., Murphy, E. *et al.* (1982). Natural history of 'high risk' bundle branch block: final report of a prospective study. *N. Engl. J. Med.*, **307**, 137

13. Dhingra, R. C., Palileo, E., Strasberg, B. *et al.* (1981). Significance of the HV interval in 517 patients with chronic bifascicular block. *Circulation*, **65**, 1265

14. Ezri, M., Lerman, B. B., Marchlinski, F. E. *et al.* (1983). Electrophysiologic evaluation of syncope in patients with bifascicular block. *Am. Heart J.*, **106**, 693–9

15. Wu, D., Denes, P., Amat-y-Leon, F. *et al.* (1978). Clinical, electrocardiographic and electrophysiologic observations in patients with paroxysmal supraventricular tachycardia. *Am. J. Cardiol.*, **41**, 1045

16. Wellens, H. J. J. (1978). Value and limitations of programmed electrical stimulation of the heart in the study and treatment of tachycardias. *Circulation*, **57**, 845

17. Akhtar, M., Damato, A. N., Ruskin, J. N. *et al.* (1978). Antegrade and retrograde conduction characteristics in three patterns of paroxysmal atrioventricular junctional reentrant tachycardia. *Am. Heart J.*, **95**, 22

18. Barold, S. and Coumel, P. Concealed preexcitation. *Am. J. Cardiol.*, **41**, 937

19. Coumel, P. and Attuel, P. (1974). Reciprocating tachycardia in overt and latent preexcitation: influence of bundle branch block on the rate of the tachycardia. *Eur. Heart J.*, **4**, 293

20. Brugada, P., Farre, J., Green, M. *et al.* (1984). Observations in patients with supraventricular tachycardia having a PR interval shorter than the RP interval. Differentiation between atrial tachycardia and a circus-movement tachycardia using an accessory pathway. *Am. Heart J.*, **107**, 556

21. Bardy, G. H., Packer, D. L., German, L. D. and Gallagher, J. J. (1981). Preexcited reciprocating tachycardia in patients with Wolff–Parkinson–White syndrome: Incidence and mechanisms. *Circulation*, **70**, 377

22. Gallagher, J. J. (1985). Variance of preexcitation: Update 1984. In Zipes, D. P. and Jalife, J. (eds.) *Cardiac Electrophysiology and Arrhythmias.* pp. 419–33. (New York: Grune and Stratton)

23. Mason, J. W., Anderson, K. P. and Freedman, R. A. (1987). Techniques and criteria in electrophysiologic study of ventricular tachycardia. *Circulation*, **75** (III), 125–30

10
Signal-averaged surface electrocardiography

R. VINCENT

INTRODUCTION

Signal averaging – a powerful technique for reducing unwanted noise[1] – has been used successfully since the early 1960s in neurology, cardiology and obstetrics. Practical applications in electrocardiography lie in two main areas: where the signals required are of conventional amplitude but noise is unusually obtrusive – the exercise electrocardiogram – and where the signals of interest are vanishingly small, being submerged by ordinary levels of background noise. Such micropotentials include activity derived from the sinus or atrioventricular nodes, from the His–Purkinje system, or from damaged areas of ventricular myocardium ('ventricular late potentials'). The signals in each case are at microvolt level $(0.2–10\,\mu V)$ rendering them invisible in standard electrocardiographic recordings. Amplification sufficient to allow their registration leads inevitably to overwhelming noise – and to the need for effective noise reduction. Signal averaging has become widely adopted for this purpose.

The technique of signal averaging and the signal-processing methods with which it is usually associated are outlined in the next section. A description follows of its applications to the recovery of His–Purkinje and ventricular late potentials, and the chapter concludes with a brief review of newer techniques that enhance signal averaging and begin to address some of its limitations.

METHODOLOGY

Signal averaging

The principle of signal averaging is illustrated in Figure 10.1. Successive cycles of a repeating waveform (in this case a filtered and noisy electrocardiographic trace) are added into an accumulator. For this addition, the cycles are aligned on the time axis by reference to a fixed point in

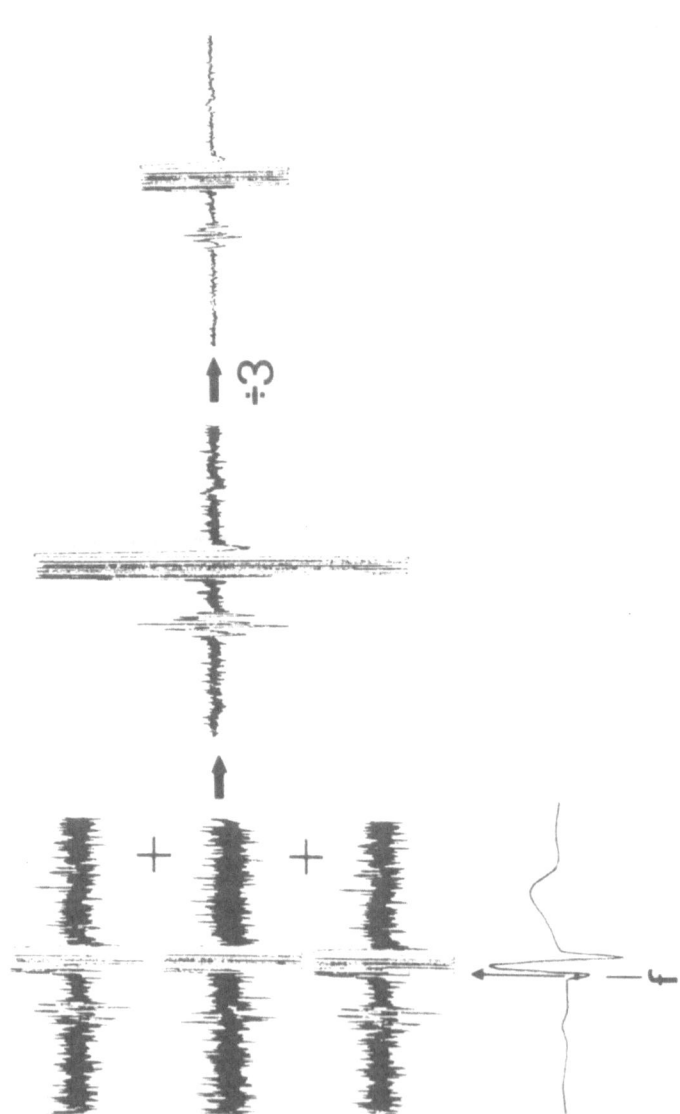

Figure 10.1 The technique of signal averaging. f indicates the position of the fiducial or trigger point

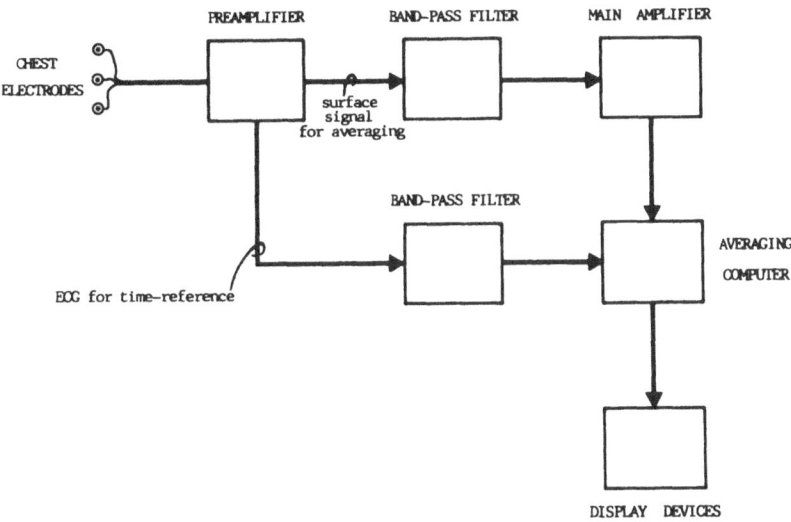

Figure 10.2 Block diagram of the major components of a signal averaging system for electrocardiography

each waveform known as the 'reference', 'fiducial', or 'trigger' point. The dependence of this method on events in time leads to the descriptive title for the technique, *'temporal* signal averaging'. The process by which the reference point is determined and influences the alignment of data in the accumulator is often referred to as 'triggering', a term adopted from early hardware devices operating in a similar manner to an oscilloscope. As the data are accumulated, random variations due to noise undergo cancellation while information synchronized to the reference point is reinforced. Division of the accumulator by the number of cycles stored results in a final signal correctly scaled, and with considerably reduced noise.

Identifying the fiducial point is a major challenge in the methodology of signal averaging. As the data themselves are too noisy for reliable triggering, a separate 'reference' waveform is derived specifically for the purpose. The reference waveform may originate from the same electrodes as the data (see Figure 10.2), or independently – but must hold a rigid temporal relationship to the signals of interest. Misalignment of the data of averaging is known as 'trigger jitter' and for cardiac micropotentials should not exceed 2 ms. (The tolerance for ST segment analysis in exercise testing is greater, perhaps 5–10 times this value.) Persistent, extended trigger jitter causes blurring and attenuation of the signals of interest; capricious malalignment due to an unexpectedly large noise spike or an aberrant QRS complex may introduce marked distortion to the averaged trace.

Defining the fiducial or trigger point has been achieved by several methods, the simplest using threshold voltage detection to identify a point on the QRS deflection of a low-gain trace. At a contrasting level of complexity are systems that are based on digital pattern-matching, or that use frequency analysis of a composite signal from multiple electrocardiographic leads. All systems incorporate some form of threshold detection or discrimination process to indicate that a correct reference point has been found. In more complex systems this process can be adjusted either by the user, or automatically by software control to reduce trigger error by rejecting especially noisy or aberrant complexes[2].

The improvement in signal-to-noise ratio achieved by averaging bears the following relationship to the number of cycles summed:

$$S/N = \sqrt{C}$$

where S and N are the signal and noise amplitude respectively and C the number of cycles included in the average.

This geometric relationship indicates that high orders of improvement in signal-to-noise relationship are increasingly 'expensive' in the number of cardiac cycles required; recording and processing time become extended and the risk of spontaneous fluctuations in morphology of the data or reference signal is increased. Most workers find little value in averaging more than 300–500 cycles, and it is preferable that noise reduction at source or by other processing techniques limits the requirement of averaging to a figure much lower than this.

Averaging for signal recovery is successful only for deflections that have a constantly repeating form; but the electrical events of the cardiac cycle fulfil this criterion and are thus well-suited to this technique. The noise from which such signals are to be recovered should, ideally, be Gaussian – that is, the instantaneous amplitude of the noise should show a Gaussian distribution. However, that this ideal is rarely achieved in practical systems seems to be no major drawback.

Associated signal processing techniques

Analog-to-digital conversion

Since signal averaging has been achieved almost entirely by digital processing, conversion of the signal from the analog to digital form is a usual pre-requisite for this technique. The conversion or *sampling rate* (digital samples per second) should, according to the Nyquist rule, be at least twice the highest frequency required in the final recording. But greater fidelity is likely to be achieved for biological signals by a sampling frequency close to five times this limit. For cardiac micropotentials a sampling frequency of 2 kHz per channel seems to offer a practical compromise between final signal fidelity and the speed/storage requirements of the processing system.

Filtering

Filtering before digitization ('analog' filtering) may be helpful as a first technique for noise reduction, and to limit any baseline drift presented to the analog-to-digital converter. But analog filters may cause unwanted effects, particularly prolongation of the signals preceding the electrocardiographic segment of interest.

In early experiments to recover cardiac micropotentials analog filters which allowed passage of only those frequencies judged to be present in the signal of interest were applied before digitization. Typical values for the chosen passband were 40–300 Hz. The relatively high value of the high-pass filter (40 Hz) ensured complete freedom from baseline drift, and a dramatic levelling of any gradual slope of the electrocardiogram (the PR, ST and TP segments) on which cardiac micropotentials were impressed. It also reduced the dynamic range (the amplitude difference between the smallest and largest signals) of the highly amplified ECG, reducing saturation or 'clipping'.

In more recent systems the trend has been to emphasize digital rather than analog processing. Digitization has been introduced at lower levels of analog gain, and analog filters used with a much broader pass-band (0.5–1000 Hz, for example.) Subsequent amplification has been achieved by software multiplication of the digitized signal, and further filtering applied using numerical techniques.

Digital filtering under software control affords considerable flexibility: it can be applied before or after averaging, or both. Complex filters can be designed to limit signal distortion in the areas of interest and their effect characterized with accuracy. Signal prolongation still occurs, but its duration can be specified exactly, allowing appropriate correction when interpreting results. Finally, different filters can be applied in sequence to a fixed set of (stored) data to optimize signal recovery in any one recording.

Other techniques

Digital processing allows ready application of additional signal manipulation including scaling (linear or non-linear), display formating, alphanumeric annotation, interactive control and data storage. Most of these techniques have been encompassed by the complete experimental or commercial signal averaging systems applied in cardiology in the last 23 years.

APPLICATIONS

His bundle electrocardiography

The possibility of recording conducting system activity at the body surface was first raised in 1973 by two independent groups working with animals[3,4]. Attempts to record surface conducting system activity in man were also reported in this year by Lazzara in the US[5] and by Stopczyk in Poland.[6] In all cases a sequence of analog high-gain amplification, filtering and digital signal averaging was used to record surface electrical activity during the PR segment that was attributed to His–Purkinje depolarization. In Berbari's work[3], the trigger for the averaging process was derived from the stimulus of atrial overdrive pacing; this provided an easily-identified event in the cardiac cycle and protected the AH interval from variations due to vagal tone; but it rendered the recording invasive, at least as far as the right atrium. Flowers and her colleagues[4] proposed that signal averaging using a QRS *trigger* was appropriate since in most cases the His–Purkinje deflection precedes ventricular activation by a constant interval. The system developed by her group using a stored reference waveform was entirely non-invasive, and paved the way for systems with clinical potential.

Early experiments in man to recover surface His–Purkinje activity showed repeatable deflections in the PR segment in 30–100% of cases, though the form and duration of the signals was variable. Verification of the source of surface PR segment activity relied on showing its close temporal association with the His bundle depolarization recorded by internal electrodes, an association that was stable in spite of varying rates of atrial overdrive pacing and of the use of drugs to alter selectively the components of atrioventricular conduction.

In these early recordings – as well as in many later studies[7,8] – external 'His' deflections often lasted well beyond the familiar internal His 'spike' (Figure 10.3). This result may seem untidy – but is consistent with the concept of continuous propagation of electrical activity from the AV node to the ventricular myocardium; moreover, a surface electrode – remote from the His–Purkinje system – may be expected to sense potentials of the distal conducting system that are out of range for intracavity electrodes.

Enthusiastic research followed the early work of Berbari, Flowers and Stopczyk. Since 1975 more than 85 reports have appeared recounting attempts to recover body surface deflections arising from the His–Purkinje system. Detailed methodology has varied, but has always been based on the general outline shown in Figure 10.2. No standard recording technique has emerged and differences in detail – including electrode position – have clearly influenced the recovery rate and clarity of the records obtained. Though no universal optimum electrode configuration has been demonstrated, it would seem that successful non-invasive 'His' recordings are often associated with a configuration in which at least one electrode is placed on the left anterior chest at about the fourth interspace and within a short distance from the left sternal edge. The surface activity due to His bundle depolarization appears to have a major vector which is 'leftward, anterior and inferior'[9]. Improved recovery results from the use of multiple electrode sites for any one recording[8].

Filtering – particularly the cutoff frequency of the high-pass filter –

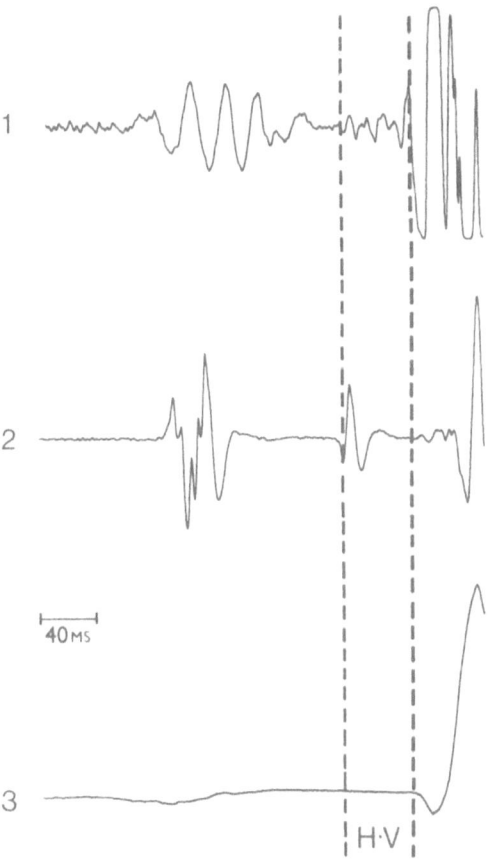

Figure 10.3 Recovery by signal averaging of activity attributed to the His–Purkinje system. Trace 1 shows a signal-averaged, high-gain recording from the chest surface of a patient undergoing conventional His-bundle electrocardiography. Multiple deflections are recorded between the time of onset of the internally-recorded His spike (trace 2) and the onset of the QRS complex. A low-gain reference waveform is shown in trace 3

profoundly influences the shape both of the atrial deflection and of the PR segment activity in the averaged waveform. Increasing the value of the high-pass filter may occasionally clarify the signals of interest, but more often they may be lost through increased attenuation at the higher setting. Low frequency components of PR segment activity that hold promise for diagnostic information unobtainable with intracardiac studies are especially vulnerable to removal by high-pass filtering.

Signal averaging has been applied to the recovery of conducting system activity by 18 research groups worldwide in studies in over 500 patients. The following are the main conclusions:

(1) Surface PR segment signals are usually of the order 0.5–2 μV in amplitude, and can be recovered non-invasively in more than half the subjects studied.

(2) No clear correlation has emerged between the pattern of deflections obtained and either any specific electrode configuration or any pathological change in the conducting system. Such a correlation may be found later with increasing clinical experience.

(3) The setting of the high-pass filter in the signal chain has an important effect on the configuration of the deflections obtained and the degree to which atrial activity encroaches into the PR segment.

(4) Atrial activity, even without the effect of high-pass filtering, may impinge on the region of His bundle activity limiting the value of the recording.

(5) Triggering for the averaging process is critical and invites careful – and flexible – system design.

(6) Late PR segment signals can often be recorded and may differ in surface vector from the 'His' deflection itself. Though these could be attributed to depolarization of the distal conducting system, this plausible and attractive idea still requires verification.

(7) The recording of multiple surface deflections in the PR segment argues for the possibility of sensing more of the continuous activation of the His–Purkinje system than is obtainable from intracavity electrodes.

(8) Failure to record clear signals has been attributed to excessive patient noise, to triggering instability or to inappropriate lead placement. Clear PR segment signals are more usually the reward of increased experience and more flexible systems for signal recording. But this is not found universally, and the reason for success or failure in individual cases is not always clear.

In spite of its early attraction, signal averaging for the recovery of surface conducting system activity has not fulfilled its promise as a useful clinical tool. It remains a research technique in which at present interest seems to be fading. The following may be blamed:

(1) Residual noise or poor signal quality in tracings obtained in spite of apparently 'optimum' recording techniques.

(2) Uncertainty over the interpretation of the surface recording particularly where residual noise or preceding atrial activity obscures the onset of the 'His' deflections.

(3) Lack of beat-to-beat information in the averaged trace.

(4) Scepticism of the value of the HV interval as a guide for prognosis.

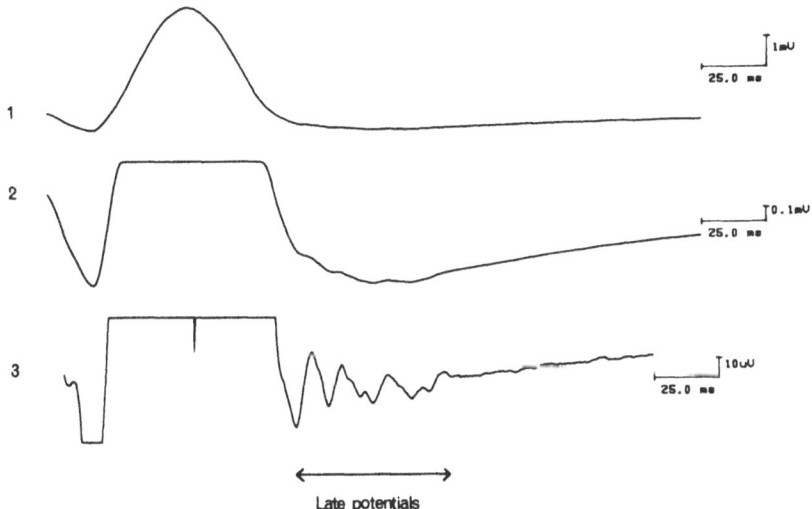

Figure 10.4 Ventricular late potentials recorded using the signal averaging technique. Traces 1, 2, and 3 show a signal averaged QRS complex and ST segment recorded from the chest surface at increasing gain. The high-gain trace (trace 3) shows abnormal activity immediately following the QRS complex

But non-invasive measurement of the HV interval, especially if this can be repeated conveniently and safely, may yet prove to be a worthwhile pursuit and further developments in recording technique are warranted.

Ventricular late potentials

Background and methodology

Fragmented electrical activity immediately following ventricular depolarization has been recorded from endocardial and epicardial sites in patients prone to sustained ventricular tachyarrhythmias[10-12]. This activity is thought by many to be closely associated with the underlying mechanisms of ventricular tachycardia – particularly local re-entry[13], though others regard late potentials as a 'bystander' phenomenon having no direct part in arrhythmogenesis[14].

Since 1978 ventricular late potentials have been recovered from the body surface by the application of signal averaging, first by Berbari and colleagues in dogs[15] and in parallel by Fontaine and co-workers in man[16]. It is of advantage in applying this technique that the QRS complex provides a readily identifiable trigger, and that the amplitude of surface late ventricular potentials is generally larger than that of signals from the His–Purkinje system (Figure 10.4).

Although no standard methodology exists, success has again followed the general pattern of signal averaging applied to highly amplified and bandpass filtered signals from a variety of electrodes on the chest surface. Settings of the high pass filter have ranged from 25 to 200 Hz with lowpass filtering in the range 300–1000 Hz. Artefact due to filter 'ringing' is again an important concern, especially as microvolt late potentials follow closely on the major deflection of the QRS. To minimize such artefact, unidirectional highpass digital filters have been designed with a rate of attenuation that is shallow or adjustable. In an alternative method named after its designer, Dr Simson[17], highpass filtering is applied in normal time order only to events early in the cardiac cycle. The remainder of the cycle, from a point 40 ms into the QRS complex, is passed through the filter in time-reversed order. Filter ringing is thereby reduced, though contrary to the impression often given in the literature, this method does not eliminate filter artefact entirely.

The definition and identification of late potential activity remains a central problem; universally accepted criteria do not exist, and many traces have been evaluated for the presence of late potentials by simple visual inspection alone. Some accept the validity of late potentials only if they appear beyond the end of a reference QRS complex at conventional gain[18]. Others – on the basis of intra-operative mapping – believe that such abnormal ventricular activity can begin within the span of the QRS complex causing overall prolongation of ventricular depolarization[13]. In this approach, total QRS duration is measured and the terminal portion of the filtered ventricular deflection examined for either its absolute amplitude, or its amplitude compared to residual noise or to the preceding ventricular activity. The groups of Simson[17], Denes[19], and Breithardt[20] have each proposed rigorous and objective definitions of late potential activity based on time/amplitude characteristics; the methodology in two[19,20] provides for automatic identification of late potentials. Unfortunately the results of the various methods proposed for identifying late potential activity correlate poorly. In a multicentre study[21] comparing four recording/interpretation methods in the same population of 109 patients, corresponding negative results were found in 68.8%, but corresponding positive results were obtained in only 5.5%.

Clinical correlations

Late potentials are rarely recorded in healthy subjects, but their incidence in patients with previously documented ventricular tachycardia or fibrillation exceeds 70%. In this group, late potentials occur most commonly in those known to have coronary artery disease. The number of false negative recordings in this group is unknown, though it should be noted that surface late potentials are recovered in less than 100% of patients with documented fractionated potentials on epicardial mapping.

The association between late ventricular potentials and recurrent ventricular tachycardia is stronger at pathological rates of less than

270/minute than in cases of ventricular fibrillation or more rapid ventricular tachycardia. The difference between these groups is also seen in the *duration* of late potentials being longer (up to 180 ms) in patients with recurrent spontaneous or inducible ventricular tachycardia and shorter in patients with previous VF. Moreover, the duration of late potentials tends to be associated with increasing ease of inducing ventricular tachycardia by provocative electrophysiological testing.

Late potentials may be recorded in patients with suspected coronary disease in the absence of previous ventricular tachyarrhythmia though with relatively low incidence (about 33%), and at low amplitude. Left ventricular contraction abnormalities, either regional or diffuse, also strongly predispose to ventricular late potentials irrespective of the distribution and extent of any underlying coronary occlusion.

Few studies have been performed in patients with acute myocardial infarction and results differ widely[18,22–27]. Their incidence ranges from 16–50% with no clear relation to infarct site or size[25]. They appear to be more strongly associated with late ventricular tachycardia and sudden death than with early ventricular fibrillation. Since late potentials may be a transient phenomenon after myocardial infarction the time of recording(s) may be critical to their recovery, and therefore to an accurate appreciation of their true incidence.

In summary, the following conditions are associated with the appearance of late potentials recovered by signal averaging:

(1) Previously documented sustained spontaneous ventricular tachycardia or fibrillation especially if the rate of the arrhythmia is less than 270/minute or if it occurs in the context of:
coronary artery disease,
previous myocardial infarction,
congestive cardiomyopathy;

(2) Readily inducible sustained ventricular tachycardia during electrophysiological testing;

(3) Contraction abnormalities of the left ventricular wall including left ventricular aneurysm;

(4) Either stable coronary artery disease or recent myocardial infarction without documented ventricular arrhythmias.

Poor correlation is found, however, between ventricular late potentials, and either the complexity of arrhythmias captured on 24 h ambulatory monitoring, the use of anti-arrhythmic drugs, or thrombolytic therapy following acute myocardial infarction even if this is associated with reperfusion arrhythmias[25].

Predictive value

In spite of the above associations, ventricular late potentials, especially in asymptomatic patients, do not prove to be a strong prognostic marker for subsequent cardiac events. Several groups have examined their predictive value in patients with ischaemic heart disease. In a study by Breithardt and colleagues[13] 511 patients admitted with either recent acute myocardial infarction or for routine angiography underwent inpatient recordings for late potential activity. Total mortality following subsequent hospital discharge was 2–3 times greater in patients with late potentials lasting 40 ms than in those with shorter or no late ventricular activity. Sudden death (within 24 h) occurred in more than four times as many patients in this same 'high risk' group. Prediction for subsequent out-of-hospital ventricular tachycardia showed a high specificity – about 63% – but the false positive rate in a minimum follow up period of 6 months was 94%. In the study population overall the predictive value of late potentials for the development of ventricular tachycardia was 5.7%. Von Leitner[26] in a study of 518 survivors of acute myocardial infaction found that late potentials had a similarly low predictive value (7.4%) for subsequent mortality.

The most encouraging prospective study so far reported is that of Denniss and colleagues[27] who recorded late potentials in 306 patients without bundle branch block during the hospital phase of acute myocardial infarction. For patients with late potentials the probability of remaining free from death or non-fatal ventricular tachycardia or fibrillation was 0.79 at 1 year, significantly lower than the corresponding figure of 0.97 for patients without late potential activity recorded early after infarction. But even in this population, late potentials showed a predictive accuracy of only 24% (sensitivity 66%, specificity 78%) for subsequent cardiac events including ventricular tachycardia/fibrillation and cardiac death.

Conclusions

It is clear that late ventricular potentials are related in some way to the mechanisms that predispose to malignant ventricular arrhythmias especially recurrent ventricular tachycardia. The recovery of late potentials may define a subset of patients warranting closer follow-up or more intensive study[28], but an improved, standardized methodology together with further prospective clinical studies is essential before the recording of this activity finds a well-defined place in routine clinical practice.

BEYOND SIGNAL AVERAGING

Temporal signal averaging is effective only when deflections of interest show a regularly repeating form, and when a time marker can be derived to which they can be synchronized accurately. It fails to provide beat-to-beat information, and functions poorly in the presence of sporadic high level noise or where the form of the signal is variable over short periods. Other techniques that may enhance or replace the averaging technique are, therefore, under scrutiny.

Limiting noise at source

The combination of ultra-low noise electronic circuits, specialized lead orientation, and the use of the Faraday cage has allowed recovery of cardiac micropotentials on a beat-to-beat basis without signal averaging. But the method is too cumbersome for routine clinical use and is only applicable to a portion of experimental subjects. A forthcoming commercial instrument is alleged to overcome these limitations[29], but awaits independent clinical assessment.

Spatial averaging

In this technique a summation is made of signals recorded separately, but simultaneously, from several sets of electrodes (usually paired). The method assumes that the form of the signal of interest presented to each electrode pair will be similar, while background noise adopts a random spatial characteritic. Spatial averaging could allow signal recovery on a beat-to-beat basis or with a small number of subsequent temporal averages, especially if environmental noise is low. But the surface distribution of cardiac micropotentials is poorly understood, varies from patient to patient, and may not in practice allow identical signal morphology at each electrode pair. This approach has so far met with limited success but warrants further study.

Advanced filtering techniques

Filtering holds the key to successful signal recovery. The rejection of frequencies contributing to noise in favour of those from which the signals of interest are formed is the objective of processing throughout the work so far described. A clear understanding of the detailed differences in frequency characteristic between signal and noise should lead to a better recovery of the deflections of interest. Filters to achieve this may be designed on the basis of generally-expected signal/noise characteristics, or in a form in which their function changes specifically according to the on-line analysis of noise present in a 'quiet' area of the electrocardiogram – usually the T-P segment. Filters influenced by the sensed characteristics of the composite data (signal-plus-noise) are known as *adaptive*, and complex filters of this type may vary their behaviour in response to signal and noise characteristics during the course of each individual cardiac cycle. Early experiments with these techniques[30] have proved rewarding, approaching the goal of beat-to-beat signal recovery, but an optimum methodology has yet to be established.

SUMMARY AND CONCLUSIONS

Signal averaging is a powerful technique for noise reduction and is well suited to electrocardiographic signals. Its use in exercise testing is well established, but care in the interpretation of averaged records remains mandatory especially in regard to distortion from isolated noise spikes of capricious mis-triggering. The isolation of cardiac micropotentials by averaging has proved fruitful in research, recovering conduction system activity in the majority of patients studied and late ventricular potentials primarily in those prone to recurrent ventricular tachycardia. But signal averaging has not fulfilled the hope of 12 years ago that it would lead to a routine clinical application for non-invasive electrophysiological assessment. Remaining difficulties in both recording and interpretation limit widespread interest in this application, but advanced digital processing and further clinical experience may yet lead to the development of useful clinical tools based on averaging or allied techniques.

References

1. Rhyme, V. T. (1969). Comparison of coherent averaging techniques for repetitive biological signals. *Med. Res. Eng.* **8**, 22–6
2. Denniss, A. R., Richards, D. A., Farrow, R. H., Davison, A., Ross, D. L. and Uther, J. B. (1985). Technique for maximising the frequency response of the signal averaged Frank vectorcardiogram. *J. Biomed. Eng.*, **8**, 207–12
3. Berbari, E. J., Lazzara, R., Samet, P. and Scherlag, B. J. (1973). Noninvasive technique for detection of electrical activity during the P–R segment. *Circulation*, **48**, 1005–13
4. Flowers, N. C., Hand, R. C., Orander, P. C., Miller, K. B., Walden, M. D. and Horan, L. G. (1974). Surface recording of electrical activity from the region of the bundle of His. *Am. J. Cardiol.*, **33**, 384–9
5. Lazzara, R., Campbell, R., Berbari, E. J., Scherlag, B. J. and Myerburg, R. J. (1973). Electrocardiogram of the His–Purkinje system in man. (Abstract). *Circulation*, **48**, Supplement IV: IV–22
6. Stopczyk, M. J., Kopec, J., Zochowski, R. J. and Pieniack, N. (1973). Surface recording of electrical heart activity during the P–R segment in man by a computer averaging technique. (Abstract). *Int. Res. Commun. Syst.* **11**, 21–2
7. Berbari, E. J., Scherlag, B. J. and Lazzara, R. (1977). A computerised technique to record new components of the electrocardioram. *Proc. IEEE*, **65**, 799–802
8. Wajszczuk, W. J., Stopczyk, M. J., Moskowitz, M. S., Zochowski, R. J., Bauld, T., Dabos, P. and Rubenfire, M. (1978). Noninvasive recording of His–Purkinje activity in man by QRS triggered signal averaging. *Circulation*, **58**, 95–102
9. Berbari, E. J., Lazzara, R., El-Sherif, N. and Scherlag, B. J. (1974). Extracardiac recordings from the His–Purkinje system during normal and abnormal conduction. (Abstract). *Circulation*, **49–50**, Supplement III: III–14
10. Ostermeyer, J., Breithardt, G., Kolvenbach, R., Korfer, R., Seipel, L., Schulte, H. D. and Bircks, W. (1979). Intraoperative electrophysiological mapping during cardiac surgery. *Thorac. Cardiovasc. Surg.*, **27**, 260–70
11. Josephson, M. E., Horowitz, L. N., Spielman, S. R., Greenspan, A. M., van de Pol, C. and Harken, A. H. (1980). Comparison of endocardial catheter mapping with intraoperative mapping of tachycardia. *Circulation*, **61**, 395–404
12. Klein, H., Karp, R. B., Kouchoukos, N. T., James, T. N. and Waldo, A. L. (1979). Ventricular mapping of abnormal myocardium in patients with and without arrhythmias. (Abstract) *Circulation*, **60**, Supplement II: II–24

13. Breithardt, G. and Borggrefe, M. (1986). Pathophysiological mechanisms and clinical significance of ventricular late potentials. *Eur. Heart J.*, 7, 364–85
14. Brugada, P., Abdollah, H. and Wellens, H. J. J. (1985). Continuous electrical activity during sustained monomorphic ventricular tachycardia. Observations on its dynamic behaviour during the arrhythmia. *Am. J. Cardiol.*, 55, 401–11
15. Berbari, E. J., Scherlag, B. J., Hope, R. R. and Lazzara, R. (1978). Recording from the body surface of arrhythmogenic ventricular activity during the S–T segment. *Am. J. Cardiol.*, 41, 697–702
16. Fontaine, G., Frank, R., Gallais-Hamonno, F., Allali, I., Phan-Thuc, H. and Grosgogeat, Y. (1978). Electrocardiographie des potentiels tardifs du syndrome postexcitation. *Arch. Mal. Coeur.*, 71, 854–64
17. Simson, M. B. (1981). Use of signals in the terminal QRS complex to identify patients with ventricular tachycardia after myocardial infarction. *Circulation*, 64, 235–42
18. Ostersprey, A., Hogg, II. W., Hombach, V., Deutsch, H. J., Winter, U., Behrenbeck, D. W., Tauchert, M. and Hilger, H. H. (1983). Diagnostic and prognostic significance of ventricular late potentials in patients with coronary heart disease. In Steinbach, K. (ed.) *Cardiac Pacing – Proceedings of the VIIth World Symposium on Cardiac Pacing*. pp. 663–70. (Vienna: Steinkopf Verlag Dormstadt)
19. Denes, P., Santarelli, P., Hauser, R. G. and Uretz, E. F. (1983). Quantitative analysis of the high frequency components of the terminal portion of the body surface QRS in normal subjects and in patients with ventricular tachycardia. *Circulation*, 67, 1129–38
20. Karbenn, U., Breithardt, G., Borggrefe, M. and Simson, M. B. (1985). Automatic identification of late potentials. *J. Electrocardiol.*, 18, 123–34
21. Oeff, M., von Leitner, E-R., Sthapit, R., Breithardt, C., Borggrefe, M., Karbenn, U., Meinertz, T., Zotz, R., Clas, W., Hombach, V. and Hopp, H-W. (1986). Methods for non-invasive detection of ventricular late potentials – a comparative multicenter study. *Eur. Heart J.*, 7, 25–33
22. Kertes, P. J., Glabus, M., Murray, A., Julian, D. J. and Campbell, R. W. F. (1984). Delayed ventricular depolarisation – correlation with ventricular activation and relevance to ventricular fibrillation in acute myocardial infarction. *Eur. Heart J.*, 5, 974–83
23. Breithardt, G., Scharzmaier, J., Borggrefe, M., Haerten, K. and Seipel, L. (1983). Prognostic significance of late ventricular potentials after acute myocardial infarction. *Eur. Heart J.*, 4, 487–95
24. Gomes, J. A., Mehra, R., Barreca, P., El-Sherif, N., Hariman, R. and Holtzman, R. (1985). Quantitative analysis of the high-frequency components of the signal-averaged QRS complex in patients with acute myocardial infarction: a prospective study. *Circulation*, 72, 105–11
25. Lewis, S. J., Lander, P. T., Taylor, P., Chamberlain, D. A. and Vincent, R. (1987). The natural history of ventricular late potential activity in acute myocardial infarction. (Abstract). *Abstracts of 36th Annual Scientific Session of the American College of Cardiology*. (In press)
26. von Leitner, E. R., Oeff, M., Spielberg, C., Gast, D., Loock, D., Piesczek, C. and Jahns, B. (1984). Superiority of high resolution ECG to 24-hour monitoring to predict prognosis in post myocardial infarction patients. (Abstract). *J. Am. Coll. Cardiol.*, 3, 623
27. Denniss, A. R., Richards, D. A., Cody, D. V., Russell, P. A., Young, A. A., Cooper, M. J., Ross, D. L. and Uther, J. B. (1986) Prognostic significance of ventricular tachycardia and fibrillation induced at programmed stimulation and delayed potentials detected on the signal-averaged electrocardiograms of survivors of acute myocardial infarction. *Circulation*, 74, 731–45
28. Lindsay, B. D., Ambos, M. D., Schechtman, K. B. and Cain, M. E. (1986). Improved selection of patients for programmed ventricular stimulation by frequency analysis of signal-averaged electrocardiograms. *Circulation*, 73, 675–83
29. Omega Research Associates, Inc. (1986). Material on file. Pittsburgh, USA

30. Lander, P. T. (1986). Computer processing methods for the recovery of low amplitude ECG signals. *D. Phil. Thesis*, University of Sussex

11
Arrhythmias in children

J. A. TILL and D. E. WARD

Abnormalities of cardiac rhythm are being recognized more frequently in childhood. Monitoring of sick children on neonatal and intensive care units has resulted in an increased awareness of both the normal and abnormal variation in a child's rhythm. Increased routine monitoring of the fetus has brought to light rhythm abnormalities in fetal life and some of these are now recognized as a cause of fetal loss. The majority of abnormal rhythms encountered in childhood are similar in terms of electrocardiographic criteria to those in adults, but may differ markedly in underlying aetiology and prognosis. A minority of arrhythmias are peculiar to childhood.

SUPRAVENTRICULAR TACHYCARDIA

Wolff–Parkinson–White syndrome

The Wolff–Parkinson–White (WPW) syndrome accounts for approximately 22% of supraventricular tachycardias in childhood[1]. In about 40% of these children there is a structural cardiac defect, and most frequently the associated condition is that of Ebstein's anomaly of the tricuspid valve or atrioventricular, ventriculoarterial discordance (anatomically corrected transposition). Those children with a positive delta wave in the left-sided chest leads, so called 'type B' WPW more frequently have a structural problem[2]. The WPW syndrome is, for the great majority of children, a benign disorder. Atrioventricular re-entry tachycardia, the most commonly associated tachycardia is rarely life-threatening, however, occurrence in early infancy may rapidly result in congestive cardiac failure. The short circuit conduction time allows very fast heart rates at this early age, leading rapidly to circulatory collapse[3]. Symptoms and signs may be easily misinterpreted, and the situation may be further confounded if certain drugs (e.g. verapamil), commonly safely used in older age groups, threaten the circulation still further[4]. However, once recognized, control is relatively simply achieved in the majority of children.

Table 11.1 Classification of supraventricular tachycardias

Re-entry

Atrioventricular tachycardia (direct AV pathway)
    Wolff–Parkinson–White syndrome – overt
                                     – concealed
    Slow anomalous pathway   – long R–P'

Atrioventricular nodal tachycardia (dual AV nodal pathways)
    Slow–fast   – common
    Fast–slow   – long R–P'

Atrial flutter

Atrial fibrillation

Re-entrant atrial tachycardia   – sinoatrial
                                         – intra-atrial (e.g. postatrial surgery)

Automatic

Ectopic atrial tachycardia

His bundle tachycardia

The natural history of WPW syndrome presenting in childhood is largely unknown. Most paediatricians feel compelled to treat a child during the first year of life when attacks can have such profound consequences on the circulation, but guidelines for the subsequent treatment are not clear. It is commonly believed that children 'grow out' of the tendency to tachycardia, and studies addressing this problem support the idea. Woodrow Benson et al.[5] followed 35 children presenting with atrioventricular re-entry tachycardia in the first 2 months of life with serial oesophageal electrophysiological studies. At 1 year, spontaneous tachycardia had not been recently documented in 83% of these children. Deal et al.[2] in their retrospective study of 90 patients presenting with WPW syndrome below the age of 4 months claimed 33% experienced recurrent tachycardia after 1 year of life. Children with recurrent tachycardia were more likely to have WPW syndrome 'type B' and were more likely to have required more than one drug for initial control. Benson's study[5] showed that there were marked changes in the electrical characteristics of the accessory pathway with age, and suggested that this might be a reason for the change in the frequency of spontaneous attacks of tachycardia. Dunnigan et al.[6] studied 22 infants and eight children with frequent attacks of tachycardia using serial electrocardiograms and 24-hour ambulatory monitoring, and was able to document events involved in the initiation of attacks. They showed that the character of the initiating event changed with the age of the child. Sinus acceleration was a common initiating event in the small infant, but was uncommon in the older child. Atrial extrasystoles appeared as initiating events in all age groups, and supraventricular tachycardia in the older child more commonly commenced following atrial or ventricular extrasystoles or junctional pauses. This is an important study not only because it may help to explain the natural history, but also because knowledge of the initiating event may enable drug therapy to be tailored more successfully. However, this change of initiating event cannot fully explain the changing frequency of tachycardia as these events themselves have a natural history which does not directly reflect that of the tachycardia. For the initiation and continuation of sustained tachycardia there needs to be a complex interplay between all components of the circuit and initiating factors, all of which may alter with age. Up to 50% of children are thought to lose pre-excitation on surface electrocardiogram with increasing age. It is not known how many lose the pathway and in how many it is merely a change in the anterograde function of the accessory pathway. James[7] suggested that accessory pathways were more common in very young children because they represented part of normal cardiac morphogenesis, and the normal moulding and reshaping of the atrioventricular node and His bundle in the first year of life accounted for their disappearance in the majority of children. Benson et al.[5] showed that despite the disappearance of tachycardia in 83% of the children, evidence of an accessory pathway could still be demonstrated in 68%. However, the role of drug therapy in preventing spontaneous attacks is not made clear in this study. Care should be taken in interpreting the disappearance or appearance of pre-excitation in the individual child as the manifestation may be intermittent from day to day. The association between persistence or disappearance of pre-excitation on surface electrocardiogram and the recurrence of tachycardia is far from clear. One might expect this, as occurrence of tachycardia will depend on the retrograde characteristics of the accessory pathway, and the manifestation of pre-excitation is related to the anterograde characteristics. Lundberg et al.[8] reported that during the first year of life the occurrence of tachycardia was as frequent whether pre-excitation was overt or concealed. During the next two decades children with concealed accessory pathways were very unlikely to have attacks of tachycardia, whereas 50% of the children with overt pre-excitation continued to have attacks. Later in life adults with concealed pathways once again suffered attacks of tachycardia.

Attacks of atrioventricular re-entry tachycardia are rarely life-threatening, but sudden death is associated with this syndrome. These rare, but tragic, deaths are thought to occur when atrial flutter or fibrillation results in rapid ventricular rates due to conduction over the accessory pathway, leading to ventricular flutter/fibrillation and death. The children at greatest risk are those with a short anterograde refractory period of the accessory pathway. The refractory pathway can be assessed during an electrophysiological study, but a rough guide to the conduction characteristics of the accessory pathway can be gained from the behaviour of the delta wave on surface electrocardiogram. Pre-excitation will occur preferentially over the accessory pathway if the anterograde refractory period is short, and this will remain so throughout the 24 hours on Holter monitoring and during exercise testing even at maximum sinus heart rates[9]. Gillette suggests that in children suspected of having a short anterograde refractory period, an electrophysiological study should be undertaken to document the characteristics and exact location of the pathway so that surgical resection may be undertaken[10]. Atrial fibrillation is rare in childhood, even in association with WPW syndrome, and many feel the risk to the child does not justify such invasive therapy. However, care must be taken when treating these patients. Certain drugs such as digoxin may further shorten the refractory period of the accessory pathway and would theoretically increase the risk of sudden death, and should, therefore, be avoided in this group of children. Using a combination of surgical division and cryoablation, success rates for ablation of accessory pathways in certain specialist centres now approach 100%[11-13]. Success is dependent not only on good operative technique and experience of the surgeon but also on careful and accurate mapping. In these centres it is reasonable to consider even very young children with drug refractory or life-threatening tachycardias for surgery. Indeed some such centres advocate a surgical procedure for all young patients who require anything but the minimum therapy for treatment because of the risk and inconvenience of chronic drug therapy. Catheter ablation of accessory pathways in children remains an innovative but experimental procedure. Again careful mapping is paramount to the success of the procedure, but the associated risks, especially with accessory pathways which may only be mapped through the coronary sinus, preclude its routine use[14]. However, with further refinement this could prove to be a very valuable alternative to surgery in the future.

Long R–P' tachycardias

In 1967, Coumel et al.[15] described a narrow complex tachycardia associated with a P' wave with superior axis occurring just before the ensuing QRS complex during tachycardia, which was characteristically persistent and often drug refractory. This long R–P' tachycardia (so named because of the relationship of the R to P' wave on surface electrocardiogram during tachycardia) was more commonly seen in children than adults. The initiating event that triggered the tachycardia was sinus acceleration, and thus tachycardia characteristically continued, stopping and starting, intermittently for long periods of time. The underlying mechanism was originally thought to involve dual AV nodal pathways[16]. In the common form of AV nodal re-entry tachycardia the anterograde limb of the circuit utilizes a slowly conducting pathway and the retrograde limb a fast conducting pathway. This form of AV nodal re-entry tachycardia is a common tachycardia in older children as in adults. The

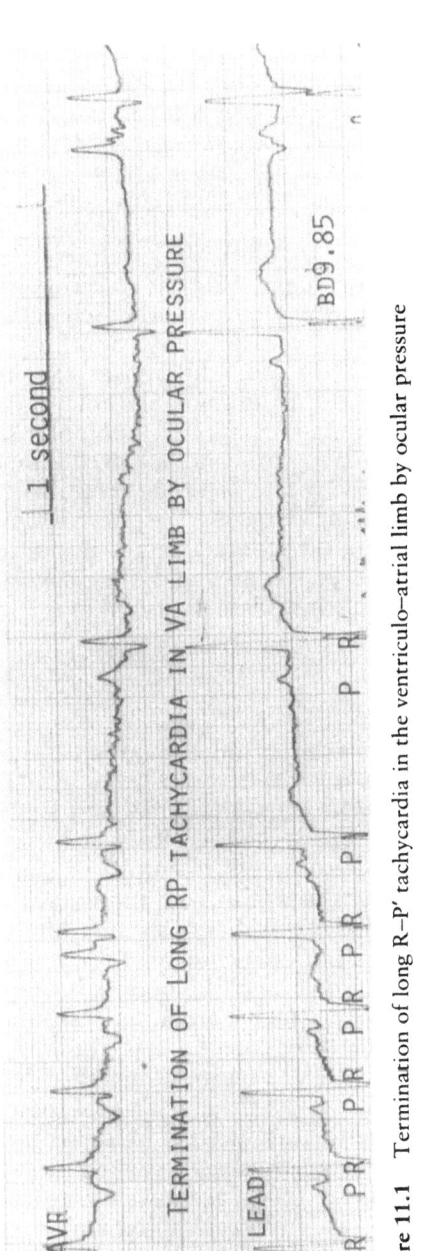

Figure 11.1 Termination of long R–P' tachycardia in the ventriculo–atrial limb by ocular pressure

unusual long R–P' tachycardia was explained by a circuit involving a fast conducting pathway in the anterograde limb and a slowly conducting pathway in the retrograde limb. In 1978, Gallagher and Sealy[17] questioned the mechanism of this tachycardia. They found evidence of a direct atrio-ventricular anomalous pathway capable of slow retrograde conduction. This accessory pathway differed from the usual direct atrioventricular pathways in that it possessed AV nodal decremental conduction characteristics, was always located in the posteroseptal region and never conducted anterogradely. There is evidence now that both these mechanisms may account for long R–P' tachycardia of childhood.

As the tachycardia is so often drug refractory other methods of management have been sought. Surgical resection has been attempted, but location of this pathway which is intimately related to the AV node has caused the surgeon some difficulty. Smith et al.[18] have recently described their attempts in four children at catheter ablation of the retrograde pathway, whilst maintaining the anterograde pathway intact. Following careful mapping they applied a unipolar shock to the area at the mouth of the coronary sinus and achieved temporary interruption of the tachycardia. However, in so doing they also caused anterograde block in two of the four patients. Despite only temporary relief of tachycardia the authors do report a better response to medical management following the procedure, and they suggest that with more experience this technique may well be useful in the future.

Ectopic atrial tachycardia

Another persistent tachycardia more commonly encountered in childhood than in later life is ectopic atrial tachycardia[1]. This tachycardia which is thought to result from an automatic focus in the atria can be difficult to differentiate from the long R–P' tachycardia, as in both the relationship of P' wave to the QRS complex is similar, and both tend to be persistent. Demonstration of continuing tachycardia in the presence of AV block confirms this diagnosis and differentiates it from the long R–P' tachycardia. Little is known of the long term prognosis of these persistent tachycardias of childhood. It is not uncommon for the older child to present with tachycardia and cardiomyopathy. It is not known whether the cardiomyopathy has resulted from the chronic abnormality of heart rate and rhythm or whether these are independent but associated problems[19]. The management of these children is further complicated by the refractory nature of these tachycardias to conventional drug therapy, and thus aggressive modes of treatment would have to be employed if the tachycardia was to be abolished. Epstein et al.[20], in a retrospective study of six children with persistent or incessant tachycardia, suggested that these tachycardias were often well tolerated. Others have reported resolution of cardiomyopathy when radical modes

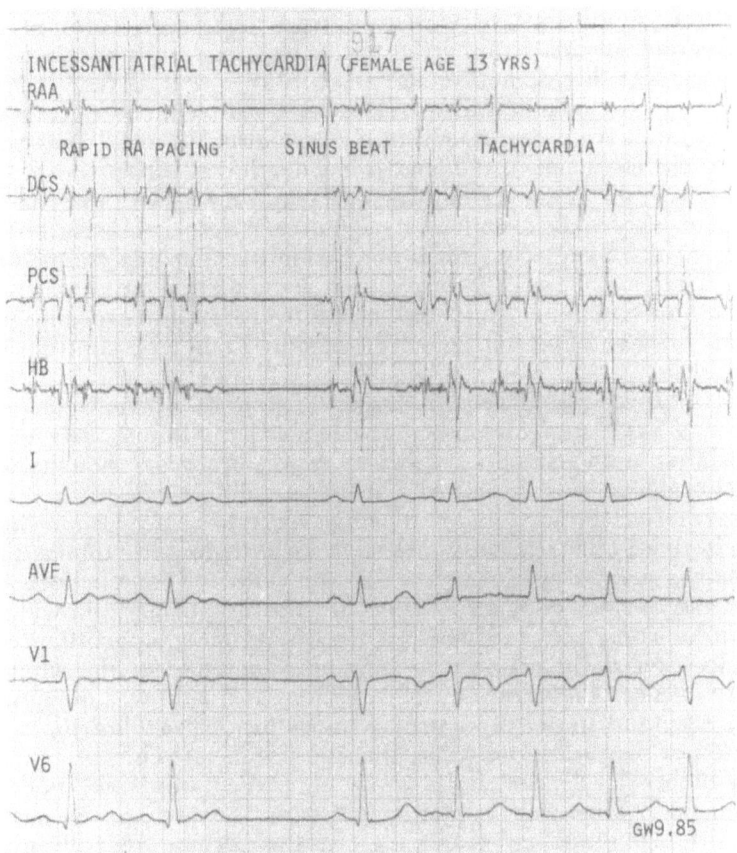

Figure 11.2 Incessant atrial tachycardia terminated by rapid atrial pacing during electrophysiological study. The tachycardia is seen to restart almost immediately. (RAA, Right atrium; DCS, distal coronary sinus; PCS, proximal coronary sinus; HB, His bundle)

of treatment finally abolish persistent tachycardia[21,22]. With improved endocardial mapping and operative techniques it may be possible eventually to manage all these children simply and safely surgically, but until this time management remains a problem.

Atrial flutter

Spontaneous atrial flutter is unusual in children without structural cardiac defects. This has recently been challenged by Dunnigan et al.[23] in a paper describing eight neonates where the diagnosis was made utilizing the technique of oesophageal recording. They suggest that the diagnosis may be easily missed in children as it may not be associated with the appearance of classical flutter waves on surface electro-cardiogram. In this group atrial flutter was frequently associated with other cardiac disease and/or the presence of a central venous pressure catheter in the atrium and was associated with a good outcome. In a collaborative study reported in 1985[24] evaluating 380 children with atrial flutter, the incidence of sudden cardiac death was increased four-fold if the arrhythmia remained uncontrolled, and it was recommended that attempts were made to control atrial flutter. Direct current cardioversion is the standard acute treatment of atrial flutter, but in a recent study by Campbell et al.[25] 63–73% of children responded to atrial pacing, and the authors recommend a trial of the relatively non-invasive oesophageal pacing prior to direct current cardioversion. Long term control remains a problem.

In children who have had surgical repair of a congenital cardiac defect, atrial flutter and other atrial tachyarrhythmias may occur in association with a sinoatrial disorder. It was originally thought that the high incidence of sudden death in these children was related to late postoperative conduction defects, however, it has since been recognized that in those children with coexistent atrial tachyarrhythmias there is perhaps a greater risk from atrial flutter with 1 : 1 conduction. A high incidence of sinus node disorder occurs most frequently following atrial repair of complete transposition (atrioventricular concordance, ventriculo–arterial discordance)[26]. Originally damage to the sinus node artery during cannulation of the superior caval vein was thought to be the cause, and initial reports of a lower incidence following a modification of the procedure where the superior caval vein was cannulated at a higher level and efforts made to protect the sinus node were promising[27]. However, a later report from the same group suggested that although immediate results were improved there was still a high late occurrence of sinus node dysfunction[28]. The continuing high incidence of arrhythmia following Mustard's operation is an important consideration in the argument for the arterial switch operation. Treatment of the tachyarrhythmias with drugs may exacerbate sinus node dysfunction, and, therefore, should be undertaken with care. Gillette et al.[29] suggest that treatment with any drug other than digoxin should not be used without prior placement of a permanent pacemaker, and they have recently described successful management of children with sinoatrial disease and associated tachycardia with antitachycardia pacemakers. Sick sinus syndrome without underlying cardiac defect is rare and has been thought to be a benign condition. However, in a few children, it may represent a potentially life-threatening condition[30]. If symptomatic, permanent pacing is recommended and usually results in successful resolution of symptoms.

His bundle tachycardia

If recognized and treated promptly, few arrhythmias in children without underlying structural cardiac defect are fatal. However, the rare His bundle tachycardia first described by Coumel et al.[31] is one such tachycardia. His bundle or junctional ectopic tachycardia usually presents in early infancy when a rapid supraventricular tachycardia proves unresponsive to either direct current cardioversion or drug therapy. It is an automatic tachycardia arising from an ectopic focus within the atrioventricular junction just above the bifurcation of the bundle of His. Careful examination of a 12-lead electrocardiogram will disclose narrow complex tachycardia often with atrioventricular dissociation. This tachycardia still carries a mortality of 50%. Treatment with drugs is associated with limited success. Control of tachycardia rate may be achieved more readily than conversion to sinus rhythm. Digoxin may be of use to support failing ventricular function which commonly accompanies this arrhythmia. Gillette et al.[32] have reported late sudden death in a child even after adequate control of tachycardia rate, and these authors advocate transcatheter His bundle ablation with implantation of a permanent pacemaker. Further follow-up is required before this aggressive approach will be universally accepted.

The aetiology of this rare condition is unknown. A similar, but less severe, tachycardia is seen post cardiac surgery[33] and here, as in the one reported case following cardiac catheter, trauma has been suggested as the cause. However, this latter tachycardia behaves differently in that it usually resolves within days of its starting and only occasionally requires vigorous treatment. Brechenmacher et al.[34] reported a child who died from His bundle tachycardia. At postmortem extensive degeneration of the His bundle was found, the mid-portion of which was split into several thin and irregular longitudinally orientated strands. This child and one other in the literature have had a blood relative with His bundle tachycardia, raising the question of a familial inheritance. It has been suggested that this may be a congenital abnormality of the His bundle, possibly arising from a defect in the reshaping and remoulding process described by James. Congenital abnormalities of the conduction system have been implicated in a number of perinatal arrhythmias. Yen Ho et al.[35] recently described defects in the conduction system resulting in fatal perinatal arrhythmias in three patients. Bharati and Lev.[36] have reported a statistically significant increased number of left-sided bundles of His in children dying of sudden infant death syndrome, and suggests that this may be a disadvantageous position for the bundle with less protection from haemodynamic stress. The full role of congenital conduction system defects in sudden infant death and in perinatal deaths due to arrhythmias remains to be fully elucidated, and will probably only become so with more careful studies of the conduction system after death.

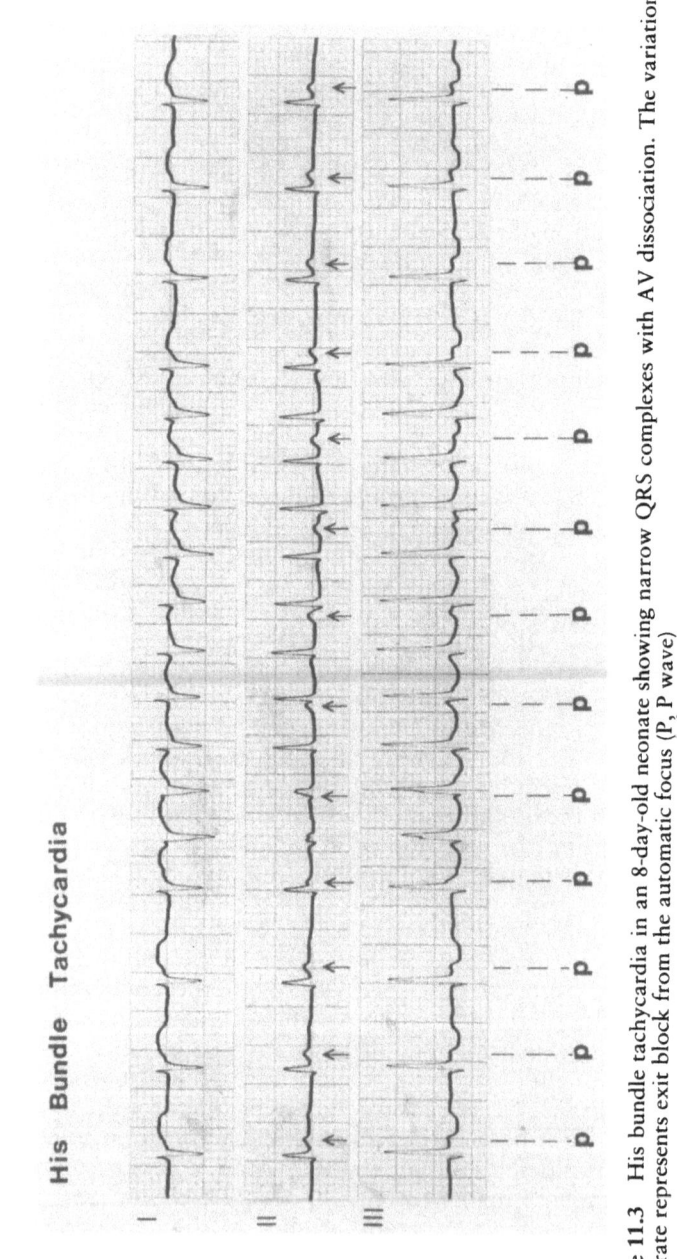

Figure 11.3 His bundle tachycardia in an 8-day-old neonate showing narrow QRS complexes with AV dissociation. The variation in QRS rate represents exit block from the automatic focus (P, P wave)

Diagnosis of tachycardias

Alongside the increased awareness of occurrence of arrhythmia in child-hood came the development of techniques applicable to children for diagnosis and treatment. The advent of smaller ambulatory monitoring equipment allowed recording of tachycardia frequency in these small patients who could not report episodes of palpatations. Telemetry is proving highly useful in the differential diagnosis of syncopal or near syncopal attacks. Electrophysiological studies may now be performed in even the smallest patient, but risks associated with the study may be expected to be greater in the child with small veins, difficult venous access and intolerance of arrhythmia[37]. Transoesophageal study utilizing the close proximity of the infant's oesophagous to the heart may over come some of these problems. Woodrow Benson et al.[38] describe the use of this technique both in the diagnosis and the treatment of rhythm disorders in children. However, the success of these elegant techniques depends on practised operators, who at present are not generally available.

With careful recording of initiation and termination of tachycardia an accurate diagnosis of the underlying mechanism can be made without resorting to invasive techniques. We have recently described the use of the short acting compound adenosine for the diagnosis and treatment of supraventricular tachycardia in children[39]. Adenosine has proved highly efficacious in our initial studies for the termination of re-entry tachycardia, interrupting re-entry tachycardias by its transient action on the AV node. Following termination of tachycardia the delay in AV nodal conduction may result in preferential conduction over an accessory pathway, thus revealing evidence of pre-excitation on the surface electrocardiogram. It is both rapid and simple and side-effects are few.

COMPLETE ATRIOVENTRICULAR BLOCK

Congenital complete atrioventricular block may be associated with structural cardiac defect or occur in isolation. The incidence is reported[40] to be approximately 1 : 20 000, and 25% of these children will have structural defects where it arises as a result of distortion of the con-duction axis. Well documented is the association between isolated con-genital complete heart block and maternal connective tissue disease[41,42]. The connective tissue disease may not be clinically apparent, and in some cases documentation of heart block in the baby has led to the diagnosis in the mother. Anti-Ro antibodies (antibodies to soluble tissue ribonucleoprotein antigens) are thought to cross the placenta and directly attack the conduction system[43]. It has recently been suggested that the defect in the conduction system in babies born of mothers with anti-Ro antibodies may occur in an anatomically distinct position compared with complete heart block due to other causes[44]. Children in

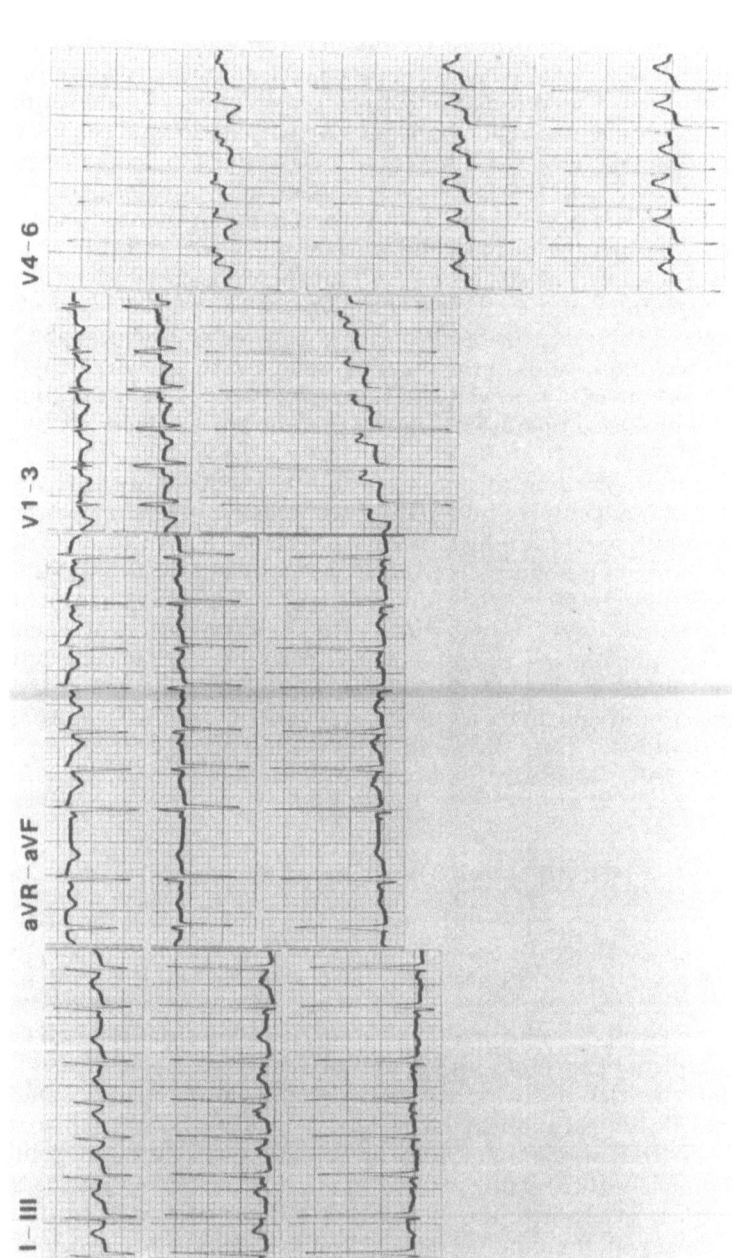

Figure 11.4 Ectopic atrial tachycardia in a 3-month-old child. P waves of small amplitude and rapid heart rates in children can make diagnosis difficult from the surface electrocardiogram

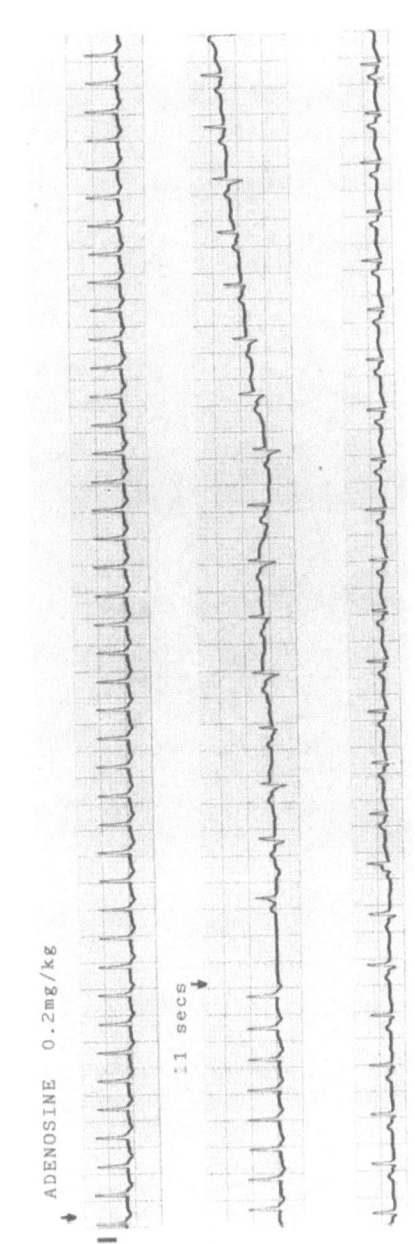

Figure 11.5 Termination of AV re-entry tachycardia with intravenous adenosine in a 1-month-old child with concealed Wolff–Parkinson–White syndrome. Following termination there is evidence of pre-excitation, disclosed on surface electrocardiogram for the first time

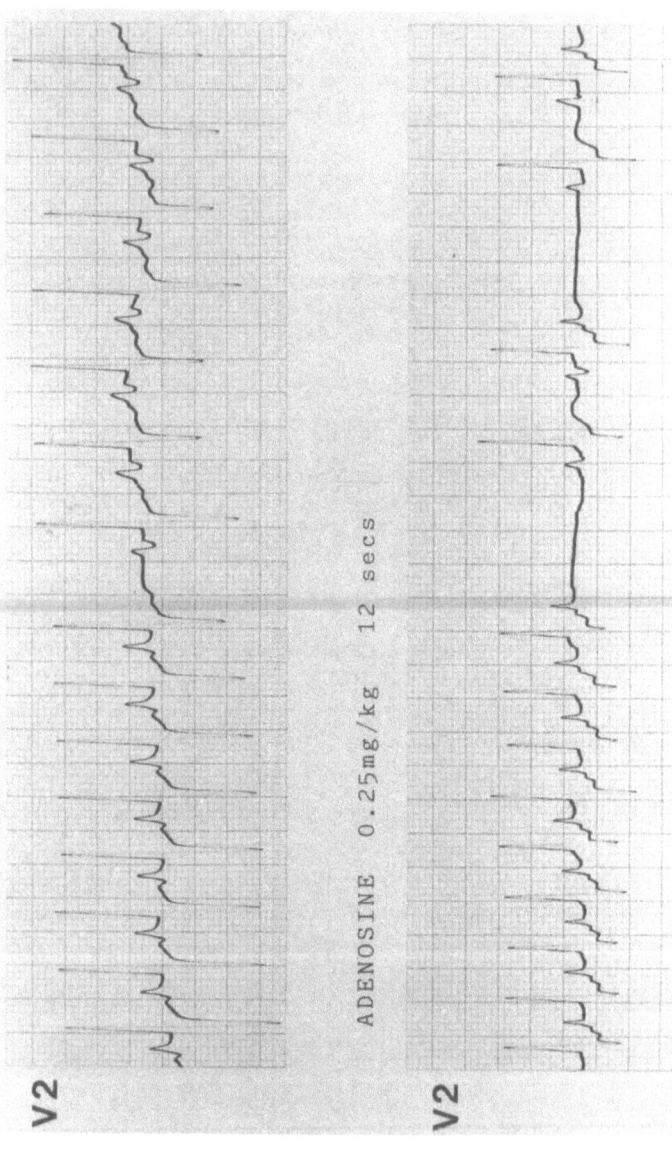

Figure 11.6 Termination of AV re-entry tachycardia in an 8-day-old neonate with intravenous flecainide and adenosine showing the different modes of action of the drugs on the re-entry circuit. Flecainide terminates the tachycardia in the retrograde limb, whereas adenosine terminates the tachycardia in the AV nodal limb of the circuit. Following termination with adenosine, atrial 'echoes' can be seen on the surface electrocardiogram suggesting the underlying mechanism of tachycardia is that of AV re-entry involving an accessory pathway

the former group had atrial-axis discontinuity, whereas one child in the latter group had absence of a segment of the His bundle. This remains to be confirmed in a larger series of patients.

Congenital complete heart block is generally well tolerated. Mortality is highest during the fetal and neonatal period, but after this time most children are asymptomatic. A minority are at risk of late sudden death and for most the risk is in early adult life. In children who are symptomatic permanent pacing, whatever age, is now possible. Improving technology has produced smaller generators with greater capability, leads less likely to dislodge or fracture and with improved care and follow-up pacing is becoming less of a problem in the small child[45,46]. The guidelines for asymptomatic children, however, remain far from clear. Few physicians are willing to undertake permanent pacing lightly, and we are as yet unable to reliably identify those at risk of late sudden death. Dewey et al.[47] addressed the problem of the long term natural history of congenital complete heart block, and prospectively followed 27 children for a mean of eight years. These authors suggest that the identification of junctional instability is a good guide to prognosis. Those children with a 'mean' heart rate of < 50 bpm, frequent episodes of junctional exit block or a flat junctional response to physical activity were more likely to succumb to sudden death or develop symptoms requiring pacing. They also suggest that the few children with a slow junctional rate and paroxysmal tachyarrhythmias are at risk because of the slow junctional recovery time which may occur following an episode of tachycardia.

Children who develop complete atrioventricular block at surgery rarely tolerate it. They have a higher risk of sudden death and are more prone to developing congestive cardiac failure. These children are, therefore, almost universally paced although methods of pacing vary widely from centre to centre.

VENTRICULAR ARRHYTHMIAS

Ventricular tachycardias in 'normal' hearts

Ventricular arrhythmias in children are rare and differ from those in adults because of their very varied underlying aetiology. Their prognosis and management varies accordingly. In childhood as in adult life ventricular arrhythmias may arise as a result of systemic disturbance, myocarditis or cardiomyopathy. A few older children have the characteristics typical of right ventricular dysplasia. In infancy, in an otherwise well child, ventricular tachycardia is very rare, but Garson et al.[48] have described a group of infants presenting with incessant ventricular tachycardia characteristically refractory to medical control. In this group no abnormality was detectable using 2D echocardiography or angiography, but at surgery small areas of fibrosis were found, visible to the naked eye. At microscopy, collections of giant cells resembling Purkinje cells were seen. These so-called Purkinje cell tumours are thought to be the substrate for the ventricular arrhythmia, and their removal has exacted a cure in all cases. Garson has termed this 'idiopathic incessant ventricular tachycardia of infancy'.

Some children, when clinically assessed, are found to have a completely normal heart, but continue to have ventricular arrhythmias. Previously, ventricular arrhythmias in these children have been considered to have a good prognosis. However, a small minority within the group die suddenly. In previous reports the criteria for a 'normal' heart on clinical assessment were not uniformly defined. Garson et al.[49] suggest that some children with right ventricular dysplasia and congestive cardiomyopathy are probably erroneously diagnosed as 'normal' if cardiac catheterization and electrophysiological study are not included in the assessment. If these children are excluded, ventricular arrhythmia and a truly normal heart may indeed have a good prognosis.

Long Q–T syndrome

It is very important to recognize and treat those children with the long QT syndrome and ventricular arrhythmia, since management is specific and may be life saving. Classically these children have a long QT interval on ECG, abnormally shaped T waves and bradycardia. T wave alternans may follow excitement, loud noises or exercise which may then evolve into a ventricular tachycardia with unusual morphology, *torsades de pointes*. This is usually self-terminating, but on occasion will lead to death. Two distinct syndromes were originally recognized. The Jervell, Lange–Neilsen syndrome where the electrophysiological abnormalities are associated with congenital deafness, an inherited autosomal recessive disorder, and Romano–Ward syndrome where there were identical cardiac electrophysiological defects associated with normal hearing, inherited as an autosomal dominant. However, this once clear dichotomy has recently become more confused with many cases appearing sporadically in the population and variants of the clinical syndrome described. Schwartz[50] has set up both a retrospective and prospective worldwide registry and has outlined criteria for diagnosis and given guidelines for therapy. He suggests that the condition arises as a result of a sympathetic imbalance, with a relative overactivity of the left stellate sympathetic ganglion and a relative underactivity of the right stellate ganglion. This theory is supported by animal experiments, where it is possible to mimic the condition by performing right stellectomy or by stimulating the left stellate ganglion. Whatever the aetiology, the registry has shown that effective treatment significantly reduces the associated mortality. Untreated, 71% of these children will die, whereas with adequate sympathetic β-blockade mortality is decreased to 6%. In those patients who continue to have syncopal attacks despite β-blockade left stellate ganglionectomy appears to be highly effective. Out of 57 patients resistant to β-blockade with stellate ganglionectomy there were only four deaths over a period of 8 years (Schwartz, personal communication). Ventricular or atrial pacing is also known to be effective in these patients[51]. Itoh et al.[52] have recently reported a close linkage between the locus for Romano–Ward syndrome and the HLA locus, and it is hoped that this may lead to a better understanding of the genetic inheritance.

Ventricular arrhythmias following repair of tetralogy of Fallot

An ever increasing group of children with ventricular arrhythmia are those following surgical repair of congenital cardiac defect. Despite a low early operative mortality there is an unacceptably high risk of late sudden death following repair of tetralogy of Fallot[53,54]. It was initially thought that late complete AV block was responsible, but in recent years it has become apparent that most of these deaths are related to ventricular arrhythmia[55,56]. The cause of arrhythmia in this group is unknown, and it is not yet possible to predict which children are at risk and which require treatment. Microre-entry circuits in the right ventricular outflow tract, the ventriculotomy site and on the right ventricular septum at the site of the ventricular septal defect have been implicated in the pathogenesis, possibly related to areas of fibrosis[57,58]. In this context it is interesting that the incidence of ventricular arrythmia and that of sudden death increases with increased age at operative repair and with the number of years postrepair. Other authors have correlated an increased risk of sudden death with high right ventricular systolic pressure following repair[59]. Garson et al.[60] have reported that treatment of all children with ventricular arrhythmia following repair has decreased the incidence of sudden death at his centre. However, the design of this study does not allow firm conclusions to be drawn. Chronic drug therapy is not without problems, and many feel reluctant to adopt such an aggressive policy for all children postrepair, especially when evidence is lacking. Further rigorously devised and properly conducted prospective studies are required to study the value of electrophysiological testing to assess risk, and the value of treatment in diminishing the risk, however it is assessed.

FETAL ARRHYTHMIAS

With more frequent routine fetal monitoring an increasing number of irregularities of rhythm have been recognized. Recent advances in echo doppler techniques have made it possible to detect, investigate and treat arrhythmias in fetal life. Utilizing these techniques it has become possible to examine the sequential relationship of atrial to ventricular contraction and in this way elucidate the mechanism of the arrhythmia[61,62]. More recently Strasburger et al.[63] have described a technique using doppler echocardiography to elucidate the mechanism of arrhythmia. An unknown percentage of these arrhythmias will be associated with a structural anomaly. Fetal bradycardia is more often associated with a structural defect than atrial or ventricular premature beats, which result in an irregular heart rate and are frequently a benign finding associated with a structurally normal heart. However, a structural anomaly should be sought in every case, and arrhythmia assessment combined with a 2-dimensional structural assessment.

When fetal bradycardia is found complete heart block should be excluded. Complete atrioventricular block may be well tolerated by the fetus, but its recognition prior to delivery is important not only so that associated complex cardiac defect may be identified and arrangements made for suitable place of delivery, but also so that bradycardia is not mistakenly diagnosed as fetal distress thus precipitating premature delivery. In the event of complete heart block fetal well-being during labour can be monitored by fetal blood sampling rather than cardiotocography.

Tachyarrhythmias are potentially life-threatening with the risk of non-immune hydrops and sudden death. Diagnosis may be complicated by the intermittent nature of the rhythm disturbance. In recent years the prognosis has improved. Drugs have been used to treat the fetus *in utero*, and there are better facilities and greater expertise should premature delivery be necessary. Digoxin has been used to treat the fetus with supraventricular tachycardia, and can be administered to the mother to attain therapeutic levels in the fetus[64]. This has resulted in conversion of supraventricular tachycardia to sinus rhythm, but may also be used simply to control ventricular response or congestive cardiac failure. Animal work has shown that digoxin crosses the placenta by passive diffusion, and in animals the levels in the mother and fetus are similar and predictable[65]. Cord digoxin levels measured at delivery are similar to maternal levels. However, doses higher than normal are required to achieve therapeutic levels in the mother. Other agents such as propranolol, verapamil, procainamide[65] and amiodarone[66] have recently been used in a small number of patients, but more experience is required before these drugs can be recommended for use in this situation.

References

1. Gillette, P. and Garson, A. (1981). *Paediatric Cardiac Dysrhythmias*, (New York: Grune and Stratton)
2. Deal, B., Keane, J., Gillette, P. and Garson, A. (1985). Wolff–Parkinson–White syndrome and supraventricular tachycardia during infancy: management and follow-up. *J. Am. Coll. Cardiol.*, 5, 130
3. Gikonyo, B., Dunnigan, A. and Woodrow Benson, D. (1985). Cardiovascular collapse in infants: association with paroxysmal atrial tachycardia. *Paediatrics*, 76, 922
4. Garson, A. (1987). Medicolegal problems in the management of cardiac arrhythmias in children. *Paediatrics*, 79, 84
5. Woodrow Benson, D., Dunnigan, A. and Benditt, D. (1987). Follow-up evaluation of infant paroxysmal atrial tachycardia: transoesophageal study. *Circulation*, 75, 542
6. Dunnigan, A., Benditt, D. and Woodrow Benson, D. (1986). Modes of onset

(initiating events) for paroxysmal atrial tachycardia in infants and children. *Am. J. Cardiol.*, **57**, 1280

7. James, T. (1970). Cardiac conduction system: fetal and postnatal development. *Am. J. Cardiol.*, **25**, 213

8. Lundberg, A. (1973). Paroxysmal tachycardia in infancy: follow-up study of 47 subjects ranging in age from 10 to 26 years. *Paediatrics*, **51**, 26

9. Bricker, J., Porter, C., Garson, A., Gillette, P., McVey, P., Traweek, M. and McNamara, D. (1985). Exercise testing in children with Wolff–Parkinson–White syndrome. *Am. J. Cardiol.*, **55**, 1001

10. Gillette, P. (1985). Supraventricular arrhythmias in children. *J. Am. Coll. Cardiol.*, **5**, 122B

11. Campbell, R., Hammon, J., Echt, D. and Graham, T. (1987). Surgical treatment of paediatric cardiac arrhythmia. *J. Paediatr.*, **110**, 501

12. Ott, D., Gillette, P., Garson, A., Cooley, D., Reul, G. and McNamara, D. (1985). Surgical management of refractory supraventricular tachycardia in infants and children. *J. Am. Coll. Cardiol.*, **5**, 124

13. Holmes, D., Danielson, G., Gersh, B., Osborn, M., Wood, D., McLaren, C., Sugrue, D., Porter, C. and Hammill, S. (1985). Surgical treatment of accessory pathways and symptomatic tachycardia in children and young adults. *Am. J. Cardiol.*, **55**, 1509

14. Ward, D.E. and Camm, A.J. (1987). *Clinical Electrophysiology of the Heart*, (London: Edward Arnold)

15. Coumel, P., Cabrol, C., Fabiato, A., Gourgon, R. and Slama, R. (1967). Tachycardie permanante par rhythme reciproque. I Preuves du diagnostic par stimulation auriculaire et ventriculaire. *Arch. Malad. Coeur*, 1830

16. Wolff. G., Sung, R., Pickoff, A., Garcia, O., Werblin, R., Ferrer, P., Tamer, D. and Gelband, H. (1979). The fast–slow form of atrioventricular nodal reentrant tachycardia in children. *Am. J. Cardiol.*, **43**, 1181

17. Gallagher, J.J. and Sealy, C.W. (1978). The permanent form of junctional reciprocating tachycardia: further elucidation of the underlying mechanism. *Eur. J. Cardiol.*, **8**, 413

18. Smith, R., Gillette, P., Massumi, A., McVey, P. and Garson, A. (1986). Transcatheter ablative techniques for treatment of the permanent form of junctional reciprocating tachycardia in the young patients. *J. Am. Coll. Cardiol.*, **8**, 385

19. Gallagher, J. (1985). Tachycardia and cardiomyopathy: The chicken–egg dilemma revisited. *J. Am. Coll. Cardiol.*, **6**, 1172

20. Epstein, M. and Benditt, D. (1981). Long-term evaluation of persistent supraventricular tachycardia in children: Clinical and electrocardiographic features. *Am. Heart J.*, **102**, 80

21. Gillette, P., Smith, R., Mullins, C., Gutgesell, H., Goh, T., Cooley, D. and McNamara, D. (1985). Chronic supraventricular tachycardia a curable cause of congestive cardiomyopathy. *J. Am. Med. Assoc.*, **253**, 391

22. Kugler, J., Baisch, S., Cheatham, J., Latson, L., Pinsky, W., Norberg, W. and Hofschire, P. (1984). Improvement of left ventricular dysfunction after control of persistent tachycardia. *J. Paediatr.*, **105**, 543

23. Dunnigan, A., Woodrow Benson, D. and Benditt, D. (1985). Atrial flutter in infancy: diagnosis, clinical features, and treatment. *Paediatrics*, **75**, 725

24. Garson, A., Bink-Boelkens, M., Hesslein, S.P., Hordof, J.A., Keane, F.J., Neches, H.W. and Porter, J.C. (1985). Atrial flutter in the young: a collaborative study of 380 cases. *Paediatr. Cardiol.*, **6**, 871

25. Campbell, R., Dick, M., Jenkins, J., Spicer, R., Crowley, D., Rocchini, A., Snider, A., Stren, A. and Rosenthal, A. (1985). Atrial overdrive pacing for conversion of atrial flutter in children. *Paediatrics*, **75**, 730

26. Hayes, C.J. and Gersony, W.M. (1986). Arrhythmias after the mustard operation for transposition of the great arteries: a long-term study. *J. Am. Coll. Cardiol.*, **7**, 133

27. El-Said, G., Gillette, P., Cooley, D., Mullins, C. and McNamara, D. (1976). Protection of the sinus node in mustards operation. *Circulation*, **53**, 788

28. Duster, M., Bink-Boelkens, M., Wampler, D., Gillette, P., McNamara, D. and Cooley, D. (1985). Long term follow-up of dysrhythmias following the Mustard procedure. *Am. Heart J.*, **109**, 1323

29. Gillette, C. P., Wampler, G. D., Shannon, C. and Ott, D. (1986). Use of cardiac pacing after the Mustard operation for transposition of the great arteries. *J. Am. Coll. Cardiol.*, **7**, 138

30. Scott, O., Macartney, J. F. and Deverall, B. P. (1976). Sick sinus syndrome in children. *Arch. Dis. Child.*, **51**, 100

31. Coumel, P., Fidell, J., Huel, P., Brechenmacher, C., Balune, A., Bretagne, J., Clematy, J., Gerard, R., Grolleau, R., Hualt, G., Mouy, J., Kachaner, J., Ribiere, M. and Toumieux, M. C. (1975). Tachycardies focales hissienes congenitales. *Arch. Malad. Coeur.*, **69**, 899

32. Gillette, P., Garson, A., Porter, C., Ott, D., McVey, P., Zinner, A. and Blair, H. (1983). Junctional automatic ectopic tachycardia: New proposed treatment by transcatheter His bundle ablation. *Am. Heart J.*, **106**, 619

33. Kerr, C. and Mason, M. (1985). Incidence and clinical significance of accelerated junctional rhythm following open heart surgery. *Am. Heart J.*, **110**, 966

34. Brechenmacher, C., Coumel, P. and James, T. (1976). De subitaneis mortibus. XV. Intractable tachycardia in infancy. *Circulation*, **53**, 377

35. Yen Ho, S., Mortimer, G., Anderson, R., Pomerance, A. and Keeling, J. (1985). Conduction system defects in three perinatal patients with arrhythmia. *Br. Heart J.*, **53**, 158

36. Bharati, S. and Lev, M. (1986). Congenital abnormalities of the conduction system in sudden death in young adults. *J. Am. Coll. Cardiol.*, **8**, 1096

37. Ward, D. (1986). The management of arrhythmias in children; are electrophysiological studies of value? *Int. J. Cardiol.*, **11**, 149

38. Woodrow Benson, D., Sanford, M., Dunnigan, A. and Benditt, G. D. (1984). Transesophageal atrial pacing threshold: role of interelectrode spacing, pulse width and catheter insertion depth. *Am. J. Cardiol.*, **53**, 63

39. Clarke, B., Till, A. J., Rowland, E., Ward, E. D., Barnes, J. P. and Shinebourne, A. E. (1987). Rapid termination of supraventricular tachycardia in children by adenosine. *Br. Heart J.*, **57**, 584

40. Roberts, K. N. (1983). Cardiac Arrhythmias in the Neonate Infant and Child. Ed Roberts and Gelband. 233

41. McCue, C., Mantakas, M., Tingelstad, J. and Ruddy, S. (1977). Congenital heart block in newborns of mothers with connective tissue disease. *Circulation*, **56**, 82

42. Litsey, S., Noonan, J., O'Connor, W., Cottrill, C. and Mitchell, B. (1985). Maternal connective tissue disease and congenital heart block. *N. Engl. J. Med.*, **312**, 98

43. Scott, J., Maddison, P., Taylor, P., Esscher, E., Scott, O. and Skinner, P. (1983). Connective-tissue disease, antibodies to ribonucleoprotein, and congenital heart block. *N. Engl. J. Med.*, **309**, 209

44. Yen Ho, S., Esscher, E., Anderson, R. and Michaelsson, M. (1986). Anatomy of congenital complete heart block and relation to maternal anti-Ro antibodies. *Am. J. Cardiol.*, **58**, 291

45. Ward, D., Jones, S. and Camm, A. (1985). Long term endocardial pacing in congenital heart disease. *Clin. Prog. Electrophysiol. Pacing*, **3**, 133

46. Gillette, P., Shannon, C., Blair, H., Garson, A., Porter, C. and McNamara, D. (1983). Transvenous pacing in paediatric patients. *Am. Heart J.*, **105**, 843

47. Dewey, R., Capeless, M. and Levy, A. (1987). Use of ambulatory electrocardiographic monitoring to identify high-risk patients with congenital complete heart block. *N. Engl. J. Med.*, **316**, 835

48. Garson, A., Smith, R., Moak, J., Ross, B. and McNamara, D. (1985). Ventricular arrhythmias and sudden death in children. *J. Am. Coll. Cardiol.*, **5**, 130B

49. Garson, A. (1986). Ventricular arrhythmias in the young: differences and similarities to adults. *Clin. Progr. Electrophysiol. Pacing*, **4**, 175

50. Schwartz, P. (1985). Idiopathic long QT syndrome: Progress and questions. *Am. Heart J.*, **109**, 399

51. Wilmer, C., Stein, B. and Morris, D. (1986). Atrioventricular pacemaker placement in Romano–Ward syndrome and recurrent Torsades de Pointes. *Am. J. Cardiol.*, **59**, 171

52. Itoh, S., Munemura, S. and Satoh, H. (1982). A study of the inheritance pattern of Romano–Ward syndrome. *Clin. Pediatr.*, **21**, 20

53. Garson, A., Nihill, M., McNamara, D. and Cooley, D. (1979). Status of the adult and adolescent after repair of Tetralogy of Fallot. *Circulation*, **59**, 1232

54. James, F., Kaplan, S. and Chou, T. (1975). Unexpected cardiac arrest in patients after surgical correction of Tetralogy of Fallot. *Circulation*, **52**, 691

55. Gillette, P., Yeoman, M., Mullins, C. and McNamara, D. (1977). Sudden death after repair of Tetralogy of Fallot. Electrocardiographic and electrophysiologic abnormalities. *Circulation*, **56**, 566

56. Webb Kavey, R., Blackman, M. and Sondheimer, H. (1982). Incidence and severity of chronic ventricular dysrhythmias after repair of Tetralogy of Fallot. *Am. Heart J.*, **103**, 342

57. Deanfield, J., McKenna, W. and Rowland, E. (1985). Local abnormalities of right ventricular depolarisation after repair of Tetralogy of Fallot: A basis for ventricular arrhythmia. *Am. J. Cardiol.*, **55**, 522

58. Horowitz, L., Vetter, V., Harken, A. and Josephson, M. (1980). Electrophysiologic characteristics of sustained ventricular tachycardia occurring after repair of Tetralogy of Fallot. *Am. J. Cardiol.*, **46**, 446

59. Chen, D. and Moller, J. (1987). Comparison of late clinical status between patients with different haemodynamic findings after repair of Tetralogy of Fallot. *Am. Heart J.*, **113**, 767

60. Garson, A., Randall, D., Gillette, P., Smith, R., Moak, J., McVey, P. and McNamara, D. (1985). Prevention of sudden death after repair of Tetralogy of Fallot: Treatment of ventricular arrhythmias. *J. Am. Coll. Cardiol.*, **6**, 221

61. Crowley, D., Dick, M., Rayburn, W. and Rosenthal, A. (1985). Two-dimensional and M-Mode echocardiographic evaluation of fetal arrhythmia. *Clin. Cardiol.*, **8**, 1

62. Steinfeld, L., Rappaport, H., Rossbach, H. and Martinez, E. (1986). Diagnosis of fetal arrhythmias using echocardiographic and doppler techniques. *J. Am. Coll. Cardiol.*, **9**, 1425

63. Strasburger, F. J., Huhta, C. J., Carpenter, J. R., Garson, A. and McNamara, G. D. (1986). Doppler echocardiography in the diagnosis and management of persistent fetal arrhythmias. *J. Am. Coll. Cardiol.*, **7**, 1386

64. Allan, D. L., Crawford, C. D., Anderson, H. R. and Tynan M. (1984). Evaluation and treatment of fetal arrhythmias. *Clin. Cardiol.*, **7**, 467

65. Dumesic, D., Silverman, N., Tobias, S. and Golbus, M. (1982). Transplacental cardioversion of fetal supraventricular tachycardia with procainamide. *N. Engl. J. Med.*, **307**, 1128

66. Arnoux, P., Seyral, P., Llurens, M., Djiane, P., Potier, A., Unal, D., Cano, J., Serradimigni, A. and Rouault, F. (1987). Amiodarone and digoxin for refractory fetal tachycardia. *Am. J. Cardiol.*, **59**, 166

12
Special aspects of arrhythmias in the elderly

A. MARTIN

INTRODUCTION

There are several important changes that occur in cardiovascular function with advancing age. These changes involve the whole of the conducting system of the heart as well as the autonomic control of the heart rhythm. In addition, elderly people are exposed to the processes of degenerative changes which occur in virtually all systems with advancing years as well as the change caused by disease. Thus the elderly would be expected to show not only a different pattern of rhythm disorders, but an altered response to these in terms of symptoms and clinical signs compared with younger persons. Since the elderly account for between 10% and 15% of the total population of the Western world, the magnitude of the problem, and the importance of its understanding, cannot be overemphasized.

The results of ambulatory monitoring studies in younger people cannot be applied to the elderly in whom such diagnostic evaluation is most frequently performed. A further difficulty concerns the definition of the ranges of 'normality' in the elderly[1,2]. There are now large numbers of studies on the incidence of arrhythmias in the elderly, but it has proved difficult to isolate the two, quite separate, effects of disease from ageing *per se*. From a clinical point of view it is probably most useful to study the results of 'typical' or unscreened elderly populations. Finally, the investigation of dysrhythmias should be linked to meticulous invasive and non-invasive studies followed-up over long periods; unfortunately these are both very difficult and often impractical.

THE SINUS NODE AND THE HEART RATE

The dominant role of the sinus pacemaker diminishes with age, and this may be explained by the progressive loss of cells in the node with advancing age[3]. In addition, there is a decline in autonomic nervous system function, not only in diseases such as diabetes[4], but as a function of ageing[5]. Thus the heart rate variability is reduced in old age[1,5] and respiratory-induced changes in heart rate are diminished[1,6]. The increase

201

in heart rate that occurs on standing in the young is also reduced in the elderly[7]. Although there is an increase in the circulating levels of adrenaline and noradrenaline in the elderly[8], there is a diminution of the cardiovascular reflexes mediated by the adrenergic system[9]. The haemodynamic response to stress in the elderly has many of the features of that due to β-blockade, with a higher cardiac output during exercise maintained by a slower heart rate, a greater stroke volume and increased end-diastolic and end-systolic volumes[10].

Thus it would appear that sinus bradycardia cannot be regarded as a 'normal' function of ageing. In our own study of a typical elderly group aged 75 years and over living in the community[1] we found that sinus bradycardia (defined as a heart rate of less than 50 bpm) occurred in 10%. We also found that the mean heart rates were slower in men (70 bpm) than in women (76 bpm); Fleg and Kennedy reported similar findings in their group of elderly people free of known heart disease[11].

The term *Sick Sinus Syndrome* (SSS)[3] is appropriately applied to people with severe degrees of sinus node dysfunction, and embraces severe sinus bradycardia (less than 40 bpm), sinus arrest and exit block, atrial fibrillation (AF) and atrial flutter as well as carotid hypersensitivity with prolonged sinus arrest. The sick sinus syndrome is more likely to occur in the presence of ischaemic heart disease, and Nelson and colleagues[12] found that in a large group of elderly people with known or suspected heart disease the incidence of prolonged sinus pauses was 2%, although in studies of more healthy people prolonged pauses have not been reported[1,11].

Before discussing the management of SSS it is important to examine the symptomatology of cardiac arrhythmias, since, in the light of our current knowledge, most asymptomatic patients should not be treated for any arrhythmia. Many symptoms referable to the heart and central nervous system may be produced in the elderly[12,13]. These include dizziness, lightheadedness, vertigo, fits, faints and falls as well as chest pain and palpitations. These symptoms are generally produced by bradycardias, although tachycardias may produce chest pain and breathlessness. Paroxysmal tachycardias, especially AF, are the commonest cause of acute dyspnoea, due to left ventricular failure, in the elderly[14]. Accidental injuries, such as femoral neck fractures, may be caused by arrhythmias[15]. The difficulty in assessing the neurological complications of arrhythmias is that the elderly suffer from multi-system disease, and symptoms such as dizziness and syncope may be due, in part or wholly, to non-cardiac causes.

SSS should only be treated if it gives rise to symptoms which may be very disabling, although rarely fatal. Bradycardic situations should be managed by permanent pacing, but several authors have recently expressed concern about the low pacing rate in the United Kingdom (UK)[16-18]. The reason for the low pacing rate in the UK, relative to similarly developed countries, is almost totally due to the failure to manage sinus node disease aggressively; both in terms of the poor availability of ambulatory monitoring and the conservative attitude of some to pacing old people[18]. We have shown, by making ambulatory monitoring widely available to the elderly, by pacing all those with symptomatic bradyarrhythmias and by setting up satellite pacemaker follow-up clinics in local hospitals, that it is quite feasible to improve the quality of life for the very old for considerable periods of time[18].

The management of tachycardias associated with the sick sinus syndrome, such as AF, is discussed below. However, on occasion it will be necessary to pace some of these patients as well as giving antiarrhythmic therapy.

SUPRAVENTRICULAR ARRHYTHMIAS

Numerous studies have demonstrated a high incidence of atrial and junctional premature contractions in both healthy and symptomatic subjects[1,11,12]. Isolated premature atrial contractions have been found in 88% of subjects free of demonstrable heart disease[11] and more frequent premature atrial contractions in about 50%[1,11,12]. There appear to be no significant differences between men and women, non-smokers and smokers or hypertensive and non-hypertensive individuals[11].

The incidence of paroxysmal atrial and junctional tachycardias found in different population surveys seems to be variable. We found that only 3% of subjects had paroxysmal supraventricular tachycardia in our 106 elderly people living at home[1], whereas Fleg and Kennedy found an incidence of 28% of benign slow atrial tachycardia in their healthy group[11]. Other authors have found an incidence of about 10% of supraventricular tachycardias in elderly asymptomatic people[19,20]. The relatively high incidence of supraventricular tachycardias found in some studies together with a low incidence of paroxysmal atrial fibrillation (PAF)[11,19,20] compared with our own findings of a high incidence of AF and PAF[1] does raise the question of electrocardiographic interpretation.

It has long been known that AF is a common finding in the elderly from resting 12-lead electrocardiographic surveys[21,22]. However, the more widespread use of ambulatory monitoring has shown that the true incidence of established, and more especially paroxysmal, AF is as high as 11% in both apparently healthy and symptomatic elderly subjects[1,12]. The vast majority of people with paroxysmal AF and atrial flutter are symptomatic, since the paroxysms are associated with a high ventricular rate[1,12,14].

The prognostic significance of AF has been the subject of some dispute, but it clearly appears, both from our work using ambulatory electrocardiography[2] and the resting electrocardiographic studies of Kulbertus and colleagues[23], that the arrhythmia is associated with a significantly higher mortality than those age-matched controls in sinus rhythm. It has long been accepted that AF associated with mitral valvular disease produces a high risk of stroke from left atrial thrombus embolization[24].

However, the majority of people with AF now being seen do not have mitral valve disease, although they may have hypertension or ischaemic heart disease[25]. There are numerous reports that suggest that non-valvular AF may also be associated with a high incidence of stroke[24,26-28], but it is questionable whether the stroke is merely related to old age, ischaemic heart disease, hypertension or associated cerebrovascular disease rather than the AF *per se*. In our long term follow-up study of apparently healthy people in the community the incidence of stroke in those with AF was lower than would have been expected in age-matched controls[25]. It has recently been shown from M-mode and 2D-echocardiographic studies that the risk of stroke may be related to the left atrial size whatever the cause of the AF[29]. Certainly, the risks of anticoagulating all people with AF on a long term basis would be unacceptable and the exercise would be prohibitively expensive[27].

The management of paroxysmal atrial fibrillation and flutter

Virtually all patients with PAF have symptoms referable to their arrhythmia because of the rapid ventricular rate[25]. Therefore, it would seem desirable to try and abolish the arrhythmia if some safe and effective means were available. Because of the natural history of PAF, which will ultimately develop into established AF[14], it may be necessary to give antiarrhythmic agents for a long time. Quinidine, procainamide and disopyramide have been shown to be effective in preventing paroxysms of AF, but their unwanted effects in the elderly are such that their clinical use on a long term basis is unwarranted in all but a few patients[25]. Amiodarone is probably the most effective drug currently assessed that will control PAF over long periods[25,30,31]. In a recent report it was shown to have controlled the symptoms in over 90% of patients in a 2 year follow-up and to abolish the arrhythmia completely in 80%. A further 10% of patients who continued to have either PAF or established AF or atrial flutter had well-controlled ventricular rates throughout the 2 year study[25]. Although verapamil has been shown to effectively cardiovert patients when given intravenously for recent-onset AF[32], it is of variable efficacy when given orally on a long term basis to control PAF[33]. Newer Class I agents, such as flecainide, may also be used effectively to control PAF, but their long term efficacy and safety have not yet been assessed[25].

When exhibiting long term treatment for PAF the unwanted effects of the drug are extremely important. Of the newer agents available disopyramide is associated with unacceptable unwanted effects, due to its anticholinergic action, and is contra-indicated in elderly men[25]. Verapamil is of marginal efficacy, and also has a significant degree of negative inotropism. Amiodarone is associated with a large number of reported unwanted effects; the commonest of which are photosensitive skin rashes, a Parkinsonian-like tremor, biochemical, and sometimes clinical, hypo- and hyperthyroidism, interstitial pulmonary fibrosis and derangement of liver function tests. Many of these unwanted effects can be minimized by keeping the dose of the drug at the lowest possible level and maintaining the serum level in the range of 0.6–1.5 μg/l[25].

In certain cases of 'refractory' PAF there may be a place for transvenous ablation of the atrioventricular mode[34, 35].

The management of established atrial fibrillation

Digoxin is still the drug of choice for the majority of patients who have an uncontrolled ventricular response to established AF[34,35]. However, up to one third of patients do not demonstrate uncontrolled heart rates and require no treatment[14]. When digoxin is used in the elderly the dose should be kept as low as possible (62.5–125 μg per day or less), since the drug is renally excreted[37]. Amiodarone may also be used effectively to control the ventricular rate[25,36], and in a significant number of patients it will chemically cardiovert them to sinus rhythm[36,38]. There may be some cases in whom the ventricular rate is difficult to control, and in these the combination of a low dose of digoxin together with a small dose of amiodarone or a β-blocker, such as pindolol (10 mg daily), may be very effective[39].

Sinus rhythm is preferable to chronic AF in the elderly since it provides the atrial 'kick' which helps to maintain cardiac output. In addition, there is the potential reduction in the risk of thrombo-embolic phenomena. Electroconversion by DC shock and chemical conversion by drugs, such as amiodarone and verapamil, may be transiently effective but, unless permanent antiarrhythmic treatment is instituted, the AF will recur. It is conventional during planned cardioversion to use anticoagulant therapy, but the risks of embolism following conversion may have been exaggerated in the past[25,38,39]. It must be remembered that amiodarone potentiates the action of warfarin, which makes anticoagulant control more difficult.

Atrial flutter is much less common than AF, and is rarely seen in healthy people[1,11]. It is, however, the commonest cause of a fixed-rate tachycardia of 150 bpm in the elderly. The management of atrial flutter may prove very difficult. In recent-onset flutter it is worth considering electroconversion and then maintaining sinus rhythm with an antiarrhythmic agent. In chronic atrial flutter digoxin may effectively block atrioventricular conduction and reduce the heart rate. Amiodarone has been shown to have the same effect, and may even effect chemical cardioversion[25]. Occasionally digoxin may reduce the atrial rate, but accelerates atrioventricular conduction thus leading to a paradoxically high heart rate.

VENTRICULAR ARRHYTHMIAS

Ventricular arrhythmias have been shown to be common in all age groups[1,23,40–42], and there is an age-related increase in the incidence of ventricular premature contractions (VPCs), which can be as high as 70–

80% in apparently healthy old people[1,11]. In studies of patients with known or suspected heart disease the overall incidence of VPCs is 73%[12]. However, the complexity of VPCs does appear to increase in patients who are symptomatic (63%) compared with those subjects who have no palpitations (22%)[1,12]. More potentially serious ventricular arrhythmias, such as paroxysmal ventricular tachycardia, have been shown to occur in 4% of apparently healthy individuals[1,11], whereas in patients with known or suspected heart disease the incidence rises to 17%[12]. Tea and coffee consumption seem to be irrelevant to the production of ventricular arrhythmias in the elderly[1,19], but there is some divergent evidence for the role of tobacco-smoking in the generation of ventricular arrhythmias[1,11,19].

The prognostic significance of ventricular arrhythmias has been the subject of speculation for two decades and has led to the formulation of prognostic criteria by Lown and Wolf[43]. There is now little doubt of the potential risk of sudden death in those with VPCs in the post-infarction period[44,45], but in apparently healthy populations of non-elderly subjects there is no convincing evidence that VPCs are potentially life-threatening[46], although they may be a predictor of underlying ischaemic heart disease[47].

There is virtually no information concerning the prognostic significance of VPCs in the apparently healthy elderly from ambulatory monitoring studies other than our own[2]. We found that there was a relationship between the number of VPCs found in our original 106 people living in the community and the increased risk of death in the ensuing 5 years. In those who originally had a VPC rate of greater than 10 per hour the crude mortality rate was 67% compared to the 36% in those that had less than 10 VPCs per hour[2]. This study also confirmed the consistency of repeated ambulatory monitoring findings, in that 92% of those who were free of VPCs on the original examination were also free from them 5 years later[2].

The management of ventricular arrhythmias

Frequent and complex VPCs usually give rise to symptoms, and these should, therefore, be treated with a Class I agent, for example flecainide, or a Class III agent, such as amiodarone. Flecainide tends to have higher and more variable peak concentrations in the elderly (Martin; unpublished work), and the dose level should be reduced in the old. Other drugs that may be effective and reasonably well-tolerated in the elderly are tocainide and mexiletine. Asymptomatic VPCs do not require treatment in the current state of our knowledge, unless they occur after myocardial infarction, when they should be treated as in younger people.

BUNDLE BRANCH BLOCK

The incidence of bundle branch block is reported as being present in 5–10% of the elderly in the community[1,48]. The usual cause of His–Purkinje disease is fibrosis or sclerosis of the conducting system rather than ischaemic heart disease[49,50]. Right bundle branch block appears to have no adverse effect of prognosis[51], but interference with left bundle conduction is associated with a higher risk of death compared with age-matched controls[23,52]. We found that eight of our 106 elderly people in the community had His–Purkinje disease[1]. In the follow-up study 5 years later three of these had died. Of the 90 people with normal conduction, 41 had died and a further six had developed bundle branch block. Thus 28% of the survivors had His–Purkinje conduction block by the age of 80 years or more[2]. 'High risk' bundle branch block was not seen in any of our apparently healthy subjects[1], and may be associated with ischaemic heart disease resulting in a higher mortality[53]. The same authors found that in those without obvious ischaemic heart disease the risks of heart block and death from a bradyarrhythmia were low[53].

ATRIOVENTRICULAR BLOCK

The incidence of first degree heart block increases with advancing age[23]. Reports of the incidence of first degree block in the elderly in general show from between 5 and 10%[21,22]. However, by the age of 90 years or more the incidence is as high as 38%[54]. First degree block is not usually associated with clinical heart disease[22], and when found as an isolated abnormality does not appear to affect the prognosis[55]. Higher degrees of heart block are rarely found in the apparently healthy elderly[1,11], but those elderly patients with complete heart block nearly always have significant symptoms due to their bradyarrhythmia, and should be paced irrespective of their symptomatic status[18].

It has been suggested that the appropriate level of pacemaker implantation should be in the range of 150–200 per million per year[56]. However, these figures do not take into account the proportion of the elderly to the total population, for example 10% and 15% in the USA and the UK, respectively. There is a wide discrepancy in the pacing rates in various countries; that in the USA probably being too high[57], and that in the UK too low[17,56]. Since the elderly comprise the vast majority of those at risk from symptomatic bradyarrhythmias of all kinds, we have suggested that it would be more appropriate to express the optimum pacemaker implantation rate in terms of the 75 years of age and over population, and this should probably be between 1 and 2 per thousand per year[18].

CONCLUSIONS

There are special aspects of arrhythmias in the elderly that are not generally encountered in younger people. These arrhythmias are modified by both degenerative ageing changes and the increased prevalence of multisystem disease. Sinus node disease leads to a loss of the normal dominant cardiac pacemaker, and may cause severe brady-arrhythmias and troublesome paroxysmal tachycardias. Since these arrhythmias may be frequent and symptomatic an aggressive approach should be taken in their management. This includes an active approach to the diagnosis and evaluation of arrhythmias by the widespread availability of ambulatory monitoring and an increase in the pacing rate in some countries, in particular the United Kingdom. Because of the inability of the elderly to handle chemotherapeutic agents as well as their younger counterparts, drug therapy in the elderly can give rise to special problems. All these matters have been fully discussed. However, there is a need for further research into the arrhythmias of the elderly, and the quest for more effective and safer chemotherapy should continue.

References

1. Camm, A. J., Evans, K. E., Ward, D. E. and Martin, A. (1980). The rhythm of the heart in elderly active subjects. *Am. Heart J.*, **99**, 598–603
2. Martin, A., Benbow, L. J., Butrous, G. S., Leach, D. and Camm, A. J. (1984). Five year follow-up of 101 elderly subjects by means of long-term ambulatory cardiac monitoring. *Eur. Heart J.*, **5**, 592–6
3. Davies, M. J. (1984). Pathology of the ageing heart. In Martin, A. and Camm, A. J. (eds.) *Heart Disease in the Elderly*. (Lancaster: MTP Press)
4. Smith, S. A. (1982). Reduced sinus arrhythmia in diabetic autonomic neuropathy: diagnostic value of an age-related normal range. *Br. Med. J.*, **285**, 1599–601
5. O'Brien, I. A. D., O'Hare, P. and Corrall, R. J. M. (1986). Heart rate variability in healthy subjects: effect of age and the derivation of normal ranges for tests of autonomic function. *Br. Heart J.*, **55**, 348–54
6. Smith, S. E. and Smith, S. A. (1981). Heart rate variability in healthy subjects measured with a bedside computer-based technique. *Clin. Sci.*, **61**, 379–83
7. Collins, K. J., Exton-Smith, A. N., James, M. H. and Oliver, D. J. (1980). Functional changes in autonomic nervous responses with ageing. *Age Ageing*, **9**, 17–24
8. Rowe, J. W. and Troen, B. R. (1980). Sympathetic nervous system and aging in man. *Endocrinol. Rev.*, **1**, 167–79
9. Lakatta, E. G. (1980). Age-related alterations in the cardiovascular response to adrenergic mediated stress. *Fed. Proc.*, **39**, 3173–7
10. Lakatta, E. G. (1986). Diminished beta-adrenergic modulation of cardiovascular function in advanced age. *Cardiol. Clin.* **4**, (2) 185–200
11. Fleg, J. L. and Kennedy, H. L. (1982). Cardiac arrhythmias in a healthy elderly population. *Chest*, **81**, 302–7
12. Nelson, R. D., Ezri, M. D. and Denes, P. (1984). Arrhythmias and conduction disturbances in the elderly. In Messerli, F. (ed.) *Cardiovascular Disease in the Elderly*. pp. 83–107. (The Hague: Martinus Nijhoff Publ.)
13. Camm, A. J. and Ward, D. E. (1984). Clinical electrocardiography. In Martin, A. and Camm, A. J. (eds.) *Heart Disease in the Elderly*. pp. 149–86. (Chichester: John Wiley)
14. Martin, A. (1974). The natural history of atrial fibrillation in the elderly. *MD Thesis*: University of London

15. Abdon, N. J. and Nilsson, B. E. (1980). Episodic cardiac arrhythmia and femoral neck fracture. *Acta Med. Scand.*, **208**, 73–6
16. Shaw, D. B. and Kekwick, C. A. (1978). Potential candidates for pacemakers. Survey of heart block and sinoatrial disorder (sick sinus syndrome). *Br. Heart J.*, **40**, 99–105
17. Rickards, A. F. (1984). Where's the block? *Br. Med. J.*, **288**, 737–8
18. Martin, A., Nathan, A. W. and Camm, A. J. (1985). Cardiac pacing in an elderly population with a satellite clinic in a district general hospital. *Age Ageing*, **14**, 333–8
19. Clee, M. D., Smith, N., McNeill, G. P. and Wright, D. S. (1979). Dysrhythmias in apparently healthy elderly subjects. *Age Ageing*, **8**, 173–6
20. Rai, G. S. (1982). Cardiac arrhythmias in the elderly. *Age Ageing*, **11**, 113–15
21. Mihalick, M. J. and Fisch, C. (1977). Electrocardiographic findings in the aged. *Am. Heart J.*, **87**, 117–21
22. Fisch, C., Genovese, P. D., Dyke, R. W., Laramore, W. and Marvel, R. J. (1957). The electrocardiogram in persons over 70. *Geriatrics*, **12**, 616–19
23. Kulbertus, H. E., de Leval-Rutten, F., Albert, A., Dubois, M. and Petit, J. (1981). Electrocardiographic changes occurring with advancing age. In Wellens, H. J. J. and Kulbertus, H. E. (eds.) *What's New in Electrocardiography*. pp. 300–14. (The Hague: Martinus Nijhoff Publ.)
24. Wolf, P. A., Kerzner, L. J., Hiltbrunner, A. V. and Kannel, W. B. (1984). Stroke resulting from nonvalvular atrial fibrillation. *J. Am. Geriat. Soc.*, **32**, 751–7
25. Martin, A., Benbow, L. J., Leach, C. and Bailey, R. J. (1986). Comparison of amiodarone and disopyramide in the control of paroxysmal atrial fibrillation and atrial flutter. *Br. J. Clin. Pract.*, **40**(4) (Suppl. 44)
26. Wolf, P. A., Dawber, T. R., Thomas, Jr, H. E. and Kannel, W. B. (1978). Epidemiologic assessment of chronic atrial fibrillation and risk of stroke: the Framingham study. *Neurology (Minneap.)*, **28**, 973–7
27. Wilson, D. B. (1985). Chronic atrial fibrillation in the elderly: risks vs benefits of long-term anticoagulation. *J. Am. Geriat. Soc.*, **33**, 298–302
28. Treseder, A. S., Sastry, B. S. D., Thomas, T. P. L., Yates, M. A. and Pathy, M. S. J. (1986). Atrial fibrillation and stroke in elderly hospitalised patients. *Age Ageing*, **15**, 89–92
29. Caplan, L. R., D'Cruz, I., Hier, D. B., Reddy, H. and Shah, S. (1986). Atrial size, atrial fibrillation, and stroke. *Ann. Neurol.*, **19**, 158–61
30. Ward, D. E., Camm, A. J. and Spurrell, R. A. J. (1980). Clinical anti-arrhythmic effects of amiodarone in patients with resistant paroxysmal tachycardias. *Br. Heart J.*, **44**, 91–5
31. Lloyd, E. A. and Mabin, T. A. (1983). Amiodarone in the treatment of patients with refractory symptomatic ventricular and supraventricular arrhythmias. *SA Med. J.*, **63**, 759–63
32. Shamroth, L. (1971). Immediate effects of intravenous verapamil on atrial fibrillation. *Cardiovasc. Res.*, **5**, 419–24
33. Klein, G. J., Twum-Barima, Y., Gulamhusein, G., Carruthers, S. G. and Donner, A. P. (1984). Verapamil in chronic atrial fibrillation: variable patterns of response in ventricular rate. *Clin. Cardiol.*, **7**, 474–83
34. Nathan, A. W., Bennett, D. H., Ward, D. E., Bexton, R. S. and Camm, A. J. (1984) Catheter ablation of the atrioventricular junction. *Lancet*, i, 1280–4
35. Ward, D. E., Hellestrand, K. J., Nathan, A. W. and Camm, A. J. (1983). Transvenous ablation of atrioventricular conduction – clinical experience in patients with refractory supraventricular tachycardias. *J. Am. Coll. Cardiol.*, **1**, 635–8
36. McCarthy, S. T., McCarthy, G. L., John, S., Chadwick, D. and Wollner, L. (1986). Amiodarone as a treatment for atrial fibrillation refractory to digoxin therapy. *Br. J. Clin. Pract.*, **40**, 4 (Suppl. 44)
37. Dall, J. L. C. (1970). Maintenance digoxin in elderly patients. *Br. Med. J.*, **2**, 705–6
38. Rowland, E., McKenna, W. J. and Krikler, D. M. (1986). Amiodarone for the conversion of established atrial fibrillation and flutter. *Br. J. Clin. Pract.*, **40**, 4 (Suppl. 44)

39. Wang, R., Camm, A. J., Ward, D., Washington, H. and Martin, A. (1980). Treatment of chronic atrial fibrillation in the elderly, assessed by ambulatory electrocardiographic monitoring. *J. Am. Geriat. Soc.*, **28**, 529–34
40. Southall, D. P., Johnston, F., Shinebourne, E. A. and Johnston, P. G. B. (1981). 24-hour electrocardiographic study of heart rate and rhythm patterns in population of healthy children. *Br. Heart J.*, **45**, 281–4
41. Brodsky, M., Wu, D. and Denes, P. (1977). Arrhythmias documented by 24-hour continuous electrocardiographic monitoring in 50 male medical students without apparent heart disease. *Am. J. Cardiol.*, **39**, 390–5
42. Clarke. J. M., Hamer, J., Shelton, J. R., Taylor, S. and Venning, G. R. (1976). The rhythm of the normal human heart. *Lancet*, **2**, 508–11
43. Lown, B. and Wolf, M. (1971). Approaches to sudden death in coronary heart disease. *Circulation*, **44**, 130–5
44. The Coronary Drug Project Research Group (1973). Prognostic importance of premature beats following myocardial infarction. *J. Am. Med. Assoc.*, **226**, 1116–24
45. Kotler, M. N., Tabatznik, B., Mower, M. M. and Tominaga, S. (1973). Prognostic significance of ventricular ectopic beats with respect to sudden death in the late postinfarction period. *Circulation*, **47**, 959–66
46. Crow, R., Prineas, R. and Blackburn, H. (1981). The prognostic significance of ventricular ectopic beats among the apparently healthy. *Am. Heart. J.*, **101**, 244–8
47. Rabkin, S. W., Mathewson, F. A. L. and Tate, R. B. (1981). Relationship of ventricular ectopy in men without apparent heart disease to occurrence of ischaemic heart disease and sudden death. *Am. Heart J.*, **101**, 135–42
48. Campbell, A., Caird, F. I. and Jackson, T. F. M. (1974). Prevalence of abnormalities of the electrocardiogram in old people. *Br. Heart J.*, **36**, 1005–9
49. Lev, M. (1964). Anatomic basis for atrioventricular block. *Am. J. Med.*, **37**, 742–50
50. Lenegre, J. (1964). Etiology and pathology of bilateral bundle branch block in relation to complete heart block. *Progr. Cardiovasc. Dis.*, **6**, 409–13
51. Fleg, J. L., Das, D. N. and Lakatta, E. G., (1983). Right bundle branch block: long-term prognosis in apparently healthy men. *J. Am. Coll. Cardiol.*, **1**, 887–93
52. Caird, F. I., Campbell, A. and Jackson, T. F. M. (1974). Significance of abnormalities of the electrocardiogram in old people. *Br. Heart J.*, **36**, 1012–16
53. McAnulty, J. H., Rahimtoola, S. H., Murphy, E., DeMots, H., Ritzman, L., Kanarek, P. E. and Kauffman, S. (1982). Natural history of 'high-risk' bundle branch block. *N. Engl. J. Med.*, **307**, 137–43
54. Bowers, D. (1969). Electrogram of nonagenarians. *Geriatrics*, **24**, 89–93
55. Rodstein, M., Brown, M. and Wolloch, L. (1968). First degree atrio–ventricular heart block in the aged. *Geriatrics*, **23**, 159–62
56. Sowton, E. (1976). Use of cardiac pacemakers in Britain. *Br. Med. J.*, **2**, 1182–4
57. Selzer, A. (1982). Too many pacemakers. *N. Engl. J. Med.*, **307**, 183–4

13
Normal and abnormal responses of cardiac rhythm to spontaneous physiological manoeuvres

D. MEHTA, D. E. WARD AND A. J. CAMM

INTRODUCTION

The autonomic nervous system plays an important role in the regulation of the rate of cardiac impulse formation, rate of spread of excitation and the contractility of the atria and ventricles. Both the sympathetic and the parasympathetic nerves influence the SA node, AV node, atrial and ventricular myocardium. The anatomy of the autonomic innervation of the heart has been described, in detail, elsewhere (Chapter 4). The myocardium and conduction system in addition respond directly to circulating catecholamines.

By virtue of its rich autonomic supply, the heart responds to varied physiological manoeuvres which reflexly alter the autonomic tone. At times, the cardiac responses to these physical manoeuvres, mediated by alteration of autonomic tone, are so exaggerated as to directly cause symptomatic arrhythmias. In this chapter, the possible mechanism and clinical significance of the changes in cardiac rhythm associated with common physical manoeuvres of daily living are discussed. Abnormal responses of cardiac rhythm to these physical manoeuvres are reviewed. Although carotid sinus stimulation and eye ball pressure affect cardiac rhythm, they are not part of day to day living and have not been included in this review.

CHANGE OF POSTURE

Changes in posture can precipitate and aggravate disturbances of cardiac rhythm by reflex alterations in the blood pressure and heart rate. Assumption of an upright posture during sinus rhythm leads to diminished central blood volume and reduction of cardiac output by 20–30%. This is due to the venous pooling in the lower limbs and results in a reflex increase in sinus rate, vasoconstriction of the resistance vessels, reduction of peripheral blood flow and maintenance of the blood supply to essential organs[1-3]. The above responses are mediated by increased sympathetic drive[4], and parasympathetic withdrawal, both of which enhance AV nodal conduction.

During supraventricular tachycardia the above responses are exaggerated. Assumption of an upright posture during tachycardia causes a more marked fall in blood pressure, and thus reflexly more marked enhancement of AV nodal conduction as shown by a shortening of the AH interval[5]. As AV nodal conduction velocity is a major determinant of the rate of AV re-entrant tachycardia, marked acceleration occurs upon standing. Curry et al.[5], showed that in such patients, raising the head end of the patient by 45° increased the tachycardia rate and shortened the AH interval, while the atrial and ventricular conduction times were essentially unchanged. Hammill et al.[6], demonstrated that in two of their patients re-entrant supraventricular tachycardia was only sustained in the upright position. Saksena et al.[7], reported a patient with automatic right atrial tachycardia that could only be sustained during the sitting or standing position. Patients with supraventricular tachycardia who are not symptomatic in the supine position might become syncopal or near syncopal on assuming the upright position. This is related to the postural decrease in cardiac output which is exaggerated by decrease in ventricular filling time caused by an increase in rate on standing. In a series of 59 patients with supraventricular tachycardia investigated by Hammill et al.[6], almost all patients developed symptoms of lightheadedness, near syncope or syncope in an upright position, which was associated with an increase in tachycardia rate and relative hypotension.

Recumbent body position is associated with increased venous return and blood pressure and a reflex bradycardia[1-3]. The reflex change in heart rate is mediated by increased vagal tone and a decreased sympathetic drive (in response to increase in blood pressure). In patients with nodal or atrioventricular tachycardias these changes in autonomic tone result in a decrease of rate and at times termination of tachycardia. Haemodynamic changes immediately after the onset of tachycardia also favour its termination. With the onset of an attack there is an initial fall in blood pressure followed by a reflex increase before it stabilizes[8,9]. The fall, and thus the reflex response, is more pronounced in the upright position. The phase of reflex increase in blood pressure results in a baroreceptor-mediated vagotonia which also decreases the rate and might terminate a tachycardia[10]. The likelihood of spontaneous termination is greatest if the tachycardia starts in a upright position and the patient lies down soon after the onset of the attack[10].

Atrial and ventricular arrhythmias have been reported to be precipitated or terminated by a change of posture, although this seems to be a rare phenomenon as indicated by few case reports. Atrial tachyarrhythmia caused by lying in the left lateral position has been reported in two patients both with mitral valve prolapse syndrome[11,12].

Peters and Penner[13] reported a case of ventricular tachycardia in whom arrhythmia occurred only in a standing position. Interestingly, Ohe *et al.*[14], have reported a case in whom ventricular tachycardia was initiated in the supine position and terminated by standing. Tachy-arrhythmias initiated with change of posture could be related to changes in autonomic tone or cardiac output. Ohe *et al.*[14], in their patient found that initiation of tachycardia was associated with an increase in left ventricular size. Volume overloading causing stretching was postulated as precipitating ventricular tachycardia. Manoeuvres which were associated with decrease in cavity size as judged echocardiographically, e.g. standing and phase II of Valsalva, terminated the attack. As atropine did not modify the arrhythmia, a reflex vagal mechanism seemed unlikely.

Conduction disturbances have also been reported with a change of posture. A prolonged PR interval (> 0.2 s) in the supine position which becomes normal on standing is seen in a small percentage of a healthy young population. Manning *et al.*[15] found the incidence to be 0.3% in a series of 19 000 healthy young air crew applicants. In an earlier publication they reported four cases with a PR interval of greater than 0.24 seconds in a recumbent position which normalized on standing without any significant change in heart rate[16]. It seems to be an innocent phenomenon possibly related to increased vagal tone as atropine also reduced the PR interval to normal in these subjects[15]. Increased sympathetic tone on standing might also enhance AV nodal conduction. Interestingly, there is one report in the literature of second degree heart block precipitated by standing, so-called 'postural heart block'[17]. The patient presented with orthostatic syncope and was found to have second degree heart block only on standing. At electrophysiology study he was found to have a prolonged HV time, thus the delay in conduction was infra-Hisian and unlikely to be related to vagal tone.

In patients with ventricular pre-excitation, the delta wave on the electrocardiogram may become diminished or more pronounced on standing[18]. Increased sympathetic tone on standing may enhance conduction in both the anomalous pathway and the normal pathway, thereby altering the degree of fusion.

RESPIRATION

In normal individuals respiration is accompanied by variation in the frequency of pacemaker discharge from the sinoatrial node. The heart rate accelerates during inspiration and slows during expiration with little or no alteration in the P wave morphology, PR interval or QRS complex. If the variation between the longest and the shortest cycles exceeds 0.12 s sinus arrhythmia is said to be present[19,20]. These changes have been found to be due to the rhythmic fluctuations in sympathetic and vagal tone, the latter being mediated by Bainbridge's reflex[20,21]. Sinus arrhythmia is a normal finding in children and young adults, and tends to decrease or disappear with advancing age[19]. The variation in heart rate with respiration increases with factors which increase vagal tone. This has been used as a non-invasive method of testing the integrity of the parasympathetic control of the heart[22]. In animals division or cooling of the vagi abolishes respiratory sinus arrhythmia. It is also absent in the transplanted human hearts as they lack innervation[23].

At times deep inspiration has been noticed to lead to ectopic atrial rhythms (Figure 13.1). By reflex enhancement of vagal tone which occurs during expiration deep breathing helps in terminating supraventricular tachycardias. Termination of tachycardia with respiration has been uniformly noted to occur during the expiratory phase[24]. This is probably related to expiratory enhancemeht of vagal tone due to two mechanisms. First, during inspiration pulmonary stretch receptors cause a reduction in the efferent vagal tone, expiration reverses this process[21]. Second, compared to inspiration there is a relative rise in blood pressure during expiration[25], this enhances vagal tone via carotid baroreceptors. The rise in blood pressure is more during supine body position. Waxman et al.[24], while studying the effects of deep respiration on paroxysmal supraventricular tachycardias, demonstrated consistent termination of tachycardia in eight of 11 patients. As expected all terminations occurred during expiration.

In some patients with anomalous pathways and intermittent pre-excitation, the latter has been noticed to be present only during deep inspiration. This is thought to be due to the increase in vagal tone at end-inspiration which either delays AV conduction, thereby allowing more ventricle to be activated by the accessory pathway, or by vagal activation of accessory pathway conduction[18].

EXERCISE

Physical exercise can precipitate disturbances of cardiac rhythm and in other instances abolish cardiac arrhythmias that are present at rest[27]. As exercise precipitates clinical arrhythmias in some patients, exercise testing has become a routine stress manoeuvre for the investigation of arrhythmias (Figures 13.2 and 13.3).

In a series of 625 patients, Jelinek and Lown[28] found that exercise increased the prevalence of supraventricular premature beats 3-fold, and atrial tachycardias, atrial flutter and atrial fibrillation 2-fold. The occurrence of ventricular couplets and ventricular tachycardia was increased by a factor of 8, while the detection of isolated ventricular premature beats was increased by a factor of 1.7. Although both atrial and ventricular arrhythmias can be induced by exercise, the primary emphasis has always been laid on exercise-induced ventricular arrhythmias which are more frequent and are closely related to ischaemic heart disease, cardiomyopathy and decreased long term survival.

The precise mechanism responsible for exercise-induced cardiac

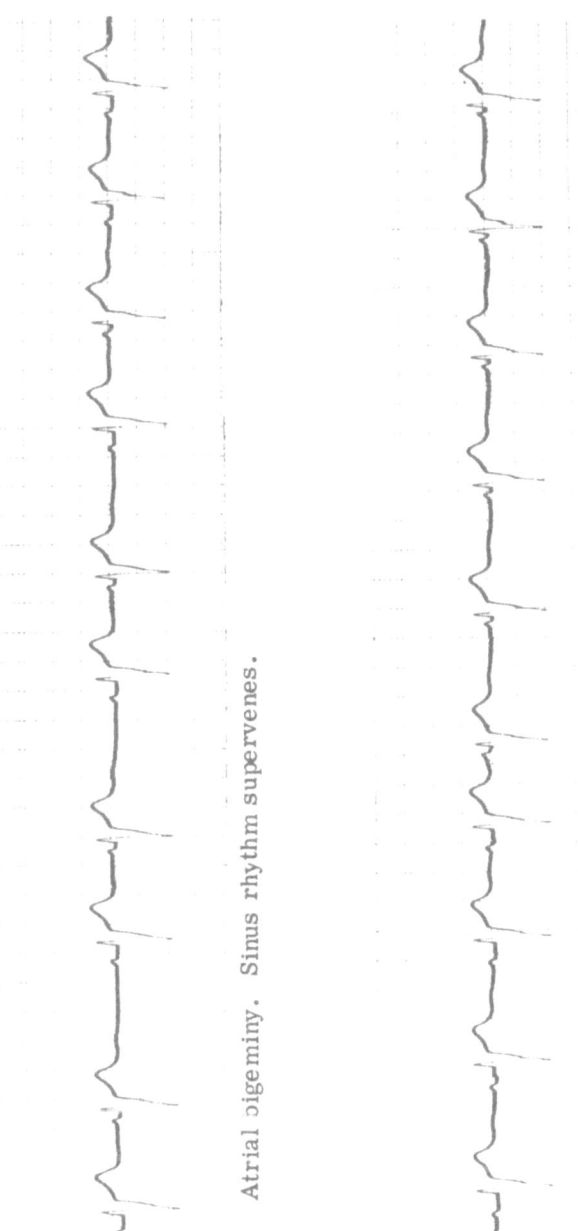

Atrial bigeminy. Sinus rhythm supervenes.

Deep inspiration results in emergence of an idio-atrial rhythm.

Figure 13.1 Top trace shows frequent atrial premature beats (2nd, 4th and 6th). Deep inspiration (lower trace) results in emergence of atrial rhythm as identified by a change in P wave morphology and a shorter PR interval. This is unlikely to be functional rhythm with iso-rhythmic dissociation of P waves as first beat of ectopic rhythm is premature

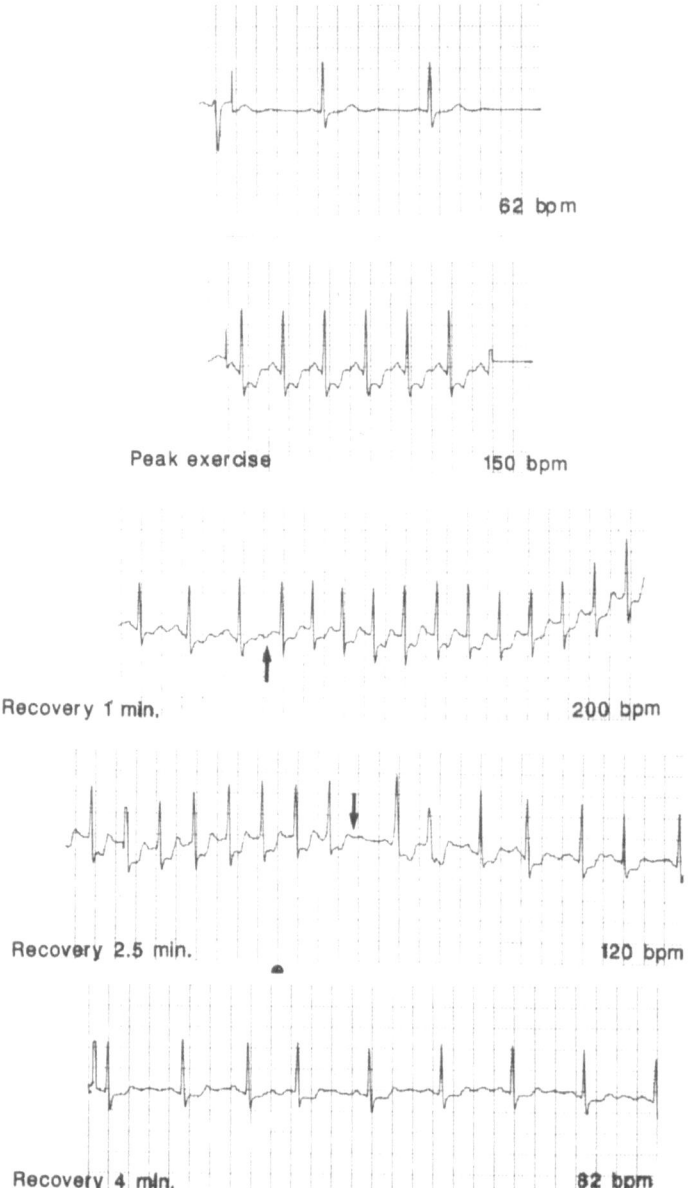

62 bpm

Peak exercise   150 bpm

Recovery 1 min.   200 bpm

Recovery 2.5 min.   120 bpm

Recovery 4 min.   82 bpm

Figure 13.2 Exercise induced paroxysmal supraventricular tachycardia. Tachycardia starts 1 min into recovery and stops spontaneously. Onset and termination are shown by arrows

216

EXERCISE INDUCED VENTRICULAR ARRHYTHMIAS

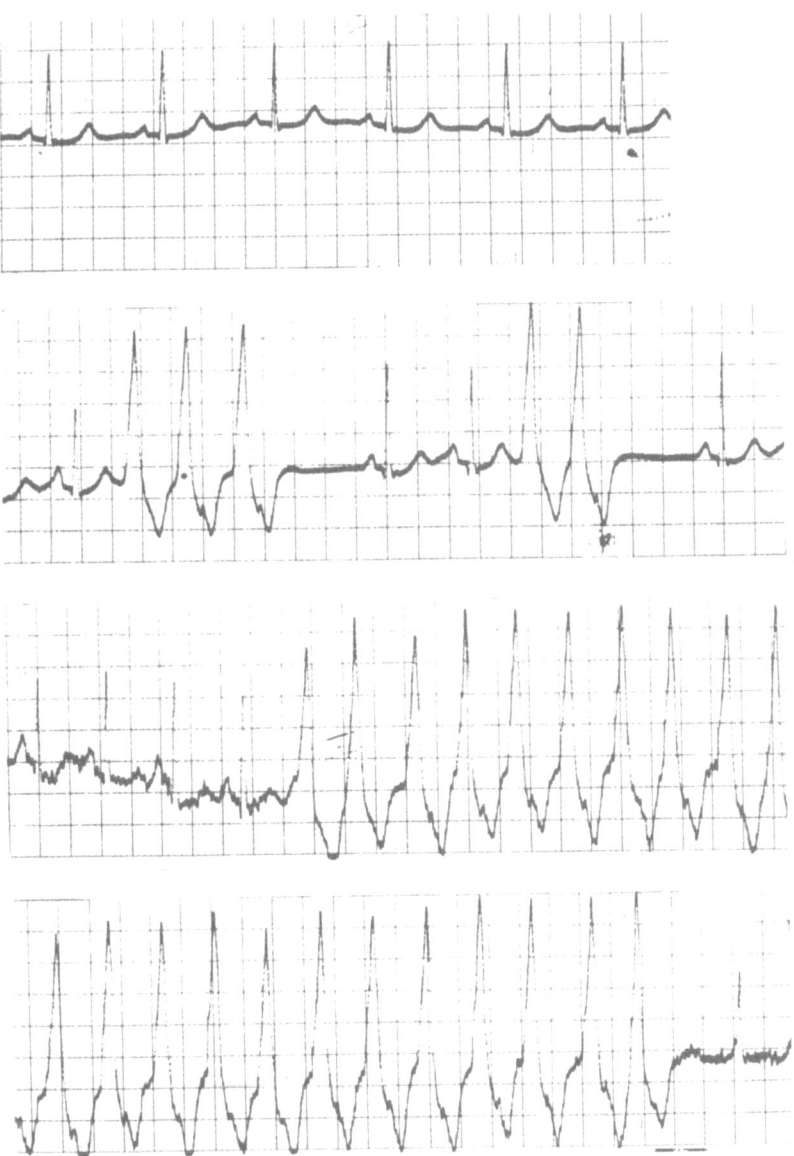

Figure 13.3 Exercise results in frequent couplets and triplets of ventricular premature beats and finally ventricular tachycardia. Tachycardia stops spontaneously during the recovery phase (bottom trace)

rhythm disturbances remains uncertain. However, from the available data the following mechanisms seem likely[29]:

(1) Exercise is associated with increased sympathetic and decreased parasympathetic activity. Increased sympathetic tone enhances phase 4 depolarization of the cardiac action potential which provokes spontaneous discharge and increases automaticity[30-32]. Arrhythmias related to this mechanism cannot usually be initiated by programmed electrical stimulation but isoprenaline infusion might precipitate them. Myocardial ischaemia caused by coronary artery disease may predispose to increased automaticity.

(2) Increased heart rate, systolic blood pressure and cardiac contractility during exercise increase myocardial oxygen demand and might result in relative myocardial hypoxia, especially in patients with ischaemic artery disease. Non-uniform ischaemia, as in coronary heart disease, may result in regional blocks in conduction and/or temporal dispersion of depolarization and repolarization, predisposing to re-entry[33].

(3) Triggered activity related to delayed after-depolarizations has also been suggested as a possible mechanism for exercise-induced ventricular tachycardias[34].

Paroxysmal atrial tachycardia (Figure 13.2), atrial flutter and fibrillation have all been reported to be occasionally precipitated by exercise[27]. Gooch[35], reported provocation of sustained atrial arrhythmias in only five out of 3000 patients who underwent exercise testing. Levy and Broustet[36], exercised 42 of their patients with Wolff–Parkinson–White syndrome, who were known to have supraventricular tachycardia, and they were able to precipitate tachycardia only in four patients (9.5%). In two cases tachycardia occurred during exercise and two during recovery. One patient developed atrial fibrillation with pre-excitation during exercise testing. However, Strasberg et al.[37], could not provoke any tachycardia in 54 patients with Wolff–Parkinson–White syndrome who were known to have re-entrant tachycardias. In both the studies it was noticed that, in this group of patients, exercise progressively abolished pre-excitation. This phenomenon is thought to be due to increased β-sympathetic tone and vagolysis both leading to increased AV nodal contribution to ventricular activation. On the other hand sudden normalization of the QRS complex early during exercise in patients with pre-excitation is usually due to sinus tachycardia exceeding the long refractory period of the anomalous pathway[36,37].

In patients with primary sinus node disease the heart rate response to exercise has been shown to be attenuated compared to normal subjects[38,39]. Thus, exercise testing may help in identifying patients with suspected sinus node disease in whom the disorder is of extrinsic origin, as the rate response to exercise is relatively normal in these individuals[40].

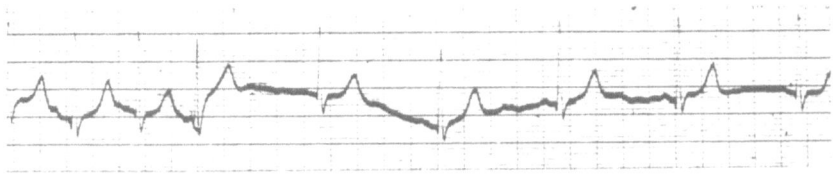

2:1 SINO-ATRIAL BLOCK OCCURRING ON EXERCISE

Figure 13.4   Exercise-induced sinoatrial block: Apparent sinoatrial block occurs after the third sinus beat. The RR interval before the block is 0.46 seconds and after the block is 0.92 seconds. This was seen during an exercise test

Unlike atrial arrhythmias induced by exercise which are usually not associated with an identifiable morphological lesion, an underlying cause such as coronary artery disease, cardiomyopathy or mitral valve prolapse is frequently found with exercise-induced ventricular arrhythmias[41]. The diagnosis of coronary artery disease is almost certain when exercise induced arrhythmia is preceded by marked ST segment alterations. Goldschlager *et al.*[42], found significant coronary artery disease in 89% of their patients with exercise-induced ventricular premature beats. In another study of 360 patients, 117 had exercise-induced ventricular arrhythmias of which 68% were found to have coronary artery disease[43]. The occurrence of ventricular arrhythmia during exercise in patients with coronary artery disease suggests multivessel disease and/or impaired left ventricular function[43-45], and is associated with an increased risk of cardiac events and decreased survival[45, 46.]

In patients with hypertrophic cardiomyopathy most sudden deaths are related to ventricular arrhythmias. Exercise was shown to provoke arrhythmias in 66 and 70% of these patients in two separate studies[47,48]. The frequency of exercise related arrhythmias was found to be significantly higher in patients with obstructive lesions, and thus exercise, like Holter monitoring, helps in identifying patients with more severe disease and those at greater risk.

Exercise related conduction abnormalities, though known, are a rare phenomenon. First degree heart block has occasionally been observed during the immediate postexercise period and is probably related to increased vagal tone[27]. Meytes *et al.*[49], found three healthy athletes in a group of 126 who developed Wenckebach atrioventricular block during vigorous exercise. This has also been thought to be related to increased vagal tone[49,50]. We have seen a patient who developed a transient 2:1 sinoatrial block on exercise, possibly by a similar mechanism (Figure 13.4). Development of Mobitz type II and bundle branch block during exercise is also known, the latter being more common. Exercise-induced bundle branch block is usually a rate-related phenomenon, and when seen can often be reproduced by atropine administration. Its significance in relation to diseases of the conduction system is not known.

It is a common observation that atrial and ventricular premature

219

beats present at rest might be abolished by exercise. This may be related to the phenomenon of overdrive suppression[51], or changes in automaticity caused by sinus tachycardia.

DIVING/FACE IMMERSION

Submersion of the nose or mouth in water produces a complex cardiovascular reflex response (diving reflex) which comprises peripheral vasoconstriction, decreased heart rate, decreased cardiac output and some increase in blood pressure[52-54]. It is an adaptive response in vertebrates which conserves oxygen when availability is low, as in the submerged state. It has been extensively studied in ducks, where the responses are particularly marked allowing a diving time of up to 15 min[52-55]. In man diving, or apnoeic facial immersion, produced a response identical to that in ducks, although less intense, resulting in 15–30% decrease in heart rate (compared to 80% decrease in heart rate seen in ducks and seals) and a proportionate decrease in cardiac output. As expected these physiological responses are associated with some electrocardiographic changes. Sinus bradycardia, sinus arrhythmia, atrioventricular block, atrioventricular nodal rhythm and idioventricular rhythm, all of which indicate vagotonic response, have been recorded in apparently normal divers[56].

Facial wetting seems to be an essential sensory component of the reflex, as the response is absent if the face is covered by polyethylene before submersion[53,57]. The site of application of a wet cold stimulus is important in the genesis of this bradycardic response, as illustrated by the cold pressor test where immersion of hands in cold water produces a tachycardia[58]. Detailed studies of the heart rate response to facial immersion have shown that there is an initial tachycardia lasting a few seconds which is followed by a bradycardia, and there is an inverse relationship between water temperature and the degree of bradycardia[59,60]. The afferent impulses for this reflex are carried by the trigeminal nerve, and bilateral section of this nerve in ducks has been shown to abolish all cardiovascular responses to diving[61]. The efferent response leading to bradycardia is associated with a peripheral pressor response and is primarily mediated by the vagus. These vagotonic actions (bradycardia and increased blood pressure) may effect a termination of supraventricular tachycardias. In contrast, carotid stimulation causes bradycardia accompanied by decreased vasomotor tone.

The diving reflex has been used for the termination of supraventricular tachycardias (Figure 13.5). It is safer than carotid sinus massage which is associated with a danger of diminished cerebral blood flow, hypotension and ventricular arrhythmias[62]. Wildenthal et al.[63], were able to terminate supraventricular tachycardias in all seven patients in whom facial submersion was tried. Whayne and Killip[58], tried facial submersion in six patients with premature ventricular contractions, no change in frequency was seen in four, ventricular premature contractions were

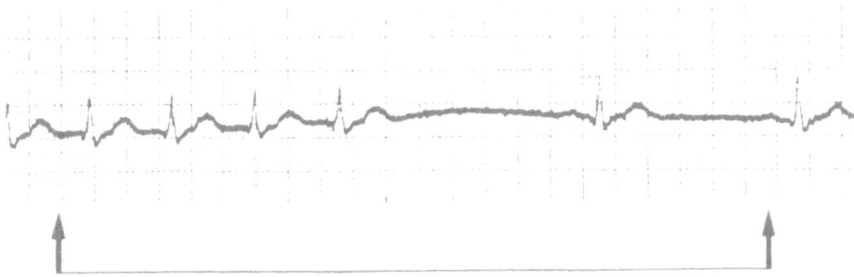

THE DIVING REFLEX TERMINATING ATRIOVENTRICULAR
REENTRANT TACHYCARDIA

Figure 13.5 Termination of a supraventricular tachycardia during face immersion: Duration of face immersion is indicated by arrows

abolished in one and increased in frequency in the other. In the clinical setting facial submersion has not been associated with dangerous untoward effects although periods of sinus arrest of up to 4 s and nodal rhythm and escape beats, have been described during apnoeic manoeuvres of various types[64,65]. Wolf[65], speculated that the reflex response to immersion may be implicated as a cause of sudden death in patients with heart disease. He suggested that individuals with abnormalities of AV nodal conduction may be highly susceptible to immersion in water and other facial stimuli.

COUGHING

Coughing is a protective reflex caused by an irritant stimulus to the respiratory passages below the level of the pharynx. In normal subjects it produces changes in cardiac rhythm similar to those seen with the Valsalva manoeuvre. Syncope due to bradyarrhythmias is a well-documented complication of this protective reflex[66-72]. In addition there are isolated case reports in the literature of coughing terminating tachyarrhythmias.

Cough syncope is usually seen after a prolonged bout of violent coughing especially in patients with chronic obstructive lung disease[73]. In the cases reported in the literature the aetiology of decreased cerebral perfusion has been found to be pulmonary, vascular or cardiac. Sharpey-Shafer[74], noted a markedly raised intrathoracic pressure during coughing in his patient with cough syncope, and concluded that this syndrome resulted from raised intrathoracic pressure causing a reduced venous return and decreased cardiac output. McIntosh et al.[66] suggested that the raised intrathoracic pressure was transmitted to the cerebrospinal fluid, increasing intracranial pressure and thus squeezing blood out of the cerebral circulation. Strauss et al.[69], reported a patient with cough syncope in whom decreased cerebral blood flow during coughing was due to bilateral carotid stenosis. Wenger *et al.*[70], have described a case of hypersensitive carotid sinus syndrome who presented with cough syncope – denervation of the carotid sinus relieved symptoms. In two separate case reports cough syncope has been proved to be directly due to atrioventricular block, the symptoms were abolished by pacing[71,72] (Figure 13.6). In these cases the underlying mechanism was postulated to be a vagal reflex, because atrioventricular block during coughing was abolished by atropine. The vagus carries afferents from the pulmonary stretch and pain receptors[75], and it seems likely that hypersensitive bronchopulmonary reflexes during coughing cause excessive stimulation of the vagus and result in atrioventricular block. However, in the case reported by Hart *et al.*[71], vagal manoeuvres such as Valsalva, carotid massage and eye ball pressure did not reproduce the heart block. Possibly, in these patients the hypersensitivity was limited to the afferent limb of the reflex arc, for example over-sensitive pulmonary stretch receptors. We have also observed heart block during vomiting (Figure 13.7). Two similar cases in whom symptomatic heart block followed nausea and vomiting were reported by Talwar *et al.*[76], who also postulated a vagally mediated reflex, because in one of their patients atropine reversed the heart block.

Termination of tachyarrhythmias with coughing has also been reported. Wei *et al.*[77], reported a patient in whom coughing repeatedly terminated a drug resistant ventricular tachycardia. In a large retrospective study Caldwell *et al.*[78], found that coughing terminated ventricular tachycardias in six patients. Interestingly, Francis *et al.*[79], reported a patient with junctional tachycardia with functional bundle branch block in whom coughing did not affect the tachycardia but interrupted aberrancy.

VALSALVA MANOEUVRE

The Valsalva manoeuvre is reproduced during numerous daily activities such as lifting, coughing, pushing, vomiting, defaecation etc. Changes in cardiac rhythm are common during manoeuvres involving Valsalva-like straining, though these changes often go unnoticed and are not usually symptomatic[80-82]. In a study involving 75 French horn players changes suggestive of wandering atrial pacemaker were noticed in 37, and one subject developed second degree heart block whilst blowing the instrument[83]. None of these changes was associated with any symptoms. Due to the reflex cardiovascular changes during the Valsalva manoeuvre which are dependent on an intact autonomic nerve supply it has become an important investigative tool in cardiology.

The manoeuvre involves a strain phase and a relaxation phase. During the strain phase intrathoracic pressure is increased due to the contraction of expiratory muscles against closed airways. This increased pressure is transmitted to the right atrium and large veins resulting in a decrease in venous return and a fall in stroke volume. The systemic arterial

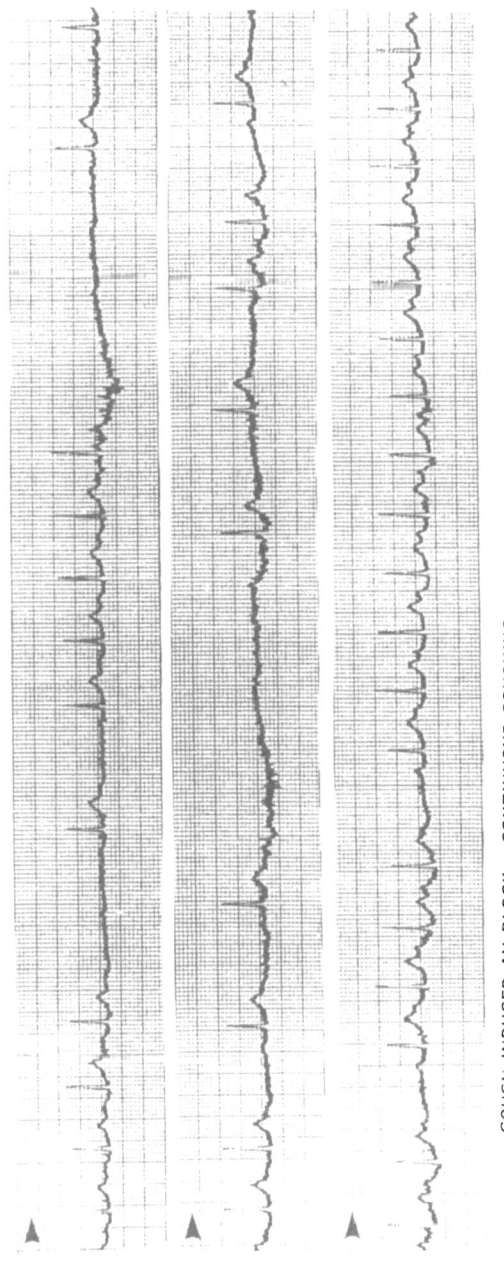

COUGH INDUCED AV BLOCK.   CONTINUOUS COUGHING

Figure 13.6 Electrocardiagram of a patient with cough syncope during a bout of coughing. Arrows indicate continuous recording. There is a gradual accommodation of the reflex as atrioventricular block subsides with continuous coughing

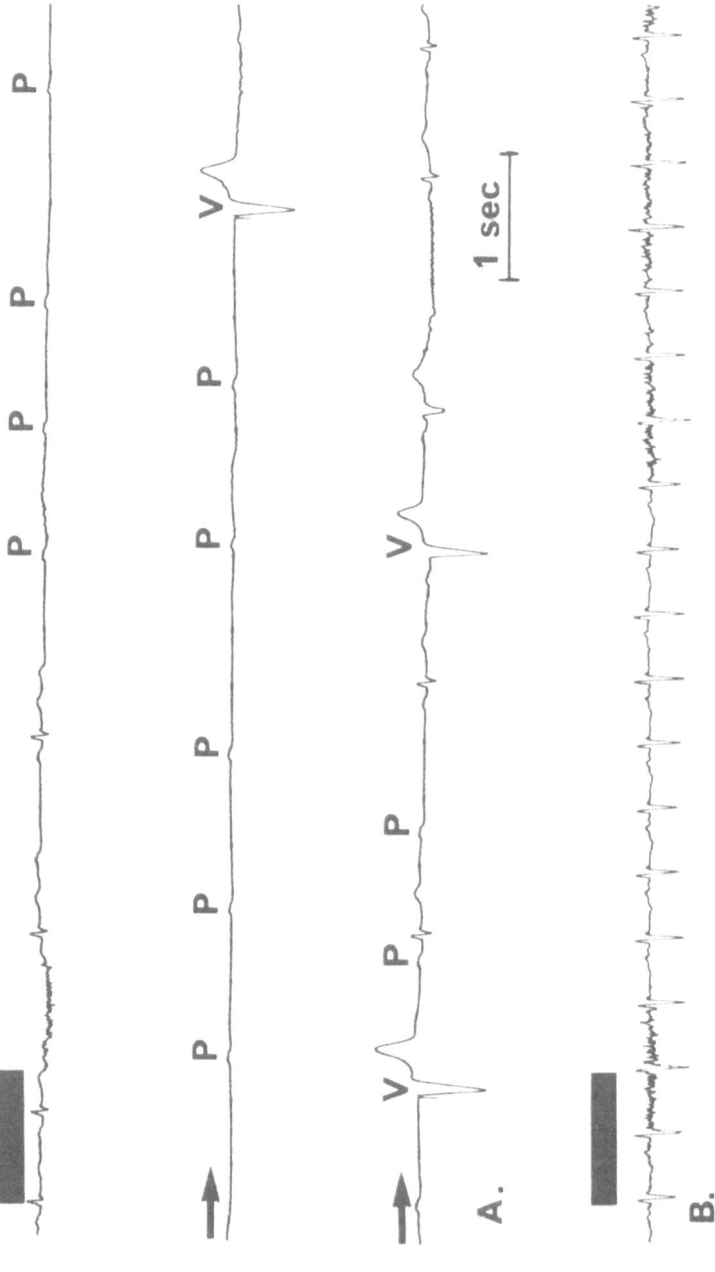

Figure 13.7 **A:** Electrocardiogram during induced vomiting. Arrows indicate continuous recording. Onset of vomiting (bar) is associated with complete atrioventricular block, sinus bradycardia and ventricular asystole. Fixed rate ventricular pacing was started after 15 sec, (P= p waves, V= ventricular paced beats). **B:** Induced vomiting after prior administration of atropine fails to show conduction abnormality

(systolic and pulse) pressures fall, and within 6–7 seconds there is a baroreceptor-mediated increase in heart rate and an increase in peripheral vascular resistance[84]. Due to decreased venous return the heart size decreases, which has been shown radiologically, angiographically[85] and echocardiographically[86,87]. Robertson *et al.*[86], have shown a 11.2% decrease in left ventricular end-diastolic and a 9.4% decrease in end-systolic volumes, with a 29% decrease in stroke volume during the strain phase of the Valsalva manoeuvre.

During the relaxation phase the circulatory changes of the strain phase are reversed. An increase in venous return causes an increase in stroke volume and arterial pressure[84]. Within 5 seconds of release there is an overshoot of arterial pressure due to increased cardiac output, whilst vasoconstriction persists. This results in stimulation of aortic and carotid baroreceptors and a reflex vagus-mediated cardiac slowing and inhibition of vasoconstriction. Pressure overshoot during this phase is a qualitative index of vasoconstrictor tone. A pulse pressure of greater than control within 5 seconds of release of the strain is considered to represent a normal response[88].

Autonomic reflex responses prevent the fall of blood pressure during the strain phase and cause a post release overshoot of blood pressure and reflex bradycardia. There is a direct relationship between the changes in rate and blood pressure during the strain and the release phases[88]. If the autonomic system is diseased, as in diabetic neuropathy[89], or is pharmacologically blocked by atropine and propranolol[84], the decrease of blood pressure during the strain phase is exaggerated and reflex tachycardia is absent. If only atropine is given the vagal bradycardia is prevented and the sympathetic reflex rise of arterial pressure is increased and prolonged[84]. Transplanted denervated hearts lack reflex heart rate, and blood pressure changes seen with the Valsalva manoeuvre indicating that the above changes are neurologically mediated[23].

The Valsalva manoeuvre has proven to be an easy non-invasive means of assessing autonomic function[90], and has been used to evaluate rate-related phenomena such as bundle branch blocks which appear during the strain phase of the manoeuvre when the heart rate is increased, and then disappear during the relaxation phase when the rate slows. During the Valsalva manoeuvre supraventricular tachycardias may slow or terminate. This effect has diagnostic and therapeutic significance. Usually the tachycardia terminates during the parasympathetic pre-dominant (relaxation) phase, but occasionally termination occurs during the strain phase. When used clinically to terminate supraventricular tachycardia, during the relaxation phase the patient should be recumbent to minimize sympathetic tone and optimize the chance of success[91].

Although termination of a tachycardia with the Valsalva manoeuvre was previously used to differentiate wide QRS complex supraventricular tachycardias from ventricular tachycardias it has recently been documented that ventricular tachycardias may also terminate with the Valsalva manoeuvre[92]. Termination of ventricular tachycardias has been noticed to occur during strain phase, and is thought to be related to the decrease in heart size. Waxman et al.[92], reported successful termination of ventricular tachycardia in nine of their 11 patients in whom it was tried, all terminations occurred during the strain phase and were associated with a decrease in left ventricular size at echocardiography.

SWALLOWING

Swallowing in normal subjects produces a transient acceleration of the cardiac rate[93]. Symptomatic tachycardias and bradycardias have been reported with this reflex function. Limited investigations available in the reported cases give clues to the possible mechanisms of these rhythm disturbances.

Bradycardia has been more frequently reported. There are about 30 cases in the literature of this well established, albeit rare, complication of swallowing frequently called 'swallowing syncope' or 'deglutition syncope'. Most cases have been due to atrioventricular block[94-98], with a few being due to sinus bradycardia[99,100], sinus arrest or sinoatrial block[101]. Interestingly, most cases have been associated with oesophageal diseases such as diverticulae[94,101], strictures and spasms[94], hiatus herniae[95,98], or carcinomatosis[100]. Distension of the oesophagus seems to be the precipitating event, as cardiac slowing in some of the reported cases has been reproduced by inflating a balloon in the oesophagus[96,99,101]. It seems to be a vagally-mediated reflex, as atropine abolishes the bradyarrhythmia. It is likely that this reflex is initiated by an active afferent barrage of impulses from the oesophagus due to distension, leading to a cardiac vagotonic response. His bundle recordings in a patient with atrioventricular block on swallowing have showed that the level of block was supra-Hisian, consistent with a vagal mechanism[95]. An identical mechanism is thought to be responsible for the bradycardia reported with episodes of pain in glossopharyngeal neuralgia – a crossover of intense afferent impulses from the glossopharyngeal nerve to the vagus leading to a vagotonic response[102,103]. Levin and Posner[104], in a case of swallowing syncope, found demyelination of the vagus and infiltration of the glossopharyngeal nerve. This patient also showed recent right coronary occlusion. In a case of AV block on swallowing following acute myocardial infarction Ragaza et al. postulated that the acute infarction sensitized the conduction system to normal vagal activity[97].

Correcting the oesophageal abnormality seems to be an obvious treatment, but has met with only limited success[105-107]. Atropine or ephedrine provide temporary control, but in cases where the symptoms are persistent pacemaker therapy is appropriate. However, in five patients reported recently by Armstrong et al.[98], only two needed pacemakers.

A more unusual event associated with swallowing is tachycardia (Figure 13.8). After its first description by Sakai and Mori[108] in 1926

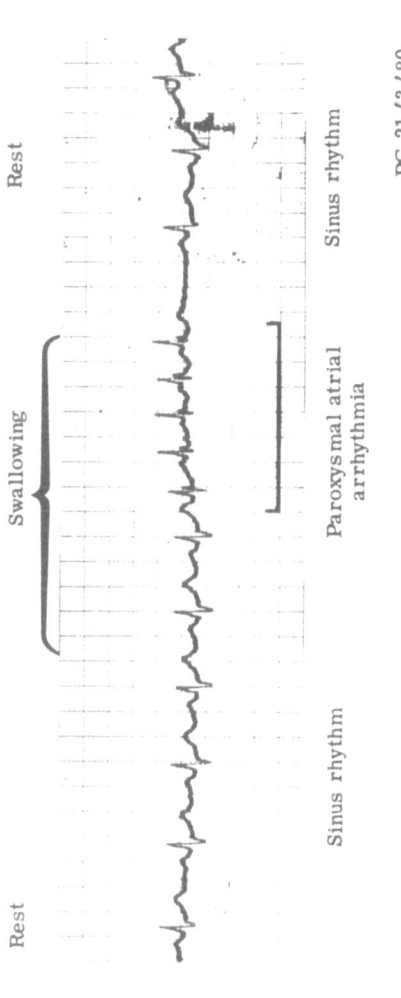

Rest

Swallowing

Rest

Sinus rhythm

Paroxysmal atrial
arrhythmia

Sinus rhythm

PG 21/3/80

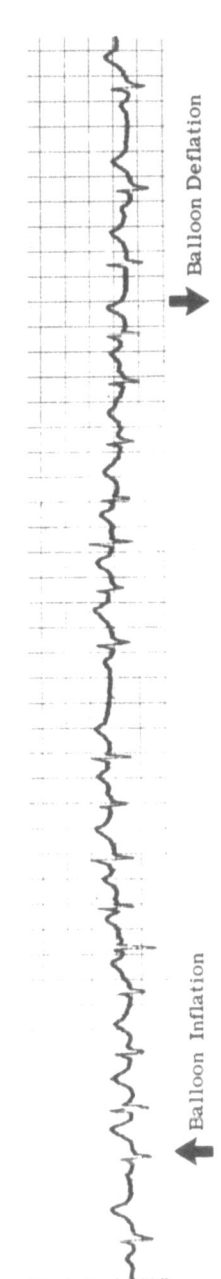

← Balloon Inflation

Balloon Deflation →

P. C.

Figure 13.8 Swallowing-induced short bursts of tachycardia: supraventricular tachycardia was induced by swallowing (top trace) and inflation of a balloon in the oesophagus (bottom trace). At electrophysiology this tachycardia was shown to be of right atrial origin

who called it 'schlucktachycardie', 11 cases have been reported in the literature[109–118]. Paroxysmal atrial tachycardia with or without aberrant conduction has been most frequently seen[109–116]. There are isolated reports of atrial fibrillation[116,117], and premature ventricular beats[118]. Unlike deglutition syncope none of these cases have been associated with oesophageal or cardiac lesions. From the data presently available, the mechanism of 'schlucktachykardie' appears to be less well understood than deglutition syncope.

Tachycardia appears to be unrelated to the alteration in autonomic tone which occurs on swallowing, as both atropine and β-blockers have failed to prevent its occurrence. As inflation of a balloon in the oesophagus was, in a few cases, shown to start and sustain the tachycardia[109,110,116,117] (Figure 13.8), local pressure on the left atrium was postulated but has not been successful in initiating tachycardia in other reported cases[113]. Studies to localize the origin of tachycardia have not revealed consistent results. While Schroeder et al.[114], and Bexton et al.[115] localized it to the high right atrium in their patient, Engel et al.[112] localized the origin to left atrium in their patient. In these cases the tachycardia showed features of an automatic focus, i.e.:

(1) Tachycardia began with premature P waves arising throughout the range of diastole[112–114].

(2) A gradual abbreviation of the cycle lengths was seen in the first few beats – 'warm up period'.

(3) Tachycardia could not be initiated or terminated by a timed atrial beat[112,114].

(4) A Wenckebach block during continued tachycardia precluded the atrioventricular node as a part of the circuit.

Atrial micro re-entry caused by temporal dispersion of the atrial refractory period in a non-uniform manner is also postulated[111,113]. A case of swallowing-induced atrial tachycardia and atrial fibrillation has also been reported in a patient with Wolff–Parkinson–White syndrome[116].

Administration of quinidine[108,111–115] and procainamide[109,110] have proved to be the most successful in controlling this unusual rhythm disturbance. Therapy with a vagolytic drug (atropine), a vagotonic drug (digoxin) and β-blockers has not proved helpful in this form of tachycardia. In one reported case, reserpine[116], and in another case disopyramide[115], were found to be totally effective in preventing swallowing-induced atrial tachycardia.

MICTURITION

Loss of consciousness during or soon after micturition is a rare though well known phenomenon[119–124]. It is almost exclusively reported in healthy males, and is related to voiding in the standing position[124]. In a typical case, the individual retires after moderate drinking, gets up at night to urinate, feels dizzy and briefly loses consciousness during or soon after voiding. Recovery is rapid and complete and episodes are usually not repeated. The mechanism of this neurophysiological event is not clearly understood, but the following mechanisms have been postulated:

(1) *Vasovagal reaction:* Straining during micturition produces a Valsalva-like manoeuvre which increases both intra-abdominal and intrathoracic pressure. Increased intrathoracic pressure decreases venous return which leads to decreased cardiac output. This, together with vagally-induced bradycardia, could result in syncope. Alcohol contributes by causing vasodilatation and a further decrease in cardiac output[119,124]. Eberhart and Morgan[122] suggested that a functional bladder neck obstruction might induce an intense Valsalva response. It is also suggested that the lordotic posture assumed during voiding further decreases cardiac output.

(2) *Hypotension:* Sleeping causes a decrease in blood pressure[125], when the subject gets up at night his blood pressure further decreases due to postural hypotension and vagal stimulation, the latter caused by the act of voiding[120].

(3) A form of *temporal lobe epilepsy* has been implicated[126].

(4) *Atrioventricular block.* Schoenberg *et al.*[127], reported a case where straining caused intermittent heart block possibly due to a vagal mechanism. As the phenomenon is not reproducible, data on electrocardiographic changes during micturition syncope are not often available.

It seems likely that micturition syncope is a symptom-complex arising as a result of several mechanisms. It is not a diagnostic problem as in almost all reported cases no abnormality was found, and electrocardiograms and encephalograms were normal after the episode. Usually no therapeutic manoeuvre is necessary as it does not tend to recur. A related disorder 'defaecation syncope' is seen in constipated elderly patients on straining or after manual disimpaction[128]. This could be due to a Valsalva-related atrioventricular block or sinus bradycardia.

CONCLUSION

Changes in heart rate and rhythm seen with physiological manoeuvres in healthy subjects are largely due to the associated haemodynamic changes and reflex alterations in autonomic tone caused by them. These changes are a good non-invasive means of assessing cardiac autonomic innervation. Decrease in heart rate is mediated by vagal stimulation and increase by sympathetic activation.

Vagal influence on the heart is reflexly altered by stimulation of other afferent connections of the vagus such as those from lungs, gastrointestinal tract and carotid baroreceptors. As a result of these connections an increase in vagal tone with Valsalva (relaxation phase), deep inspiration, swallowing and facial immersion makes these manoeuvres, to some extent, effective in terminating re-entrant atrioventricular tachycardias. From the limited studies into the mechanism of these responses it appears that at times hypersensitive vagal reflexes are responsible for excessive bradycardia and associated symptoms. Sinus bradycardia and atrioventricular block as seen with some of the reported cases of cough syncope, swallowing syncope and postural symptoms are possibly related to a common efferent response to one of the vagal afferents. The mechanism of tachyarrhythmias reported with spontaneous physiological manoeuvres is less well understood. They could be related to increased sympathetic activity, especially the arrhythmias precipitated by exercise. Dispersion of repolarization of cardiac muscle, due to autonomic imbalance could lead to re-entry circuits. Ventricular stretching has been postulated as a precipitating factor.

Thus, in susceptible individuals certain activities may provoke cardiac arrhythmias. These tachyarrhythmias and bradyarrhythmias can be attributed to sympathetic and parasympathetic stimulation respectively, and formal testing of the autonomic function usually helps in demonstrating their autonomic bases. In selected cases, electrophysiological studies may further elucidate the underlying mechanisms.

References

1. Robinson, B. F., Epstein, S. E., Beiser, G. D. and Braunwald, E. (1966). Control of heart rate by the autonomic nervous system: Studies in man on inter-relation between baroreceptor mechanism and exercise. *Circ. Res.*, **19**, 400–11
2. Wang, Y., Marshall, R. J. and Shepard, J. T. (1960). The effect of change of posture and of graded exercise on the stroke volume in man. *J. Clin. Invest.*, **39**, 1051–61
3. Loeppky, J. A., Greene, E. R., Hoekenga, D. E., Caprihan, A. and Luft, U. C. (1981). Beat-by-beat stroke volume assessment by pulsed Doppler in upright and supine exercise. *J. Appl. Physiol.*, **50**, 1173–82
4. Rosenthal, T., Birch, M., Osikowaska, B. and Sever, P. S. (1978). Changes in plasma noradrenaline concentrations following sympathetic stimulation by gradual tilting. *Cardiovasc. Res.*, **12**, 144–7
5. Curry, P. V. L., Rowland, E., Fox, K. M. and Krikler, D. M. (1978). The relationship between posture, blood pressure and electrophysiological properties in patients with paroxysmal supraventricular tachycardias. *Arch. Mal. Coeur*, **71**, 293–9
6. Hammill, S. C., Holmes, D. R., Wood, D. L., Osborn, M. J., Mclaran, C., Sugrue, D. D. and Gersh, B. J. (1984). Electrophysiological testing in the upright posture: Improved evaluation of patients with rhythm disturbances using tilt table. *J. Am. Coll. Cardiol.*, **4**, 65–71
7. Saksena, S., Siegel, P. and Rathyen, W. (1983). Electrophysiologic mechanisms in postural supraventricular tachycardia. *Am. Heart J.*, **106**, 151–4
8. Curry, P. V. L. (1979). The hemodynamic and electrophysiological effects of paroxysmal tachycardia. In Narula, O. S. (ed.) *Cardiac Arrhythmias: Electrophysiology, Diagnosis and Management.* pp. 364–381. (Baltimore: Williams and Wilkins)
9. Goldreyer, B. N., Kastor, J. A. and Kershbaum, K. L. (1976). The hemodynamic effects of induced supraventricular tachycardia in man. *Circulation*, **54**, 783–9
10. Waxman, M. B., Sharma, A. D., Cameron, D. A., Huerta, F. and Wald, R. W.

(1982). Reflex mechanisms responsible for early spontaneous termination of paroxysmal supraventricular tachycardia. *Am. J. Cardiol.*, **49**, 259–72

11. Desser, K. B., DeSa'Neto, A. and Benchimol, A. (1979). Hearts that go thump in the night: Positional atrial flutter in a patient with mitral valve prolapse. *N. Engl. J. Med.*, **300**, 717–18

12. Oliven, A. and Abinader, E. (1981). Postural-related supraventricular tachyarrhythmia in mitral valve prolapse syndrome. *Am. Heart J.*, **102**, 130–1

13. Peters, M. and Penner, S. L. (1946). Orthostatic ventricular tachycardia. *Am. Heart J.*, **2**, 645–52

14. Ohe, T., Tomobuchi, Y. and Shimomura, K. (1985). Induction and termination of ventricular tachycardia by changing body posture. *Am. J. Cardiol.*, **56**, 800–1

15. Manning, G. W. and Sears, G. A. (1962). Postural heart block. *Am. J. Cardiol.*, **9**, 558–63

16. Manning, G. W. and Stewart, C. B. (1945). Alerations in PR interval associated with change in posture. *Am. Heart J.*, **30**, 109–17

17. Seda, P. E., McAnulty, J. H. and Anderson, C. J. (1980). Postural heart block. *Br. Heart J.*, **44**, 221–3

18. Butrous, G. B., Kaye, G. C., Nathan, A. W., Banim, S. O. and Camm, A. J. (1984). Respiratory modulation of atrioventricular pathway conduction. *Circulation*, **70**, II–217

19. Marriot, H. J. L. and Myerburg, R. J. (1984). Recognition and treatment of cardiac arrhythmias and conduction disturbances. In Hurst, J. W. (ed.) *The Heart*. 4th edn., p. 644. (McGraw Hill)

20. Levy, M. N., Degeest, H. and Zieske, H. (1966). Effects of respiratory centre activity on the heart. *Circ. Res.*, **18**, 67–78

21. Glick, G. and Braunwald, E. (1965). Relative roles of the sympathetic and parasympathetic nervous systems in the reflex control of heart rate. *Circ. Res.*, **16**, 363–75

22. Katona, P. G. and Jih, F. (1975). Respiratory sinus arrhythmia: non-invasive measure of parasympathetic cardiac control. *J. Appl. Physiol.*, **39**, 801–5

23. Shaver, J. A., Leon, D. F., Gray, S., Leonard, J. J. and Bahnson, H. T. (1979). Hemodynamic observations after cardiac transplantation. *N. Engl. J. Med.*, **281**, 822–7

24. Waxman, M. B., Bonet, J. F., Finley, J. P. and Wald, R. W. (1980). Effects of respiration and posture on paroxysmal supraventricular tachycardia. *Circulation*, **62**, 1011–20

25. Sharpey-Schafer, E. P. (1965). Effect of respiratory acts on the circulation. In Hamilton, W. F. and Dow, P. (eds.) *Handbook of Physiology*. Vol. III, pp. 1875–86. (Washington: American Physiological Society)

26. Wilson, F. N. (1915). A case in which vagus influenced the form of the ventricular complex of the electrocardiogram. *Arch. Intern. Med.*, **16**, 1008–11

27. Cheung, E. K. (ed.) (1983). Exercise induced cardiac arrhythmias. In *Principles of Cardiac Arrhythmias*. 3rd edn., p. 619. (Baltimore, London: Williams and Wilkins)

28. Jelinek, M. V. and Lown, B. (1974). Exercise stress testing for exposure of cardiac arrhythmias. *Prog. Cardiovasc. Dis.*, **16**, 497–522

29. Sung, R. J., Shen, E. N., Morady, F., Scheinman, M. M., Hess, D. and Botvinich, E. H. (1983). Electrophysiologic mechanism of exercise-induced sustained ventricular tachycardia. *Am. J. Cardiol.*, **51**, 525–30

30. Cranefield, P. F. (1977). Action potentials, afterpotentials and arrhythmias. *Circ. Res.*, **41**, 415–23

31. Vassalle, M., Levine, M. J. and Stuckey, J. H. (1968). On the sympathetic control of ventricular automaticity. The effects of stellate ganglion stimulation. *Circ. Res.*, **23**, 249–58

32. Vassalle, M., Stuckey, J. H. and Levine, M. J. (1969). Sympathetic control of ventricular automaticity. Role of the adrenal medulla. *Am. J. Physiol.*, **217**, 930–7

33. Han, J. and Moe, G. K. (1964). Nonuniform recovery of excitability of ventricular muscle. *Circ. Res.*, **14**, 44–52

34. Wu, D., Kou, H. and Hung, J. (1981). Exercise-triggered paroxysmal ventricular tachycardia. A repetitive rhythmic activity possibly related to afterdepolarization. *Ann. Intern. Med.*, **95**, 410–14
35. Gooch, A. S. (1972). Exercise testing for detecting changes in cardiac rhythm and conduction. *Am. J. Cardiol.*, **30**, 741–6
36. Levy, S. and Broustet, J. P. (1981). Exercise testing in Wolff–Parkinson–White syndrome. *Am. J. Cardiol.*, **48**, 976
37. Strasberg, B., Ashley, W. W., Wyndham, C. R. C., Bauernfeind, R. A., Swiryn, S. P., Dhingra, R. C. and Rosen, K. M. (1980). Treadmill exercise testing in Wolff–Parkinson–White syndrome. *Am. J. Cardiol.*, **45**, 742–8
38. Abbott, J. A., Hirschfield, D. S., Kunkel, F. W. and Scheinman, M. M. (1977). Graded exercise testing in patients with sinus node dysfunction. *Am. J. Med.*, **62**, 330–8
39. Holden, W., McAnutly, J. C. and Rahimtoola, S. H. (1978). Characterisation of heart rate response to exercise in the sick sinus syndrome. *Br. Heart J.*, **40**, 923–30
40. Agruss, N. S., Rosin, E. Y., Adolph, R. J. and Fowler, N. O. (1972). Significance of chronic sinus bradycardia in elderly people. *Circulation*, **46**, 924–30
41. Sandberg, L. (1961). The significance of ventricular premature beats or runs of ventricular tachycardia developing during exercise tests. *Acta Med. Scand.*, **169**, (Suppl. 365) 62–77
42. Goldschlager, N., Cake, C. and Cohn, K. (1973). Exercise induced ventricular arrhythmias in patients with coronary artery disease: Their relation to angiographic findings. *Am. J. Cardiol.*, **31**, 434–40
43. McHenry, P. L., Morris, S. N. and Kavalier, M. (1974). Exercise induced arrhythmias: Recognition, classification and clinical significance. In Fisch, C. (ed.) *Complex Electrocardiography*. 2nd edn., p. 235. (Philadelphia: F. A. Davies & Co)
44. Helfant, R. H., Pine, R., Kabde, V. and Banka, V. S. (1974). Exercise related ventricular premature complexes in coronary heart disease. Correlations with ischemia and angiographic severity. *Ann. Intern. Med.*, **80**, 589–92
45. Califf, R. M., McKinnis, R., McNeer, F., Marrell, F. E., Lee, K. L., Pryor, D. B., Waugh, R. A., Harris, P. J., Rosati, R. A. and Wagner, G. S. (1983). Prognostic value of ventricular arrhythmias associated with treadmill exercise testing in patients studied with cardiac catheterization for suspected ischaemic heart disease. *J. Am. Coll. Cardiol.*, **2**, 1060–7
46. Udall, J. A. and Ellestad, M. H. (1977). Predictive implications of ventricular premature contractions associated with treadmill stress testing. *Circulation*, **56**, 985–9
47. McKenna, W. J., Chetty, W., Oakley, C. M. and Goodwin, J. F. (1980). Arrhythmias in hypertrophic cardiomyopathy: Exercise and 48 hours ambulatory electrocardiographic assessment with and without beta adrenergic blocking therapy. *Am. J. Cardiol.*, **45**, 1–5
48. Savage, D. D., Seides, S. F., Maron, B. J., Myers, D. J. and Epstein, S. E. (1979). Prevalence of arrhythmias during 24-hour electrocardiographic monitoring and exercise testing in patients with obstructive and nonobstructive hypertrophic cardiomyopathy. *Circulation*, **59**, 866–75
49. Meytes, I., Kaplinsky, E., Yahini, J. H., Hanne-Paparo, N. and Neufeld, H. N. (1975). Wenckebach A–V block: A frequent feature following heavy physical training. *Am. Heart J.*, **90**, 426–30
50. Rozanski, J. J., Castellanos, A. and Sheps, D. (1980). Paroxysmal second degree atrioventricular block induced by exercise. *Heart Lung*, **9**, 887–90
51. Alanis, J. and Benitez, D. (1967). The decrease in the automatism of the Purkinje pacemaker fibres provoked by high frequency stimulation. *Jpn. J. Physiol.*, **17**, 556–62
52. Andersen, H. T. (1966). Physiological adaptations in the diving vertebrates. *Physiol. Rev.*, **46**, 217–43
53. Bergman, S. A., Campbell, J. K. and Wildenthal, K. (1972). 'Diving reflex' in man: its relation to isometeric and dynamic exercise. *J. Appl. Physiol.*, **33**, 27–31

54. Strauss, M. B. (1970). Physiological aspects of mammalian breath holding and diving, a review. *Aerospace Med.*, **41**, 1362–81
55. Yonce, L. R., Folkow, B. and Hill, C. (1970). The integration of cardiovascular response to diving. Editorial. *Am. Heart J.*, **79**, 1–4
56. Oslen, C. R., Fanestil, D. P. and Scholander, P. E. (1962). Some effects of breath holding and apneic underwater diving on cardiac rhythm in man. *J. Appl. Physiol.*, **17**, 461–6
57. Hunt, H. G., Whitaker, D. K. and Willmott, N. J. (1975). Water temperature and diving reflex (letter). *Lancet*, **1**, 572
58. Whayne, T. F. and Killip, T. (III). (1967). Simulated diving reflex in man: Comparision of facial stimuli and response in arrhythmia. *J. Appl. Physiol.*, **22**, 800–7
59. Arabian, J. M., Furedy, J. J., Morrison, J. and Szalai, J. P. (1983). Treatment of PAT: Bradycardiac reflexes induced by dive vs body-tilt. *Pav. J. Biol. Sci.*, **18**, 88–93
60. Hurwitz, B., and Furedy, J. J. (1978). The human dive reflex: an experimental topographic and physiological analysis. *Psychophysiology*, **16**, 192 (Abstr.)
61. Andersen, H. T. (1963). The reflex nature of the physiological adjustments to diving, and their afferent pathways. *Acta Physiol. Scand.*, **58**, 263–73
62. Cohen, M. V. (1972). Ventricular fibrillation precipitated by carotid sinus pressure: case report and review of literature. *Am. Heart J.*, **84**, 681–6
63. Wildenthal, K., Leshin, S. J., Atkins, J. M. and Skelton, C. L. (1975). The diving reflex used to treat paroxysmal atrial tachycardia. *Lancet*, **1**, 12–14
64. Lamb, L. E., Dermksian, G. and Sarnoff, C. A. (1958). Significant cardiac arrhythmias induced by common respiratory maneuvers. *Am. J. Cardiol.*, **2**, 563–72
65. Wolf, S. (1964). The bradycardia of dive reflex – a possible mechanism of sudden death. *Trans. Am. Clin. Climatol. Assoc.*, **76**, 192–8
66. McIntosh, H. D., Estes, E. H. and Warren, J. V. (1956). The mechanism of cough syncope. *Am. Heart J.*, **52**, 70–82
67. Aronson, D. W., Rovner, R. N. and Patterson, R. (1970). Cough syncope: Case presentation and review. *J. Allergy*, **46**, 359–63
68. Kerr, A. and Eich, R. H. (1961). Cerebral concussion as a cause of cough syncope. *Arch. Intern. Med.*, **108**, 248–52
69. Strauss, M. J., Longstreth, W. T. and Thiela, B. L. (1984). Atypical cough syncope. *J. Am. Med. Assoc.*, **251**, 1731–3
70. Wenger, T. L., Dohrmann, M. L., Strauss, H. C., Conley, M. J., Wechsler, A. S. and Wagner, G. S. (1980). Hypersensitive carotid sinus syndrome manifested as cough syncope. *Pacing Clin. Electrophysiol.*, **3**, 332–9
71. Hart, G., Oldershaw, P. J., Cull, R. E., Humprey, P. and Ward, D. E. (1982). Syncope caused by cough-induced complete atrioventricular block. *Pacing. Clin. Electrophysiol.*, **5**, 564–6
72. Saito, D., Matsuno, S., Matsushita, K., Takeda, H., Hyodo, T., Haraoka, S., Watanabe, A. and Nagashima, H. (1982). Cough syncope due to atrio-ventricular conduction block. *Jpn. Heart J.*, **23**, 1015–20
73. Crofton, J. and Douglas, A. (eds.) (1983). *Respiratory Diseases*. The Structure and Function of Respiratory Tract. 2nd edn., pp. 19 and 80. (Oxford, London, Edinburgh, Melbourne: Blackwell Scientific)
74. Sharpey-Schafer, E. P. (1953). The mechanism of syncope after coughing. *Br. Med. J.*, **2**, 860–3
75. Klassen, K. P., Morton, D. R. and Curtis, G. M. (1951). The clinical physiology of human bronchi. III. The effect of vagus section on the cough reflex, bronchial caliber and the clearance of bronchial secretions. *Surgery*, **29**, 483–91
76. Talwar, K. K., Edvardson, N. and Varnauskas, E. (1985). Paroxysmal vagally mediated AV block with recurrent syncope. *Clin. Cardiol.*, **8**, 337–40.
77. Wei, J. Y., Greene, H. L. and Weisfeldt, M. L. (1980). Cough-facilitated conversion of ventricular tachycardia. *Am. J. Cardiol.*, **45**, 174–6
78. Caldwell, G., Miller, G., Vincent, R. and Chamberlain, D. A. (1985). Simple mechanical methods for cardioversion: defence of the precordial thump and cough version. *Br. Med. J.*, **291**, 627–30

79. Francis, C. K., Singh, J. B. and Polansky, B. J. (1972). Interruption of aberrant conduction of atrioventricular junctional tachycardia by cough. N. Engl. J. Med., 286, 357–8

80. Dawson, P. M. (1943). An historical sketch of Valsalva experiment. Bull. Hist. Med., 14, 297–320

81. Porth, C. J. M., Bamrah, V. S., Tristani, F. E. and Smith, J. J. (1984). The Valsalva maneuver: mechanisms and clinical implications. Heart Lung., 13, 507–18

82. Valentinuzzi, M. E., Powell, T., Baker, L. E. and Powell, T. (1974). The heart rate response to the Valsalva maneuver. Med. Biol. Eng., 12, 817–22

83. Nizet, P. M., Borgia, J. F. and Jorvath, S. M. (1976). Wandering atrial pacemaker (Prevalence in French hornists). J. Electrocardiol., 9, 51–2

84. Korner, P. I., Tonkin, A. M. and Uther, J. N. (1976). Reflex and mechanical circulatory effects of graded Valsalva manoeuvers in normal man. J. Appl. Physiol., 40, 434–40

85. Brooker, J. Z., Alderman, E. L. and Harrison, D. C. (1974). Alterations in left ventricular volumes induced by Valsalva manoeuvre. Br. Heart J., 36, 713–18

86. Robertson, D., Stevens, R. M., Friesinger, G. C. and Oates, J. A. (1977). The effect of Valsalva maneuver on echocardiographic dimensions in man. Circulation, 55, 596–602

87. Parisi, A. F., Harrington, J. J., Askenazi, J., Pratt, R. C. and McIntyre, K. M. (1976). Echocardiographic evaluation of Valsalva maneuver in healthy subjects and patients with and without heart failure. Circulation, 54, 921–7

88. Lee, G. J., Matthews, M. B. and Sharpey-Shafer, E. P. (1954). The effects of Valsalva manoeuvre on the systemic and pulmonary artery pressure in man. Br. Heart J., 16, 311–316

89. Ewing, D. J., Campbell, I. W., Burt, A. A. and Clarke, B. F. (1973). Vascular reflexes in diabetic autonomic neuropathy. Lancet, 2, 1354-6

90. Levin, A. B. (1966). A simple test of cardiac function based upon the heart rate changes induced by Valsalva maneuver. Am. J. Cardiol., 18, 90–9

91. Bellet S. (ed.) (1972). Essentials of Cardiac Arrhythmias: Diagnosis and Management. p. 102. (Philadelphia: W. B. Saunders)

92. Waxman, M. B., Wald, R. W., Finley, J. P., Bonet, J. F., Downar, E. and Sharma, A. D. (1980). Valsalva termination of ventricular tachycardia. Circulation, 62, 843–51

93. Gandevia, S. C., McCloskey, D. I. and Potter, E. K. (1978). Reflex bradycardia occurring in response to diving, nasopharyngeal stimulation and ocular pressure, and its modification by respiration and swallowing. J. Physiol., 276, 383–94

94. Bortolotti, M., Cirignotta, F. and Labo, G. (1982). Atrioventricular block induced by swallowing in a patient with diffuse esophageal spasm. J. Am. Med. Assoc., 248, 2297–9

95. Lichstein, E. and Chadda, K. D. (1972). Atrioventricular block produced by swallowing, with documentation on His bundle recordings. Am. J. Cardiol., 29, 561–3

96. Weiss, S. and Ferris, E. B. (1934). Adams–Stokes syndrome with transient complete heart block of vasovagal reflex origin. Mechanism and treatment. Arch. Intern. Med. (Chicago), 54, 931–51

97. Ragaza, E. P., Rectra, E. H. and Pardi, M. T. (1970). Intermittent complete heart block associated with swallowing as a complication of acute myocardial infarction. Am. Heart J., 79, 396–400

98. Armstrong, P. W., McMillan, D. G. and Simon, J. B. (1985). Swallow syncope. Can. Med. Assoc. J., 132, 1281–4

99. Sapru, R. P., Griffiths, P. H., Guz, A. and Eisele, J. (1971). Syncope on swallowing. Br. Heart J., 33, 617–22

100. Tomlinson, I. W. and Fox, K. M. (1975). Carcinoma of oesophagus with 'swallow syncope'. Br. Med. J., 2, 315–16

101. James, A. H. and Oxon, D. M. (1958). Cardiac syncope after swallowing. Lancet, 1, 771–2

102. Kong, Y., Heyman, A., Entman, M. L. and McIntosh, H. D. (1964). Glossopharyngeal neuralgia associated with bradycardia, syncope, and seizures. *Circulation*, 30, 109–13
103. Khero, B. A. and Mullins, C. B. (1971). Cardiac syncope due to glossopharyngeal neuralgia, treated by transvenous pacemaker. *Arch. Intern, Med.*, 128, 806–8
104. Levin, B. and Posner, J. B. (1972). Swallow syncope: report of a case and review of literature. *Neurology*, 22, 1086–93
105. Wik, B. and Hillestad, L. (1975). Deglutition syncope. *Br. Med. J.*, 3, 747
106. Golf, S. (1977). Swallowing syncope. *Acta Med. Scand.*, 201, 585–6
107. Tolman, K. G. and Ashworth, W. D. (1971). Syncope induced by dysphagia: Correction by esophageal dilatation. *Am. J. Dig. Dis*, 16, 1026–31
108. Sakai, D. and Mori, F. (1926). Uber einen Fall Von Sog 'Schlucktachykardie'. *Z. Gesamte. Exp. Med.*, 50, 106–9
109. Kramer, P., Harris, L., Kaplan, R. and Hollander, W. (1962). Recurrent supraventricular paroxysmal tachycardia precipitated by swallowing. *Proc. N. Engl. Cardiovasc. Soc.*, 21, 21
110. Bajaj, S. C., Ragaza, E. P., Silva, H. and Goyal, R. K. (1972). Deglutition tachycardia. *Gastroenterology*, 62, 632–5
111. Lindsay, A. E. (1973). Tachycardia caused by swallowing: Mechanisms and treatment. *Am. Heart J.*, 85, 679–84
112. Engel, T. R., Laporte, S. M., Meister, S. G., and Frankl, W. S. (1976). Tachycardia upon swallowing: Evidence of a left atrial automatic focus. *J. Electrocardiol.*, 9, 69–73
113. Mirvis, D. M., Bandura, J. P. and Brody, D. A. (1977). Symptomatic swallowing-induced paroxysmal supraventricular tachycardia. *Am. J. Cardiol.*, 39, 741–3
114. Schroeder, D. P., Wooley, C. F. and Leier, C. V. (1978). An electrophysiologic study of swallowing induced tachycardia. *Chest*, 74, 314–17
115. Bexton, R. S., Nathan, A. W., Hellestrand, K. J. and Camm, A. J. (1981). Paroxysmal atrial tachycardia provoked by swallowing. *Br. Med. J.*, 282, 952
116. Keidar, S., Grenadier, E., Fleischman, P. and Palant, A. (1984). Swallowing induced atrial tachycardia and fibrillation in a patient with Wolf–Parkinson–White syndrome. *Am. J. Med. Sci.*, 288, 32–4
117. Cohen, L., Larson, D. W. and Strandjord, N. (1970). Swallowing induced atrial fibrillation. *Circulation* (Suppl. III) 42, 145 (Abstr)
118. Forsberg, C. W. (1930). Paroxysmal premature ventricular contractions induced by swallowing; case report. *Lancet*, 53, 298–302
119. Proudfit, W. L. and Forteza, M. E. (1959). Micturition syncope. *N. Engl. J. Med.*, 260, 328–31
120. Lukash, W. M., Sawyer, G. T. and Davies, J. E. (1964). Micturition syncope produced by orthostasis and bladder distention. *N. Engl. J. Med.*, 270, 341–4
121. Donker, D. N., Robles de Madina, E. O. and Kieft, J. (1972). Micturition syncope. *Electroencephalogr. Clin. Neurophysiol.*, 33, 328–31
122. Eberhart, C. and Morgan, J. W. (1960). Micturition syncope. Report of a case. *J. Am. Med. Assoc.*, 174, 2076–7
123. Lyle, C. B., Monroe, J. T., Flinn, D. E. and Lamb, L. E. (1961). Micturition syncope. Report of 24 cases. *N. Engl. J. Med.*, 265, 982–6
124. Godec, C. J. and Cass, A. S. (1981). Micturition syncope. *J. Urol.*, 126, 551–2
125. Pickering, G. (1965). Hyperpiesis: High blood pressure without any evident causes: essential hypertension. *Br. Med. J.*, 2, 959–68
126. Zivin, I. and Rowley, W. (1964). Psychomotor epilepsy with micturition. *Arch. Intern. Med.*, 113, 8–13
127. Schoenberg, B. S., Kuglitsch, J. F. and Karnes, W. E. (1974). Micturition syncope not a single entity. *J. Am. Med. Assoc.*, 229, 1631–3
128. Pathy MS. (1978). Defecation syncope. *Age Ageing*, 7, 233–6

14
Ventricular arrhythmias in acute myocardial infarction

R. W. F. CAMPBELL

INTRODUCTION

Myocardial infarction is a dynamic pathological process which begins with acute regional myocardial ischaemia and finishes with fibrotic repair. During the acute phase, ventricular arrhythmias are a common and much feared complication. Their incidence and implications depend both upon their type and their time of occurrence after the onset of symptoms of infarction. Of the many ways to group and classify these complicating arrhythmias, separating those primarily due to acute electrical instability from those which are related to infarct size is convenient and has clinical relevance.

VENTRICULAR ARRHYTHMIAS RELATED TO ACUTE ELECTRICAL INSTABILITY

The process of cell death in myocardial infarction is not instantaneous. During at least the first 4 hours and for perhaps up to 8 hours, the dramatic changes in transmembrane currents and in conduction and refractoriness which occur in the infarcting zone relative to the surrounding normal myocardium, predispose to abnormal automaticity and re-entry.

Ventricular fibrillation

Ventricular fibrillation is responsible for the substantial early mortality which occurs in acute myocardial infarction[1]. With the exception of rare instances of ventricular fibrillation spontaneously terminating or being reverted by a blow to the chest[2] or by medical therapy[3], ventricular fibrillation is fatal unless reversed by countershock. The surface ECG of ventricular fibrillation, shows disorganized rapid irregular ventricular activation, and is the same whatever the circumstances of the arrhyth-

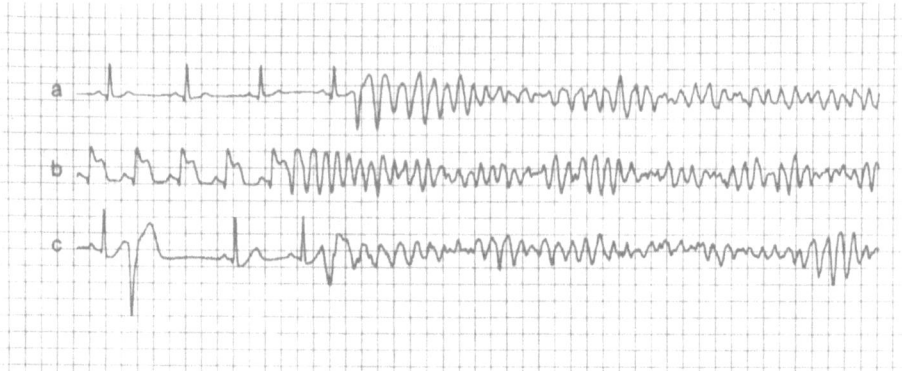

Figure 14.1 Surface ECG of ventricular fibrillation; **a:** primary VF; **b:** secondary VF; **c:** non-ischaemic VF

mia. (Figure 14.1). However, ventricular fibrillation subtypes can be defined by their clinical context.

Primary ventricular fibrillation

Primary ventricular fibrillation complicates the acute phase of infarction and occurs in the absence of shock or cardiac failure[4]. Its incidence declines exponentially from the onset of symptoms. It has been considered independent of the size and the site of infarction[5], but an excess incidence in patients with large anterior infarcts has been reported[6]. For many years, primary ventricular fibrillation was considered predictable on the basis of so-called 'warning arrhythmias'[7]. Lown et al. proposed a hierarchy of ventricular arrhythmias ranging from isolated infrequent ventricular ectopic beats to R-on-T ventricular ectopic beats which was based on their predictive value for primary ventricular fibrillation[7]. The need to detect 'warning arrhythmias' has, in part, been responsible for the increasing sophistication of ECG rhythm monitoring systems in coronary care units. Evidence now suggests that ventricular fibrillation is not predicted by premonitory arrhythmias[6,8,9]. However, there is a temporal association between R-on-T ventricular ectopic beats and primary ventricular fibrillation, both these arrhythmias having a high early incidence[9]. The possibility that an increasing frequency of R-on-T ventricular ectopic beats may predict primary ventricular fibrillation has been advanced but remains unsubstantiated[9].

Primary ventricular fibrillation should be treated by a DC shock of 200–400 joules. In over 90% of patients, sinus rhythm can be restored[10,11]. For those resuscitated, the current practice is to give lignocaine for at least 24 hours to prevent recurrences. The value of this strategy is unclear, as despite such management, ventricular fibrillation recurrence rates of up to 30% have been reported[10]. Longer term prophylaxis of recurrences using oral Class I therapy has largely been abandoned with the realization that the risk of primary ventricular fibrillation is self-limiting consequent upon the transient electrical instability of the myocardium in the early hours of infarction.

Up to 10% of patients with primary ventricular fibrillation do not survive, despite rapid and appropriate resuscitation[10,11]. This has rekindled interest in methods of preventing primary ventricular fibrillation. Of the many antiarrhythmic agents tested for this role, only lignocaine has been shown to significantly reduce the incidence of primary ventricular fibrillation[12,13]. Successful prophylaxis appears to require a dose of lignocaine high enough to cause toxicity in a sizeable proportion of treated patients. In a recent large study examining the prophylactic efficacy of intramuscular lignocaine, the incidence of primary ventricular fibrillation was significantly reduced, but at the cost of a significant increase in asystole[13]. This, and reports of toxicity in patients with suspected but later disproven infarction[14], may restrict the clinical application of lignocaine prophylaxis.

If primary ventricular fibrillation is a consequence of electrical instability and is not related to the extent of myocardial damage, then resuscitated survivors would be expected to have a good long term prognosis. Many studies have indicated this to be the case[15,16], but new data force reconsideration. Schwartz et al.[17] reported that patients with ventricular fibrillation complicating anterior myocardial infarction had a significantly poorer prognosis than patients with the same arrhythmia complicating an inferior infarct. The major difference arose in the first year of follow-up, when a 32% mortality was observed in those with anterior infarction and ventricular fibrillation. If substantiated these findings would stimulate the search for a safe effective prophylactic strategy for primary ventricular fibrillation.

Secondary ventricular fibrillation

As by definition shock or failure must be present at the time of its occurrence, secondary ventricular fibrillation is considered later with the other arrhythmias associated with infarct size.

Reperfusional ventricular fibrillation

Reperfusion of a total coronary artery occlusion, particularly if achieved within 2 hours, can cause a variety of ventricular arrhythmias, including ventricular fibrillation[18] (see Chapter 3). Thrombolytic therapy is an obvious means of provoking reperfusional ventricular fibrillation, but spontaneous natural reperfusion may also be responsible for some incidents of ventricular fibrillation seen in coronary care units. As with other subtypes of ventricular fibrillation, there is no distinguishing electrocardiographic pattern to separate this arrhythmia from primary ventricular fibrillation. Reperfusional ventricular fibrillation responds well to defibrillation. It is usually a transient and isolated event; its underlying pathophysiology rapidly disappearing with continuing reperfusion. Reflecting as it does revascularization of previously jeopardized tissue it may betoken a good long term prognosis, although this will depend upon the measures taken to prevent reocclusion.

Acute occlusional ventricular fibrillation

Acute occlusion of a coronary artery may provoke ventricular fibrillation[19]. Whilst this arrhythmia might reasonably be categorized as primary ventricular fibrillation, clinical evidence suggests it may be a separate entity. Acute occlusional ventricular fibrillation occurs within seconds or minutes of cessation of blood flow, producing near instantaneous collapse, often without time for the development of symptoms such as chest pain. Although probably very amenable to defibrillation, acute occlusional ventricular fibrillation carries a high mortality as rarely is the victim in a medically equipped environment. This is one of the forms of ventricular fibrillation seen by out-of-hospital rescue squads[20], but it probably is very rare in coronary care units. The reduction of mortality that is provided by secondary prevention with β-blockers in survivors of a first myocardial infarction may arise by prevention of acute occlusional ventricular fibrillation.

Ischaemic but non-infarction ventricular fibrillation

Out-of-hospital rescue squads resuscitate some patients in ventricular fibrillation who later are proven not to have sustained an acute myocardial infarction[21]. Until the results of serial electrocardiograms and enzyme studies are known, these patients are indistinguishable from patients with infarction complicated by primary or acute occlusional ventricular fibrillation. Initially non-infarction ventricular fibrillation was considered to have a good prognosis particularly as myocardial damage had not occurred but experience has shown that further out-of-hospital arrests are common[22]. The majority of patients with non-infarction ventricular fibrillation have severe underlying coronary artery disease[23], and it is probable that in some patients the sudden development of a zone of intense myocardial ischaemia creates the myocardial substrate which supports ventricular fibrillation. Whether non-infarct ventricular fibrillation is due to acute occlusion (spasm or microthrombosis) or to reperfusion (so early that no damage occurs) is unknown. Prophylaxis can be provided by improving and securing myocardial perfusion[24]. Antiarrhythmic drugs, including β-adrenoreceptor blocking therapy, have not proved of benefit for these patients[25].

Ventricular tachycardia

Ventricular tachycardia is an important, but ill defined, arrhythmia which if rapid and sustained will cause immediate haemodynamic upset. The majority of incidents of ventricular tachycardia complicating acute myocardial infarction barely satisfy the widely used definition of ventricular tachycardia as three or more consecutive ventricular ectopic beats at a rate equal to or greater than 120 bpm. Brief salvoes of ventricular ectopic beats (Lown grade IVb) are very common during acute myocardial infarction, but sustained ventricular tachycardia, particularly monomorphic ventricular tachycardia, is most unusual. As such, 'ventricular tachycardia' (ventricular ectopic beat salvoes) in acute infarction rarely causes symptoms or haemodynamic upset, and appears not to have either immediate or late prognostic significance[26]. Its pattern of occurrence closely follows that observed for isolated ventricular ectopic beats[9] suggesting that the pathophysiology of these two forms of ventricular arrhythmias may be similar.

Sustained ventricular tachycardia is related to the extent of the myocardial infarction and is discussed later.

Ventricular ectopic beats

Ventricular ectopic beats are a near universal accompaniment of myocardial infarction being common at all phases of injury and healing. Depending upon their frequency, their morphology, their sequential occurrence and their relationship to the preceding T wave, they may be described as infrequent, frequent, multiform, repetitive (pairs and salvoes) and as R-on-T ventricular ectopic beats[7]. With the exception of R-on-T ventricular ectopic beats which disappear within the first 4–8 hours[9] of infarction, the other forms are present throughout most of the early phase of infarction[9]. Ventricular ectopic beat frequency falls after 24–48 hours, but then increases as the patient mobilizes reaching a peak at 6–8 months postinfarction before again decreasing. None of these ventricular ectopic beats (except perhaps R-on-T) have immediate implications. They rarely produce symptoms and cause little or no haemodynamic upset, and no feature of their expression during the acute infarct phase has been associated with late prognostic implications.

VENTRICULAR ARRHYTHMIAS ASSOCIATED WITH INFARCT SIZE

Some ventricular arrhythmias are related to the extent of myocardial damage sustained during infarction. Not surprisingly therefore, these ventricular arrhythmias are of prognostic importance.

Secondary ventricular fibrillation

Secondary ventricular fibrillation occurs in the setting of shock or cardiac failure[4]. It can occur at any time during the process of infarction and does not share primary ventricular fibrillation's predilection for the early hours after the onset of symptoms. Secondary ventricular fibrillation has a grave immediate and late prognosis[16]. Only about 30% of afflicted patients can be resuscitated and the outlook for survivors is a 50% one year mortality. By definition secondary ventricular fibrillation is a complication of severe myocardial damage and prognosis may more reflect this than any independent contribution of the arrhythmia itself. Surprisingly, very little research has been undertaken to determine the optimal management for survivors of secondary ventricular fibrillation, which for the present remains empirical and individual.

Late ventricular fibrillation

There are probably many mechanisms by which late ventricular fibrillation arises. A group of patients at particularly high risk of this arrhythmia are those who have sustained an anterior infarction and whose electrocardiogram shows right bundle branch block and axis shift[27]. The risk of developing late ventricular fibrillation appears concentrated within the 6 weeks from the onset of symptoms of infarction. Optimal management may be to hospitalize the patient during this period of time[28] as antiarrhythmic prophylaxis is of unproven efficacy.

Sustained ventricular tachycardia

Sustained ventricular tachycardia is a dangerous arrhythmia. It can cause hypotension and may degenerate to ventricular fibrillation. Sustained ventricular tachycardia typically occurs 2 or more days after myocardial infarction, usually in patients who have sustained substantial anterior infarcts. There is a strong association between the development of left ventricular aneurysms and the occurrence of this arrhythmia[29]. Immediate therapy is indicated for a sustained attack, programmed stimulation, DC version or medical therapy each having a role to play. Recurrences are very common and long term prophylaxis is advisable. Drug therapy may be selected empirically or by the results of invasive electrophysiological testing. The latter is preferable, as there is strong evidence of an improved prognosis for patients who are discharged on medication which has been proved effective against programmed stimulation provocation of the clinical arrhythmia[30]. Unfortunately, a sizeable proportion of patients with sustained ventricular tachycardia prove intractable to medical therapy, and it is for them that surgical procedures (encircling endocardial ventriculotomy, subendocardial resection etc) have proved an effective management[31].

Frequent ventricular ectopic beats

Many clinical characteristics of survivors of myocardial infarction have been investigated for their potential to predict late sudden death. The identification that ventricular tachycardia and fibrillation are responsible for a major proportion of this late mortality focussed attention on the prognostic significance of ventricular ectopic beats. A positive relationship was quickly established, but whether ectopic beats had independent prognostic importance remained controversial, particularly as they were associated with severe underlying coronary artery disease or extensive myocardial damage[32]. Further work has confirmed a role for ventricular ectopic beats as identifying high risk survivors of myocardial infarction, but ventricular ectopic beat frequency is the crucial factor[33,34]. Ventricular ectopic beats are frequently found in patients with ischaemic heart disease, particularly during the first months after infarction. Only when their frequency exceeds 10 per hour are they of prognostic significance. Sustained high levels of ventricular ectopic beat activity may be detected by a rhythm strip recorded during a standard electrocardiographic recording but for accurate quantitation a dynamic electrocardiogram (Holter ECG) is necessary. The prognostic significance of ventricular ectopic beats provoked or aggravated by exercise testing is less well established, but it is likely that a similar threshold frequency exists in this setting.

Frequent ventricular ectopic beats are a marker of risk, but are not the direct mechanism by which patients die. Suppression of ventricular ectopic beats by antiarrhythmic drugs has not been rewarded by an improved prognosis[35], although the studies to date have not entirely excluded a positive role for such therapy. β-Adrenoreceptor blocking therapy does reduce late mortality, perhaps as discussed by preventing acute occlusional ventricular fibrillation. Until recently it appeared plausible to consider that high frequency ventricular ectopic beats were markers for late fatal ventricular tachyarrhythmias, and that therapy should be directed to the prophylaxis of the fatal event without it being necessary to alter the ectopic marker. Now subgroup analysis in a prophylactic trial of β-adrenoreceptor blocking therapy suggests that patients who derived prognostic benefit from the therapy were those in whom it suppressed ventricular ectopic beats[36]. If substantiated this observation would have important clinical and therapeutic implications.

CONCLUSIONS

Infarction related ventricular arrhythmias are complex (Table 15.1). They challenge our understanding of the pathophysiology of arrhythmogenesis, and present a dynamic problem for the clinician who must be aware of their immediate and late implications and decide their optimal management.

Table 14.1 Characteristics, implications and treatment of ventricular arrhythmias complicating AMI

Arrhythmia	Time window from onset of MI	Implications immediate	late	Infarct size relationship	Treatment
Primary VF	0–24 h	5–8% †	9–23% 1 year†	none	lignocaine prophylaxis
Non-infarct VF	—	?	80% recurrence	—	? CABG or angioplasty
Acute occlusional VF	0–30 min	? 90% †	?	?	? β-blockers
Reperfusional VF	30–240 min	< 8% †	? none or good	none	? any required
VEBs (any type except frequent)	0–years	none	none	possible	none required
Secondary VF	0–months	30% †	> 50% 1 year†	yes	?
Sustained VT	> 2 days	? 20% †	60% 1 year†	yes	antiarrhythmic drugs surgery or AICD
Frequent VEBs	> 2 days	none	× 2+ mortality	yes	? β-blockers
Late VF	> 2 days	? 50% †	30% 6 weeks†	yes	hospitalization

MI – myocardial infarction;
VF – ventricular fibrillation;
CABG – coronary artery bypass grafting;
AICD – automatic implantable cardioverter defibrillator;
VEBs – ventricular ectopic beats;
VT – ventricular tachycardia; † – mortality

References

1. Adgey, A. A. J., Allen, J. D., Geddes, J. S., James, R. G. G., Webb, S. W., Zaida, S. A. and Pantridge, J. F. (1971). Acute phase of myocardial infarction. *Lancet*, 2, 501–4
2. Lown, B. and Taylor, J. (1970). Thump version. *N. Engl. J. Med.*, **283**, 1223
3. Sanna, G. and Arcidicacono, R. (1973). Chemical ventricular defibrillation of the human heart with bretylium tosylate. *Am. J. Cardiol.*, **32**, 982–7
4. Oliver, M. F., Julian, D. G. and Donald, K. W. (1967). Problems in evaluating coronary care units. Their responsibility and their relation to the community. *Am. J. Cardiol.*, **20**, 465–74
5. Bigger, J. T., Dresdale, R. J., Heissenbuttal, R. H., Weld, F. M. and Wit, A. L. (1974). Ventricular arrhythmias in ischemic heart disease: mechanism, prevalence, significance and management. *Prog. Cardiovasc. Dis.*, **4**, 255–99
6. El-Sherif, N., Myerburg, R. J., Scherlag, B. J., Befeler, B., Aranda, J. M., Castellanos, A. and Lazzara, R. (1976). Electrocardiographic antecedents of primary ventricular fibrillation. *Br. Heart J.*, **38**, 415–22
7. Lown, B., Fakhro, A. M., Hood, W. B. and Thorn, G. W. (1967). The coronary care unit. New perspectives and directions. *J. Am. Med. Assoc.*, **19**, 188–98
8. Lie, K. I., Wellens, H. J. J., Downar, E. and Durrer, D. (1975). Observations on patients with primary ventricular fibrillation complicating acute myocardial infarction. *Circulation*, **52**, 755–9
9. Campbell, R. W. F., Murray, A. and Julian, D. G. (1981). Ventricular arrhythmias

in first 12 hours of acute myocardial infarction. Natural history study. *Br. Heart J.*, **46**, 351–7

10. Kertes, P. and Hunt, D. (1984). Prophylaxis of primary ventricular fibrillation in acute myocardial infarction. The case against lignocaine. *Br. Heart J.*, **52**, 241–7

11. Dubois, C., Smeets, J. P., Demoulin, C., Pierard, L., Foidart, G., Henrard, L., Tulippe C., Preston, L., Carlier, J. and Kulbertus, H. E. (1986). Incidence, clinical significance and prognosis of ventricular fibrillation in the early phase of myocardial infarction. *Eur. Heart. J.*, **7**, 945–51

12. Lie, K. I., Wellens, H. J. J., Von Capelle, F. J. and Durrer, D. (1974) Lidocaine in the prevention of primary ventricular fibrillation. *N. Engl. J. Med.*, **29**, 1324–6

13. Koster, R. and Dunning, A. J. (1985). Intramuscular lidocaine for prevention of lethal arrhythmias in the prehospitalization phase of acute myocardial infarction. *N. Engl. J. Med.*, **313**, 1105–10

14. Mogensen, L. (1970). Ventricular tachyarrhythmias and lignocaine prophylaxis in acute myocardial infarction. *Acta Med. Scand.*, **513**, 1–80

15. Kushnir, B., Fox, K. M., Tomlinson, I. W., Portal, R. W. and Aber, C. P. (1975). Primary ventricular fibrillation and resumption of work, sexual activity and driving after first myocardial infarction. *Br. Med. J.*, **4**, 609–13

16. Goldberg, R., Szklo, M., Tonascia, J. and Kennedy, H. L. (1979). Acute myocardial infarction. Prognosis complicated by ventricular fibrillation or cardiac arrest. *J. Am. Med. Assoc.*, **241**, 2024–27

17. Schwartz, P. J., Zaza, A., Grazi, S., Lombardo, M., Lotto, L., Sbressa, C. and Zappa, P. (1985). Effects of ventricular fibrillation complicating acute myocardial infarction on long term prognosis. Influence of site of infarction. *Am. J. Cardiol.*, **57**, 384–9

18. Witkowski, F. X. and Corr, P. B. (1984). Mechanisms responsible for arrhythmias associated with reperfusion of ischaemic myocardium. *Ann. NY Acad. Sci.*, **427**, 187–98

19. Williams, D. O., Scherlag, B. J., Hope, R. R., El-Sherif, N. and Lazzara, R. (1974). The pathophysiology of malignant ventricular arrhythmias during acute myocardial ischemia. *Circulation*, **50**, 1163–72

20. Liberthson, R. R., Nagel, E. L., Hirschmann, J. C. and Nussenfeld, S. R. (1974). Prehospital ventricular defibrillation. Prognosis and follow up course. *N. Engl. J. Med.*, **291**, 317–21

21. Cobb, L. A., Werner, J. A. and Trobaugh, G. B. (1980). Sudden cardiac death; a decade's experience with out of hospital resuscitation. *Mod. Concepts Cardiovasc. Dis.*, **49**, 31–6

22. Cobb, L. A., Baum, R. S., Alvarez, A. and Schaffer, W. A. (1975). Resuscitation from out-of-hospital ventricular fibrillation: 4 years follow up. *Circulation*, **52**, (Supp. III) 223–8

23. Liberthson, R. R., Nagel, E. L., Hirschmann, J. C., Nussenfeld, S. R., Blackbourne, B. D. and Davis, J. H. (1974). Pathophysiologic observations in prehospital ventricular fibrillation and sudden cardiac death. *Circulation*, **44**, 790–8

24. Tresch, D. D., Wetherbee, J. N., Siegel, R., Troup, P. J., Keelan, M. H., Olinger, G. N. and Brooks, H. L. (1985). Long-term follow-up of survivors of prehospital sudden cardiac death treated with coronary bypass surgery. *Am. Heart. J.*, **110**, 1139–45

25. Skale, B. T., Miles, W. M., Heger, J. J., Zipes, D. P. and Prystowsky, E. N. (1986). Survivors of cardiac arrest: prevention of recurrence by drug therapy as predicted by electrophysiologic testing or electrocardiographic monitoring. *Am. J. Cardiol.*, **57**, 113–19

26. de Soyza, N., Bennett, F. A., Murphy, M. L., Bissett, J. K. and Kane, J. J. (1978). The relationship of paroxysmal ventricular tachycardia complicating the acute phase of myocardial infarction to long term survival. *Am. J. Med.*, **64**, 377–81

27. Hauer, R. N. W., Lie, K. I., Liem, K. L. and Durrer, D. (1982). Long-term prognosis in patients with bundle branch block complicating acute anteroseptal infarction. *Am. J. Cardiol.*, **449**, 1581–5

28. Lie, K. I., Liem, K. L., Schuilenberg, R. M., David, G. K. and Durrer, D. (1978). Early identification of patients developing late in-hospital ventricular fibrillation after discharge from the coronary care unit. A 5.5 year retrospective study of 1897 patients. *Am. J. Cardiol.*, **41**, 674–7

29. Cohen, M., Packer, M. and Gorlin, R. (1983). Indication for left ventricular aneurysmectomy. *Circulation*, **67**, 717–22

30. Marchlinski, F. E., Waxman, H. L., Buxton, A. E. and Josephson, M. E. (1983). Sustained ventricular tachyarrhythmias during the early post infarction period: electrophysiological findings and prognosis for survival. *J. Am. Coll. Cardiol.*, **2**, 240–50

31. Di Marco, J. P., Lerman, B. B., Kron, I. L. and Sellers, T. D. (1985). Sustained ventricular tachyarrhythmias within two months of acute myocardial infarction; results of medical and surgical therapy in patients resuscitated from the initial episode. *J. Am. Coll. Cardiol.*, **6**, 759–68

32. Schulze, R. A., Humphries, J. O'N, Griffith, L. S. C., Ducci, H., Achuff, S., Baird, M. G., Mellits, E. D. and Pitt, B. (1977). Left ventricular and coronary angiographic anatomy. Relationship to ventricular irritability in the late hospital phase of acute myocardial infarction. *Circulation*, **55**, 839–43

33. Moss, A. J. (1980). Clinical significance of ventricular arrhythmias in patients with and without coronary artery disease. *Prog. Cardiovasc. Dis.*, **23**, 33–52

34. Multicenter Postinfarction Research Group. (1983). Risk stratification and survival after myocardial infarction. *N. Engl. J. Med.*, **309**, 331–6

35. May, G. S., Eberlein, K. A., Fubers, C. D., Passamani, E. R. and DeMets, D. L. (1982) Secondary prevention after myocardial infarction. A review of long term trials. *Prog. Cardiovasc. Dis.*, **24**, 331–52

36. Olsson, G. and Rehnqvist, N. (1986). Identification of long term survivors after myocardial infarction by evaluation of initial antiarrhythmic response to metoprolol. *Eur. Heart, J.*, **6**, 44 (Abst)

15
Practical cardiac pacing

E. J. PERRINS

In this chapter only cardiac pacemakers used for the treatment of bradycardias will be considered. Approximately 10 000 pacemaker implants are performed in the UK each year, which represents approx. 160 implants per million population. This contrasts with considerably higher rates in many other developed countries (USA, Canada and West Germany) of up to 500 per million[1]. In this country this almost certainly represents under-diagnosis and referral, particularly of patients suffering from sick sinus syndrome and carotid sinus syndrome.

INDICATIONS

Pacemakers are implanted either for symptomatic bradycardia or for prophylaxis against sudden death, or for both. There are only three major causes of bradycardia: (1) atrioventricular (AVB) block, (2) sick sinus syndrome (SSS), and (3) carotid sinus syndrome (CSS). Their respective incidence is shown in Figure 15.1. It is important to note that there is some overlap in diagnosis between SSS and AVB but much less between CSS and the other two.

SYMPTOMS

The symptomatology is similar regardless of aetiology.

Syncope

This is the most important symptom and is classically termed Adams–Stokes attacks[2,3]. Typically the patient loses consciousness without warning, usually falling to the ground and sustaining injury. The patient is at first very pale then becomes cyanosed. Consciousness is regained rapidly, often accompanied by facial flushing due to reactive hyperaemia. The patient is rarely confused for longer than a few minutes and then recovery is complete. The attacks coincide with either asystole or occasionally ventricular fibrillation. Although typically many patients

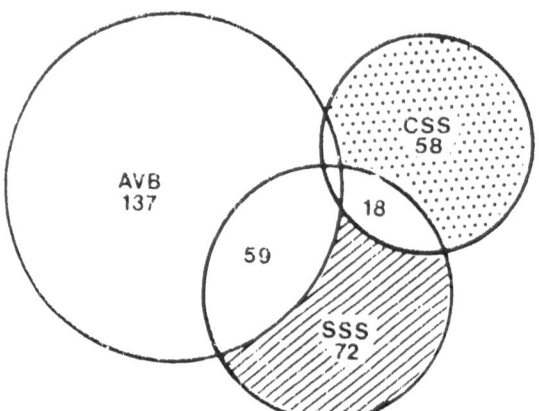

CSS only n = 58   30(2-74)months

SSS only n = 72   30(2-62)months

Figure 15.1   Venn diagram showing relative frequency of electrophysiological diagnoses in 352 patients presenting for pacing (1977–83). Note the overlap beween sick sinus syndrome (SSS) and atrioventricular block (AVB) both overlap much less with carotid sinus syndrome (CSS)

show variations of this pattern some undoubtedly do get a warning, and clonic–tonic convulsions may ensue if cerebral anoxia is prolonged, occasionally sphincter incompetence can occur, but this is rare. Similarly, confusion may be prominent but it is unusual to get a sustained neurological deficit after an attack. Attacks of prolonged unresponsiveness have been described in sick sinus syndrome and are thought to be due to persistent extreme sinus bradycardia[4]. They have been called hibernation attacks, and have been reported to last for up to one and a half hours, but they are rare and such symptoms would normally suggest an epileptic syndrome or hysteria. It must be remembered that in sick sinus syndrome there is probably an increased incidence of systemic embolism so that occasionally true cerebral ischaemic symptoms may occur in addition to bradycardia.

Dizziness

Transient dizziness is common between major attacks described above but a significant number of patients only experience dizziness, and this is more a feature of sick sinus syndrome. There are usually no features of vertigo but as with syncope neurological syndromes may co-exist with the attack leading to erroneous diagnoses of cerebral ischaemia. Dizziness is usually associated with extreme bradycardia, although it may also be caused by reflex hypotension either in patients with carotid sinus syndrome or in patients with pacemaker syndrome (see below).

Minor symptoms

Patients often complain of palpitations (which are usually tachycardias in patients with SSS). Chest discomfort is common, though rarely is it typically anginal. There is a very rare condition of true bradycardiac angina where the ischaemia only occurs during severe and sustained bradycardia. Neck pulsation is an important symptom often overlooked or attributed to hysteria (often in women) but which is due to venous cannon waves during atrioventricular dissociation. This symptom may also occur during ventricular pacing.

HEART FAILURE

Sustained bradycardia in the context of normal ventricular function never causes heart failure, however a significant number of patients with bradycardias have myocardial disease and in them the symptoms of heart failure may be exacerbated. Tiredness is a common complaint in patients unable to increase their cardiac output during exercise, and is occasionally the only symptom of bradycardia present.

A significant number of patients with bradycardias are asymptomatic, but many of these will still require pacing.

Atrioventricular block

This is the commonest reason for pacemaker implant in the UK, but worldwide the incidence of SSS is greater.

Complete heart block (CHB)

All patients with wide complex CHB require pacing for prognostic reasons irrespective of whether they have symptoms. This also applies to wide complex CHB (QRS > 0.12 ms) which is intermittent. The only possible exceptions are asymptomatic patients with narrow complex complete heart block proven to be congenital through prolonged observation and not associated with structural heart disease. Many cardiologists would still insist on thorough assessment of these patients with stress testing and Holter monitoring before finally withholding a pacemaker.

It must be stressed that patients with asymptomatic CHB must be paced unless there are overwhelming reasons not to. Saventrine therapy is now discredited and must not be used; patients receiving this drug for bradycardia should be considered for pacing.

Mobitz type 2 atrioventricular block (AVB)

All asymptomatic patients and those symptomatic patients with persisting block should be paced unless there has been a very recent myocardial infarction (MI). It may be reasonable to withhold pacing in asymptomatic patients with intermittent Mobitz type 2 block although if additional cardiac disease is present a pacemaker is probably indicated.

Mobitz type 1

Wenkebach block had been thought to be a benign arrhythmia but recent evidence would suggest this is not the case. All symptomatic patients should be paced.

Sick sinus syndrome

This condition is characterized by periods of sinus arrest or sino-atrial (SA) block causing either intermittent or sustained severe bradycardia. The bradycardia may exist alone or in combination with paroxysmal atrial flutter/fibrillation, sinus tachycardia or atrial tachycardia. There is an increased incidence of systemic embolism in this condition. All symptomatic patients benefit from pacing and this often reduces the subsequent incidence of tachycardias although some patients require additional drug therapy. There is as yet no clear evidence that asymptomatic patients with SSS derive prognostic benefit from pacing, and this should probably be withheld unless the associated tachycardias are troublesome. Drug therapy on its own for these patients will often precipitate severe bradycardia.

Carotid sinus syndrome

This condition is now being increasingly recognized as a cause of symptomatic bradycardia[5]. Its true incidence is difficult to assess but it may be as high as 30 new patients per million per year. It is caused by overactivity of the carotid sinus baroreflex arc. The exact site of the abnormality is not known although the available evidence suggests a central disorder. The reflex arc causes sinus arrest and often atrio-ventricular block due to intense vagal activity (cardio-inhibitory). In addition, peripheral vasodilation leading to hypotension may occur (vasodepressor). Some patients may have a mixed cardio-inhibitory and vasodepressor response. The condition is often overlooked as in between attacks the heart rhythm is almost invariably normal. Carotid sinus massage for 6 s with the patient resting and recumbent will often reveal the diagnosis, a pause of greater than 3.5 s being significant. It must be emphasized that the reflex can be activated spontaneously in many ways, the patient's symptoms do not normally relate to neck movement or pressure and in fact are indistinguishable from Adams–Stokes syncope. These patients are particularly susceptible to pacemaker syndrome (see below) and atrioventricular pacing is the mode of choice.

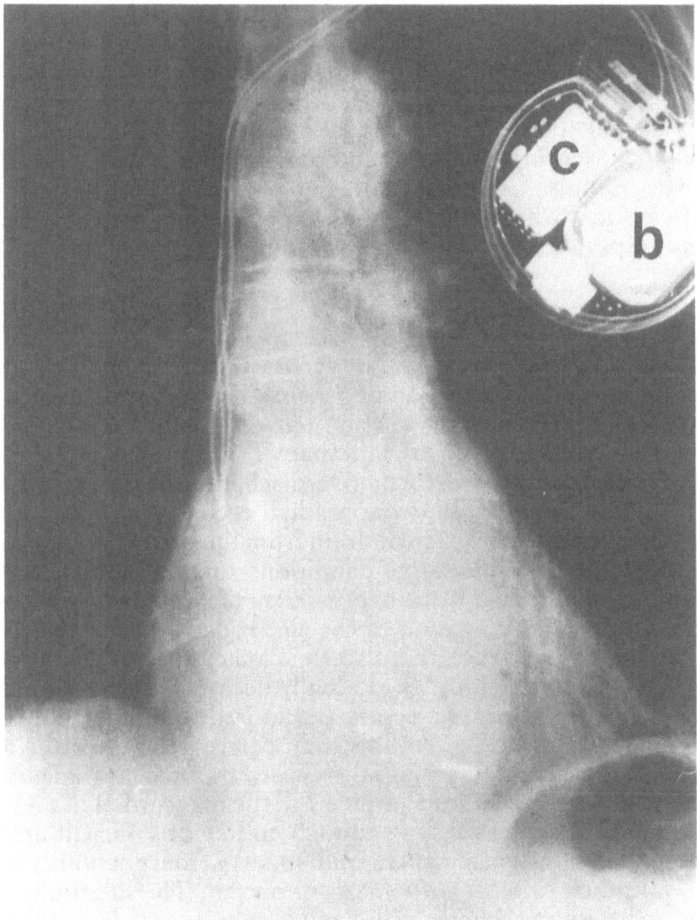

Figure 15.2 This X-ray of an implanted pacemaker clearly shows the battery (b) and the micro-circuit (c). In this older design there is a lot of empty space in the can, in newer designs specially shaped batteries and circuits allow very efficient packing of the components within the can contributing to the size reduction

PACEMAKER TECHNOLOGY

A pacemaker is an implantable electronic device consisting of a battery and an electronic circuit usually totally encapsulated in a metallic can and connected to the heart by one or more leads (Figure 15.2). The connections may be made entirely within the lead (bipolar), or alternatively the pacemaker can may form one part of the circuit (unipolar).

Pacemaker batteries are usually of the lithium iodine type which have a very high power to weight ratio. They also have extremely predictable discharge characteristics with a gradual rise in internal impedance which

251

allows accurate and safe end-of-life prediction, often with as much as a one year safety margin. In addition, the cells do not self-discharge so that if the current drawn by a pacemaker circuit is reduced this will be reflected in a longer unit life.

The pacemaker circuit is functionally divided into a central timing or control block, sensing amplifiers and output circuits which produce the pacemaker impulse. The heart of any pacemaker is the timing and control circuitry which triggers the output circuits at the appropriate time and responds to the information from the sensing circuits.

Output circuits

These form a square-wave signal of accurately defined pulse-width and amplitude, usually in the region of 5 volts. The output is electronically regulated to ensure constant energy delivery in the face of gradually falling battery voltage during the lifetime of the pacemaker. The output is generally produced by a capacitive discharge mechanism. This has two advantages: first, by allowing gradual recharging of the capacitor between output pulses the current drain from the battery is kept constant which allows optimal discharge conditions for the battery. Secondly, the capacitor minimizes DC leakage currents from flowing through the lead which can cause corrosion of the electrode surface by electrolysis. However, the capacitance, and also the capacitance of the lead/tissue interface, may allow 'ringing' (a gradually decaying oscillation) to occur after stimulation and careful design is required to minimize this effect. In addition, polarization potentials may persist long after the applied stimulus. The polarization potential is caused by ionic movements across the small gap between the lead surface and the myocardial tissues. These after-potentials may persist long enough and be of sufficient amplitude to be sensed by the pacemaker, and there is the possibility of self-inhibition leading to a dangerous loss of output. The situation is worse in two lead systems where 'cross talk' may occur, leading to false triggering or inhibition of the other channel. Many manufacturers incorporate 'recharge' circuits which apply a small potential (similar to the polarization voltage) opposite to the applied voltage after stimulation to minimize this effect. Atrial and ventricular output circuits are essentially the same. Although the timing and control blocks incorporate circuitry to limit the upper rate of the pacemaker, the output circuit will generally incorporate a further rate-limiting circuit to operate in the event of catastrophic failure of the control block. Finally, in multi-programmable devices both the pulse-width and output voltage or current may be selectable.

Sensing amplifiers

Sensing circuits are high sensitivity amplifiers which have to detect endocardial P-waves and QRS complexes reliably whilst rejecting other extraneous signals, such as radiofrequency or electromagnetic inter-ference, muscle potentials (EMG), after-potentials, T-waves and in dual chamber modes interference from the other channel. As the amplitude of P-waves is in the region of 0.5–5 mV and the QRS complex 2.5–15 mV considerable problems with interference exist and the design of the sensing circuits is correspondingly complex. Two principal mechanisms are employed to optimize sensing: (1) signal filtering, and (2) periods during which normal sensing is disabled (refractory periods). The incoming signal first passes through a RF filter to remove radiofrequency interference (low-pass filter), then a tuned filter to detect particular characteristics of the P-wave or QRS complex (band-pass filter) and finally through a noise detection circuit which if activated by high frequency noise (usually greater than 8 impulses per second) will disable sensing (see below). However, despite complex filters the high sensitivity of the amplifiers makes the removal of after-potentials and T-waves very difficult. Accordingly, a refractory period is required to disable the sensing amplifier for a short period after a paced or sensed event (150–350 ms). The operation of refractory periods is crucial to understanding complex pacemaker function and electrocardiograms. During the refrac-tory period any signal which appears at the input must not be interpreted as either a P-wave or QRS complex by the device. The simplest (and earliest) approach was to disconnect total sensing during the refractory period. However, this had the disadvantage that if, for example, a QRS complex occurred just at the end of the refractory period (in a ventricular channel) then the amplifier would be switched back on in time to detect the following T-wave: similarly, if noise occurred during the refractory period and continued when sensing was re-started it might then be detected as a QRS complex and cause inappropriate inhibition. There-fore, some modern sensing circuits continue to sense during the terminal part of the refractory period. If a sensed event occurs during this 'noise sampling period' then the refractory period is re-set but no signal is passed to the pacemaker timing circuits. If interference continues then the refractory period is continuously reset so that no sensing occurs, and the pacemaker automatically reverts to fixed rate asynchronous stimulation. This mechanism prevents continuous inhibition of the pacemaker by high levels of continuous noise. In some designs this noise sampling period is only activated by a signal from the noise detection circuitry which in addition may trigger a refractory period if noise is detected outside of the refractory period. Noise inhibition was a sig-nificant problem with early designs when pacemaker dependent patients encountered high levels of interference such as micro-wave ovens and airport security devices.

Atrial sensing requires different filtering to ventricular sensing and requires a separate atrial amplifier.

Timing circuits

These circuits define the basic escape intervals for pacemaker operation. In the earliest devices they were simple transistor oscillators. Modern designs use a highly stable crystal controlled master oscillator. The timing circuits operate by counting a pre-determined number of master clock pulses. When the count is finished (times-out) the counter signals the control circuitry. In multiprogrammable units where many individual timing intervals are adjustable this system allows easy alteration of the timing period by changing the number of pulses to be counted.

Control circuitry

In simple non-programmable VVI, VOO, AAI and AOO devices no separate control circuits were required as the operation of the device was defined by a single parameter – the escape interval of the R–R timer. In any unit incorporating programmability, and in all dual chamber or rate responsive units, control circuits are required. These circuits are extremely complex, and in multiprogrammable DDD pacemakers are of equivalent complexity to a microprocessor chip. The large development costs of these chips is causing a trend towards full microprocessor control of the pacemaker, controlled by both read only and externally programmable random access memory. New pacemaker modes and operating parameters may then be developed by changing the operating program (software) which is cheaper than building a new chip. The advent of software controlled pacemakers is bringing new problems of long-term reliability not previously encountered by so-called 'hard-wired' devices (i.e. the operation of the device is totally defined by the physical configuration of the circuit). The long-term reliability of software and of memory devices within the chip is difficult to define. Most microprocessor based pacemakers, therefore, incorporate a separate failsafe ventricular pacemaker which will maintain ventricular pacing in the event of a microprocessor malfunction. However, it must be emphasized that the large scale integrated circuits are inherently more reliable than designs using discrete components, and that the increased complexity of the DDD device does not render it more susceptible to random failure than a VVI pacemaker.

Communications

In programmable devices a communications link is required between programmer and pacemaker. Early designs[6] used various forms of electromagnetic induction, or even the simple opening and closing of a reed switch by a pulsed magnetic field to produce programming pulses. Radiofrequency digital communication is the most frequently used system now. Most systems require the transmission to the pacemaker of a long binary word which may be from 10 to 30 bits long. The mitted word will contain check digits to ensure security. In other designs the programming word is transmitted twice, and only accepted by the pacemaker if both signals match. In addition, the receiver circuitry is generally only switched on by the presence of a high magnetic field (provided by the programming 'head') which activates an internal reed switch. These features allow a very high degree of programme security and resistance to 'phantom programming'. Further refinements have included the provision of bi-directional telemetry. This allows the internal settings of the pacemaker to be read by the programming device, which in turn allows proper confirmation of programming and is essential if a malfunction is suspected. A number of units also allow the real-time telemetry of endocardial signals. Some systems use simple amplitude modulated radiofrequency signals, whilst others have opted for analog to digital conversion within the pacemaker and subsequent digital transmission. Real-time endocardial recordings may be helpful in the diagnosis of arrhythmias. In addition, some models provide timing markers which indicate when the pacemaker is sensing and pacing in atrium and ventricle. This latter feature may be helpful in ECG interpretation, and may ultimately be developed into fully automatic ECG analysis by the programmer.

Programmers

As the complexity of pacemakers has increased their size has decreased. This cannot be said of programmers which have in many cases become very large and unwieldy microcomputers (Figure 15.3). The development of really simple to operate but effective programmers is still lagging far behind pacemaker designs. As the different manufacturers' pacemakers become more and more similar, due to the adoption of microprocessor controlled circuits, it will ultimately be the programming and telemetry systems which really distinguish the different devices. At present misprogramming is far more likely to occur due to incorrect operation of the programmer than to any other cause, and very detailed records of programming operations must be kept. The ability to interrogate the pacemaker as to its programmed settings is of great assistance in this respect.

TYPES OF PACEMAKER

Pacemaker modes are described by a three letter code with optional fourth and fifth positions. The first letter is the chamber paced (V, ventricle; A, atrium; D, both; O-none). The second letter is the chamber sensed (A,V,D,O) and the third letter is the mode of sensing (I, inhibitor; T, trigger; D, trigger and inhibit; O, none). An optional fourth letter describes whether the unit has rate response (R). The fifth letter relates

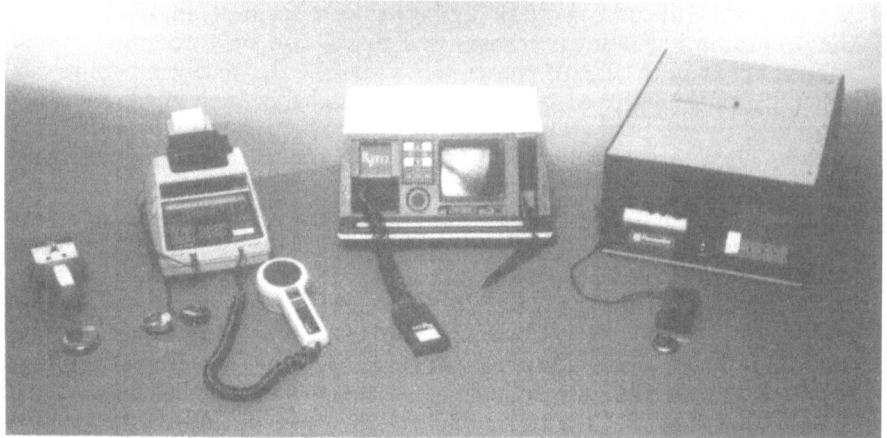

Figure 15.3 Pacemakers with their programmers. As pacemakers became smaller and more sophisticated their programmers became large and complex (left to right)

to tachycardia functions. A simple ventricular inhibited pacemaker is, therefore, VVI, a dual chamber pacemaker DDD, and a ventricular rate responsive unit VVIR.

Pacemakers conveniently divide into single chamber fixed rate devices (VVI – ventricular inhibited, AAI – atrial inhibited), dual chamber devices (DVI – AV sequential pacing, DDD, dual chamber physiological with atrial rate response) and sensor driven single chamber rate responsive units which are basically VVI pacemakers whose basic rate is altered according to some sensed parameter, e.g. Q–T interval, temperature, respiration and body activity. Other sensors are under active development such as mixed venous oxygen saturation.

A block diagram of a dual chamber pacemaker (DDD) is shown in Figure 15.4. The unit functions as an AV sequential pacemaker when the atrial spontaneous rate is below the programmed lower rate. When the atrial rate is between the low rate and the upper rate then each P-wave is followed by a QRS (either paced or sensed). If the P-wave rate is above the upper rate then the pacemaker introduces some form of AV block (often similar to Wenkebach block) to limit the upper rate (Figure 15.5).

A block diagram of a rate-responsive pacemaker is shown in Figure 15.6. The principle is the same regardless of the sensor system employed, but the complexity of the algorithm relating the sensed parameter to the predicted heart rate is very dependent on the sensor used. Q–T, for example, is very complex whereas respiration is relatively simple. The pacemaker has programmable upper and lower rates and usually has at least a slope or sensitivity adjustment which changes the rate of change of rate with exercise.

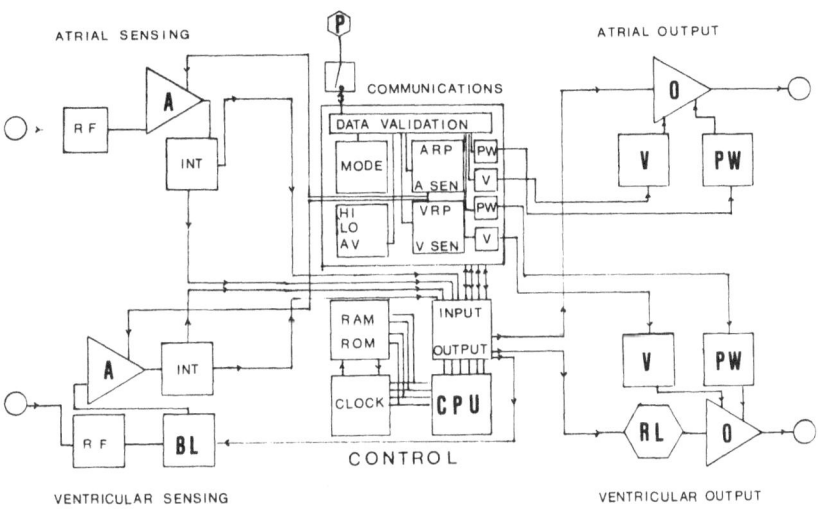

Figure 15.4 Block diagram of a multi-programmable DDD pacemaker. This is seen to be a highly sophisticated device. A, sensing amplifier; BL, blanking circuit; CPU, computer processor chip; O, output stage; V, voltage output control; PW, pulse-width output control; RL, hardware rate limiting circuit on the ventricular channel to protect against 'runaway'

It is beyond the scope of this article to go into detailed functional descriptions of each of the pacing modes.

Pacing mode selection

Many recent studies have shown clear clinical advantages of dual chamber rate responsive (DDD) pacemakers over constant rate pacemakers (VVI) in patients with AVB and SSS[7,8]. These units are selected in patients in whom it is thought will benefit particularly from the increased effort tolerance. This is influenced by financial factors (they are more expensive) and the fact that the implant is more complex. Younger patients are obvious candidates. In order to function correctly DDD pacemakers require normal sinus node function and particularly the absence of atrial fibrillation. In these patients sensor driven rate responsive pacemakers will be required. At present in the UK, about 20% of implants are with dual chamber or rate responsive units. Many cardiologists believe, however, that the majority of patients should in

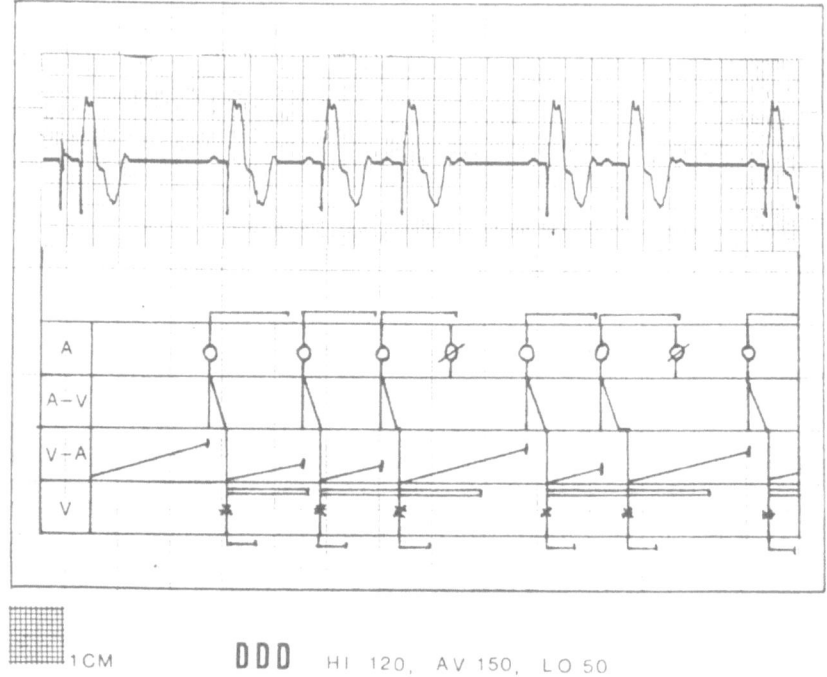

1 CM   DDD   HI 120, AV 150, LO 50

Figure 15.5 ECG and timing diagram showing Wenkebach upper rate behaviour of a DDD pacemaker. In QRS complexes 3 and 4 and 5 and 6 the P–R interval can be seen to lengthen, as the atrial rate is above the programmed upper rate of 120 bpm until the succeeding P wave is blocked by the lengthening atrial refractory period (upper line above the timing diagram). For a full discussion of pacemaker timing diagrams see Perrins *et al.* (1985) Interpretation of dual chamber electrocardiograms. *Pacing Clin. Electrophysiol.*, 8, 6–16

fact receive these complex devices so long as money is available to pay for them.

Pacemaker leads

There have been very significant advances in pacemaker lead design over the last 10 years. The lead is usually constructed from a plastic tube (silicone or polyurethane) in which there is a coiled conductor (often multi-stranded). The tip of the lead is about 10 mm^2 and may be coated with carbon or some other compound, or alternatively roughened or even porous. These 'tip technologies' result in lower threshold and superior sensing characteristics and are much superior to the older polished metallic designs. The most important advance has been 'active fixation' where at the lead tip an arrangement exists to temporarily

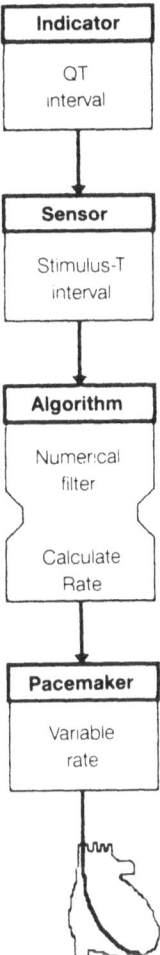

Figure 15.6 Block diagram of a rate responsive pacemaker

lodge the lead until its fibrotic attachment is complete. This may be in the form of little projections (tines or fins, Figure 15.7) which entangle in the RV trabeculae[9,10], or devices which screw into the myocardium itself. Fixation devices have dramatically reduced the complication rate, so that less than 1% of leads displace after implantation. Atrial leads have been developed to the same state of reliability as ventricular leads. In addition it is now possible to construct thin diameter bipolar leads which is leading to an increased use of bipolar systems, particularly in dual chamber pacemakers where the sensing and cross-talk characteristics are improved.

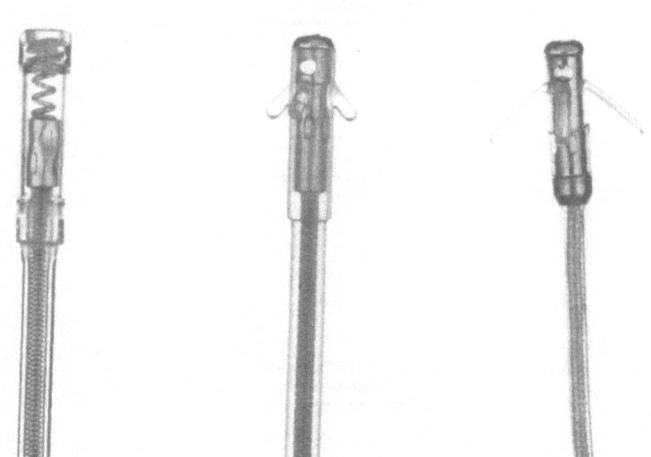

Figure 15.7   Three ventricular pacing leads showing screw and tine fixation

SURGICAL IMPLANTATION

Pacemakers are generally implanted under local anaesthetic, and the vast majority are endocardial with venous access to either the cephalic vein by cut-down or to the subclavian vein by direct puncture. The leads are threaded through the vein into the heart under fluoroscopic control and positioned at the apex of the right ventricle and in the right atrial appendage (if an atrial lead is being used). The pulse generator itself is placed in a pocket fashioned between the surface of the pectoralis major and the subcutaneous tissue. The implant procedure is extremely simple and rarely takes longer than 45 minutes. Epicardial systems are still implanted, usually in the presence of major congenital or valvular heart disease affecting the right side of the heart. Epicardial pacing generally requires a general anaesthetic and an approach to the heart which is xiphisternal. The procedure carries increased morbidity (and possibly mortality) compared to the endocardial approach. There is also unequivocal evidence that epicardial leads are less durable than endocardial ones, presumably related in part to greater mechanical stresses.

FOLLOW-UP

Once the unit is implanted and stitches have been removed the pacemaker has to be checked at 4–6 weeks, initially. At follow-up clinics (which require specialized equipment and appropriately trained technicians) the pacemaker is tested and programmed. In simple terms this involves checking adequate capture and sensing in one or both chambers and in testing the battery. Battery tests may in-part be performed by the pacemaker/programmer combination, but in addition the state of the battery is often linked to the pulse-width or basic pacing rate of the unit. In more complex devices considerable fine tuning may be required in order to maximize the haemodynamic advantages to the patient. After initial visits the pacemaker needs to be checked at 6–12 monthly intervals. The patient is advised that the pacemaker places no restrictions on him/her at all. Patients may drive once the first 4–6 weeks follow-up appointment has been deemed satisfactory, patients are no longer required to notify the Vehicle Licensing Centre in Swansea that they have been fitted with a device, although they should tell their insurance company. Modern pacemakers can be expected to last on average 7 years although many could last up to 15 years.

COMPLICATIONS

Complications during the implant are very rare and are generally related to venous access, particularly with direct puncture of the subclavian vein which can result in pneumothorax or haemothorax or even laceration of the subclavian artery. For this reason many operators prefer to use the cephalic approach where possible, although in reality a good operator must be competent at both techniques. It is possible for the pacing lead to perforate the heart acutely, often only resulting in a poor threshold, and this may go unrecognized. Acute tamponade can occur but is extremely rare. Primary infections are unusual but erosion at the site of the implant (which may or may not be infective) can occur in up to 2% of implants. Prompt management of a suspicious wound may save the patient from having to have a complete explantation and such patients should be referred back immediately to their pacemaker clinic.

Lead displacement occurs in less than 1%, but the lead may become unsatisfactory for sensing (entrance block) or pacing (exit block) acutely without displacement[11]. This is temporary in about half of cases and programmability to adjust output or sensitivity will cure the problem. Very occasionally patients consistently produce exit block and in them a new lead which slowly elutes a steroid from the tip is showing excellent results.

Occasionally pectoral or diaphragmatic stimulation is caused nearly always in unipolar pacemakers, this again can be generally remedied by programming.

Random failure of either the pacemaker or lead is excessively rare (99.9% of pacemakers survive 5 years without technical faults).

Pacemaker syndrome

This is an important condition which only affects patients with ventricular pacemakers[12,13]. It usually occurs in patients who can conduct retrogradely through the AV node (this usually implies intact antero-grade conduction and so is high in patients with SSS or CSS). The

retrogradely through the AV node (this usually implies intact antero-grade conduction and so is high in patients with SSS or CSS). The retrograde P-waves cause cannon waves in the neck which may be felt and raise the left atrial pressure, sometimes causing breathlessness. In addition, atrial stretch reflexes may be activated which cause hypotension or sometimes even syncope. The symptoms usually occur at the onset of pacing and almost always at rest. Upgrading the pacemaker to a dual chamber system will cure the patient[14]. As was mentioned above patients with carotid sinus syndrome are particularly susceptible to this disorder.

References

1. Feruglio, G. A. Steinbach K. (1983) World survey on cardiac pacing. In Steinbach *et al.* (ed.) *Cardiac Pacing.* pp. 953–68. (Darmstadt: Steinkopff)
2. Adams, R. (1827). Irregularity of breathing and remarkable slowness of pulse. *Dublin Hospital Report,* **4,** 396
3. Stokes, W. (1846). Observations on some cases of permanently slow pulse. *Dublin Q. J. Med. Soc.* **2,** 73
4. Sutton, R. and Perrins, E. J. (1979). Neurological manifestations of the sick sinus syndrome. In Busse, E. (ed.) *Cerebral Manifestations of Episodic Cardiac* dysrhythmias. pp. 174–82. (Amsterdam: Excerpta Medica)
5. Perrins, E. J. and Morley, C. A. (1985). The pathophysiology of carotid sinus syndrome. In Gomez, F. P. (ed.) *Cardiac Pacing.* pp. 200–13. (Madrid: Growz)
6. Tarjan, p. (1973). Engineering aspects of implantable cardiac pacemakers. In. Samet, P. (ed) *Cardiac Pacing* p. 47. (New York: Grune and Stratton)
7. Kruse, I. *et al.* (1982). A comparison of the acute and long term effects of ventricular inhibited and atrial synchronous ventricular inhibited pacing. *Circulation,* **65,** 846–55
8. Perrins, E. J. Morley, C. A. Chan, S. L. and Sutton, R. (1982). A randomised controlled trial of physiological and ventricular pacing. *Br. Heart J.,* **50,** 112–17
9. Mond, H. and Sloman, J. (1980). The small tined ventricular lead. Absence of displacement. PACE, **3,** 171–7
10. Messenger, J., Castellanet, M. J. and Stephenson, N. L. (1982). New permanent endocardial atrial J lead: implantation techniques and clinical performance. PACE, **5,** 767–72
11. Kertes, P., Mond, H., Sloman, G. *et al.* (1983). Comparison of lead complications with polyurethane tines, silicone rubber tined and wedge tipped leads. Clinical experience with 822 endocardial ventricular leads. *Pace,* **6,** 957–62
12. Ausubel, K. and Furman, S. (1985). The pacemaker syndrome. *Ann. Intern. Med.,* **103,** 420–9
13. Alicandri, C., Fouad, F. M., Tarazi, R. C., Castle, L. and Mourant, V. (1978). Three cases of hypotension and syncope with ventricular pacing. Possible role of atrial reflexes. *Am. J. Cardiol.,* **42,** 137–42
14. Morley, C. A., Perrins, E. J., Grant, P., Chan, S. L., McBrien, D. and Sutton, R. (1982). Carotid sinus syncope treated by pacing. Analysis of persistent symptoms and the role of atrioventricular sequential pacing. *Br. Heart J.,* **47,** 411–18

16
External electrical defibrillation and cardioversion

J. C. P. CRICK

'... fatal syncope often differs from non-fatal syncope in the super-
vention in the former case of fibrillar contraction (or delirium) in
the ventricular muscle: this seals the fate of the depressed heart by
arresting the circulation...'

So wrote John A. MacWilliam nearly 100 years ago[1], eloquently noting
four important features of the usual type of cardiac arrest:

(1) the heart is diseased of its function depressed by some prior event
or metabolic disturbance;
(2) a change of rhythm occurs to ventricular fibrillation;
(3) there is a complete loss of cardiac output and collapse of arterial
pressure;
(4) the resulting global myocardial ischaemia makes spontaneous
recovery impossible so that death is usually inevitable.

The possibility of averting this fate has only been provided during
the last 40 years by the invention of cardiopulmonary resuscitation
(CPR). Of its three main components, electrical defibrillation is the
decisive step while prior restoration of the circulation and of blood
oxygenation and pH may also be required depending on the cause and
time of course of the arrest.

Defibrillation has been lifesaving in countless patients in the early
stages of acute myocardial infarction, and has made possible many
invasive or surgical procedures in which the risk from cardiac arrest
would otherwise have been prohibitively high. The use of electricity to
convert other arrhythmias to sinus rhythm, cardioversion, has become
standard practice and has been found to be both more effective and in
many circumstances far safer than the use of drugs.

HISTORY

The story of electrical defibrillation is a remarkable illustration of the apathy and inertia with which the medical establishment often greets a powerful new technique: decades or even centuries are allowed to elapse between the exposition of its principles and possibilities and the widespread adoption of its practice.

In the eighteenth century, electrostatic and electrochemical generators capable of producing a substantial shock, as well as early work on the electrical stimulation of the locomotor system, led to an interest in the general health-restoring properties of electricity. The few published reports probably represent only a small fraction of the widespread uncontrolled use of medical electricity. Some, however, are strongly suggestive of successful defibrillation, especially the report by Hawes in 1774[2]. A child who was 'to all appearances dead' following a fall was, after other resuscitation attempts had failed, given a transthoracic shock by a Mr Squires. This restored the pulse and, after a few minutes, spontaneous breathing. Afterwards, 'a kind of stupor ... remained for several days but ... (subsequently) ... her health was restored'. The only scientific investigation of this subject at that time was by Abildgaard, who used electric shocks on chickens to produce an apparently lifeless state. He showed that a further shock when applied to the chest (but not when applied elsewhere) restored life and rapid recovery while birds left untreated remained dead. He reported this phenomenon in 1775[3a,b], but its mechanism was not demonstrated until the end of the nineteenth century. Ventricular fibrillation (VF) was first described by Erichsen in 1840[4] as a 'tremulous motion' of the ventricles produced in dogs by coronary artery ligation. It was electrically induced by Hoffa and Ludwig 10 years later[5]. By 1889 MacWilliam[1] had concluded that it was responsible for most cases of sudden death. Finally, in 1900 Prevost and Battelli reported[6] that a direct current shock applied directly to a dog's fibrillating heart successfully restored regular rhythm.

More than 30 years passed after this momentous discovery before anyone even repeated their work, and this was at the instigation of the electricity industry. Prompted by Howell, Kouweenhoven (an engineer) and Hooker (a physiologist), working in dogs, confirmed the findings of Prevost and Battelli and published the results in 1933[7]. They used alternating current (AC) of about 1 A for 1–2 seconds, and noted that recovery was achieved only if defibrillation was performed within 2 minutes. Further animal experiments were performed by Wiggers and Beck who both found that delayed defibrillation was successful provided that circulation was maintained in the interim by direct (internal) cardiac massage. These results were reported in 1936 and 1937[8,9]. Beck was the first to attempt[10] and eventually in 1947 succeeded[11] in applying this technique to humans. There followed a decade of heroic and often successful resuscitation involving emergency thoracotomy, sometimes out of hospital, with manual heart massage performed until a defibrillator could be applied directly.

In 1956 Zoll showed[12] that successful external defibrillation in humans was possible, provided it was applied within a few minutes. The application of this technique rapidly spread, although it was limited to centres where the necessary apparatus, including an external pacemaker, was immediately available. Because of the need in other circumstance for internal cardiac massage, internal defibrillation continued to be the usual practice. Kouwenhoven had earlier shown[7] that external defibrillation of dogs was possible and while working on an external device in 1958 made a chance observation that revolutionized cardiac resuscitation. He noticed that the pressure of defibrillator electrodes on the dog's chest caused a rise in arterial pressure. This rapidly led to the description by Kouwenhoven, Jude and Knickerbocker in 1960[13] of the technique of external cardiac massage and from there to full closed chest resuscitation.

Most experimental and all clinical defibrillators used alternating current until 1962 when Lown and colleagues[14] showed that direct current shocks of much shorter duration were effective and caused less myocardial damage. They also showed that shocks delivered in other arrhythmias were successful in converting to sinus rhythm and were unlikely to cause ventricular fibrillation provided the 'vulnerable period' in the T-wave of the ECG was avoided.

Over the last 25 years there has been little fundamental advance in external defibrillation and cardioversion but vast experience with the technique has proved it to be safe and effective. It has been the major stimulus to the setting up of coronary care units, proposed in 1961 by Julian[15] and mobile pre-hospital resuscitation units described by Pantridge in 1967[16]. Recent years have seen the introduction of implantable cardioverter–defibrillators, described in Chapter 20 and automatic external defibrillators, described below.

ELECTROPHYSIOLOGY

Re-entry arrhythmias

The re-entry mechanism, responsible for most cardiac arrhythmias, requires that in front of the advancing wavefront there lies excitable (not totally refractory) tissue. Usually this tissue has only just recovered from the preceding depolarization and, in part of the circuit, it is likely to be still partially refractory. This causes the slowed conduction which is necessary to keep the cycle length longer than the refractory period of the weakest link (i.e. the part with the longest refractory period).

In supraventricular tachycardia (SVT) and atrial flutter (AFL) the same course is run each time, but in atrial fibrillation (AF) and VF multiple small wavefronts spread in different directions following the least refractory path available in a generally chaotic fashion. Such a wavefront is likely on occasion to find itself surrounded by refractory tissue and, therefore, unable to continue. The chances of this happening simultaneously to all the wavefronts, causing spontaneous reversion, depends on their number; so it is not surprising that there seems to be a 'critical mass' of available myocardium required for VF to continue. MacWilliam noted[17] that sustained VF was only possible in animals larger than a cat, rabbit, monkey or small dog. In larger hearts surgical excision[18] or chemical inactivation[19] of a sufficient proportion of myocardium stops fibrillation.

Re-entry ventricular tachycardias fall somewhere between the two: there is one preferred circuit but this is often functionally rather than anatomically determined and may be altered by metabolic factors or pacing stimuli or may spontaneously drift, as exemplified by the *torsade-de-pointes* pattern.

Electrical conversion

The termination of the re-entry arrhythmia is accomplished if all the excitable tissue in the circuit is simultaneously depolarized. Resting myocardium may be depolarized by the passage of a small current (about $2 \, mA/cm^2$) across the membrane, but for partially refractory fibres the threshold is around four times higher[20] and these must also be depolarized to ensure that re-entry does not continue. This is especially the case with fibrillation where most of the excitable muscle is partially refractory.

The Weiss–Lapicque relationship between strength and duration for threshold stimulation is illustrated in Figure 16.1. The minimum energy pulse is at the 'chronaxie', the duration at which current threshold is twice that for continuous current (the 'rheobase'). For resting myocardium this is in the region 1–4 ms, as demonstrated by strength–duration curves for pacing threshold. The optimum duration for partially refractory myocardium and fibres depending on slow channel depolarization is not necessarily the same and has not been experimentally determined. For a single fibre the shape of the current pulse is probably of little consequence provided it is not too far removed from a square wave. In practice the wave-forms used have been chosen mainly for the simplicity of the electronic circuits required to generate them; they are discussed further in the section on defibrillator design.

Automatic arrhythmias

Non-re-entry arrhythmias may be generated by a variety of obscure processes and the mechanism of successful electrical cardioversion (when it occurs) is unknown, though something akin to overdrive suppression of pacemaker cells is usually assumed. It may well be that the intense stimulation of the intrinsic cardiac nerves[22] is more important than myocardial depolarization. Many of these arrhythmias, especially multifocal atrial tachycardia, recur after a short period.

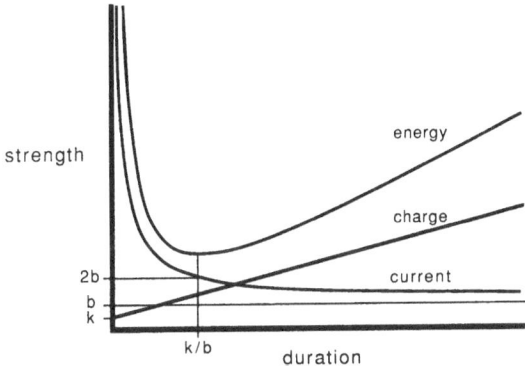

Figure 16.1 Strength–duration curves for membrane depolarization by square-wave pulses. The charge threshold Q is given by the Weiss equation: $Q = k + b.d$ where k and b are constants and d is the pulse duration. The current threshold I is given by the more familiar Lapicque equation: $I = k/d + b$ (which is equivalent as $I = Q/d$). The constant k is the minimum charge which can depolarize the membrane and is related to the membrane capacitance. The constant b is related to the membrane resistance. Lapicque referred to b as the maximum 'leakage' current which can cross the membrane without depolarizing it and so is related to the membrane resistance. Lapicque referred to b as the 'rheobase' and the duration k/b at which the current threshold threshold is twice b as the 'chronaxie'. The energy threshold is proportional (for a resistive load) to the product of the current and charge thresholds and this curve has a minimum at the chronaxie

Vulnerable period and synchronization

If a stimulus with an intensity between the resting threshold and the maximum threshold for partially refractory tissue is delivered during repolarization of a non-fibrillating region, then areas of depolarization will lie adjacent to excitable fibres. Irregular spread of depolarization into these fibres may lead to the initiation of fibrillation. This is probably the explanation for the vulnerable period during which fibrillation can easily be induced; for the ventricles it lies near the apex of the T-wave and for the atria, the T_a-wave. For defibrillation the vulnerable period of the non-fibrillating chamber should be avoided, while for cardioversion this applies to both the atria and ventricles. The vulnerable period can be avoided by triggering the shock either during diastole or early systole for the chamber concerned. In practice synchronization to the QRS complex of the external ECG, as originally proposed by Lown[14] has been universally adopted, though it should be recognized that this is less than ideal. In particular, cardioversion of SVT may result in atrial fibrillation and then a higher energy shock is usually required to restore sinus rhythm.

One of the problems with the AC defibrillators was the inability to avoid the vulnerable period with shocks of several hundred milliseconds duration so that they were only suitable for the treatment of VF.

BIOPHYSICS

The current field produced by an externally applied shock passes throughout the body which is an inhomogeneous volume conductor. The current density at a particular position depends on its distance from the electrodes, their areas and the local conductivity in relation to that of nearby tissues. Several factors related to the geometry of the field have important influences on the success of defibrillation or cardioversion.

(1) *The direction of the current flow*

Only the component of current flowing perpendicular to the membranes, i.e. the cosine fraction of the total current, has a depolarizing effect so that some fibres, orientated parallel to the field, are relatively protected. In addition, the myocardium is anisotropic as regards conductivity, 3.2 times higher in the direction parallel to the fibres[23] distorting the field towards this direction.

(2) *Uneven dose*

The current density produced is far from equal throughout the heart. In defibrillation virtually all of the excitable tissue of the atria or ventricles must be depolarized, as in remaining areas fibrillation sustained for a few hundred ms can spread back into the recovering myocardium. This factor combined with (1) means that some parts will have to receive current far in excess of threshold. The damaging effects of a high current dose may make these areas prone to spontaneous recurrence of fibrillation.

(3) *Electrode size*

For a given delivered current the current density at the skin is inversely proportional to the electrode contact area. Therefore, to minimize electrical and thermal damage to the skin and underlying structures the electrodes must be large. If, however, they are larger than the atria or ventricles a greater proportion of the total current will bypass the heart and be wasted. The size adopted is 8–9 cm diameter. The use of a larger size, 12–13 cm diameter, has been shown to make no difference to the defibrillation threshold[24].

(4) *Electrode position*

This is important in determining the pattern of the field and the region of high current density. The conventional anterolateral arrangement consists of electrodes at the upper right sternal edge and the left mid-axillary line (ECG V_6 position). For atrial defibrillation Lown suggests[25] that an anteroposterior arrangement should be preferable; although theoretical considerations would favour this, clinical experience has been conflicting: in favour[25,26], against[27] and equivocal[24]. It is likely that wide variations in chest geometry explain the individual differences and if one method fails the other should be tried. A third arrangement,

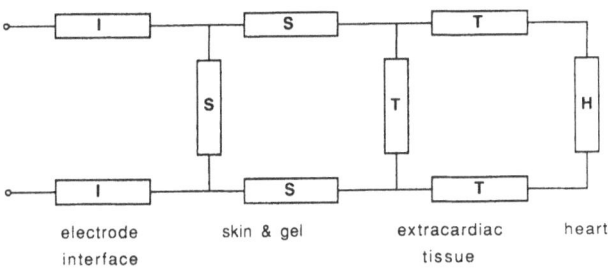

electrode   skin & gel   extracardiac   heart

interface   tissue

Figure 16.2 The components of defibrillation impedance. There is a series impedence at each of the electrode–electrolyte interfaces. The electrolyte and skin surface form a parallel impedance (which may be low if there is a 'jelly-short' between the electrodes) as well as a second series impedance. The tissue between the skin and the heart has a complex impedance with series and parallel components, the lungs having a particularly high impedance. Finally the impedance of the myocardium and the intra-cavitary blood further affects the defibrillating current

tongue to abdomen, is effective[28] and has been adopted for an automatic device, but it is not otherwise generally used.

(5) *Transthoracic impedance*

The peak current flow between the electrodes is determined, for a given stored energy setting, by the sum of the interelectrode impedance and that internal to the device, while the delivered energy is determined by their ratio. Thus a high transthoracic impedance will significantly reduce the current flow (on which defibrillation depends), while a low impedance will cause more of the stored energy to be dissipated internally. The measured overall impedance has several components, shown in Figure 16.2.

The series impedances reduce the defibrillation current. They consist of the electrode interface and skin impedance which are minimized by adequate contact pressure[29] and the use of conductive electrode gel; the extracardiac tissues, especially the left lung if it lies between the apex of the heart and the lateral electrode; and the heart itself. Anoxia causes transient ultra-structural changes in the myocardium which results in an increase in resistivity[30]. This will tend to divert current away from the myocardium, but as the increase is predominantly in the longitudinal direction there may be a beneficial reversal of the anisotropy.

The parallel impedances, if low, cause shunting of current away from the heart. Conduction across or through the skin can be a significant problem if the electrodes are placed too close together or if electrode gel forms a continuous film between them (a 'jelly short'). Pulmonary congestion or even frank pulmonary oedema develops very rapidly during a major arrhythmia, leading to a marked decrease in resistivity of the lungs. By providing a low resistance path around the heart, further current is diverted reducing the proportion of the total current flowing through the myocardium.

Defibrillator circuits are generally designed and calibrated assuming a resistive load of 50 ohm. Measured impedance with standard electrodes is rather higher, 60–80 ohm. Kerber, amongst his extensive studies on defibrillation and cardioversion, has found that smaller chest size, larger electrodes and the delivery of a previous shock were associated with lower impedance[29]. The value of these results, however, is limited as changes in parallel as well as series components are involved and are not readily separated – e.g. the lower impedance for a second shock may be due to changes in the electrode interface and skin (helpful) or the development of increasing pulmonary oedema (unhelpful). He did show that where a value greater than 100 ohm is found the energy threshold is usually substantially higher, implying an important series component[31]. He was evaluating a device which measured impedance using a small high frequency (31 kHz) current during the charging period to indicate if the electrodes should be adjusted or a higher energy set.

DEFIBRILLATOR DESIGN

Output waveform (Figure 16.3)

Although Prevost and Battelli[6] had used capacitor discharge for defibrillation, Hooker and Kouwenhoven[7] found AC shocks more successful, resulting in the early adoption of AC devices. In 1947, Gurvich and Yuniev[32] showed that capacitor discharge was made more effective when the pulse was prolonged by a coil in series with the load. This important finding was first used by Lown[14]. In the meantime McKay and Leeds[33] repeated the work, apparently with the intention of generating AC shocks from battery powered devices.

The unresisted discharge of a capacitor through a coil results in a sine-wave oscillating current. When a series resistor is added to the circuit the sine-wave is damped and decays in amplitude in successive cycles. The Lown waveform, using the transthoracic load as the resistor, is heavily damped so that the second half-cycle is much smaller than the first and there is no third half-cycle. With a resistance which just prevents a second half-cycle the system is 'critically damped' and this waveform, suggested by Edmark[34], has been most widely adopted in principle. In practice the degree of damping is as much determined by the patient's individual transthoracic resistance as by the designer's intention.

An alternative to damping the oscillation is to use a single complete cycle, a symmetrical diphasic pulse. This waveform has the theoretical advantage of depolarizing the membrane on both sides of a fibre rather than just that facing the cathode. This may lower the threshold especially of fibres not optimally orientated to the field. A diphasic pulse was first

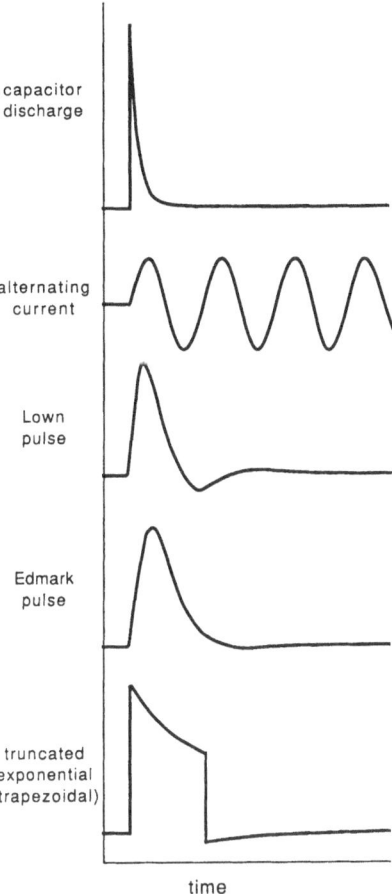

Figure 16.3 Defibrillator output pulses. The simple capacitor discharge and A.C. were used by early workers. The Lown and Edmark pulses are examples of damped capacitor/inductor discharges first used by Gurvich and Yuniev. The truncated exponential waveform is similarly effective and avoids the need for an inductor

used in an early portable defibrillator, reported by Jude, Kouwenhoven and Knickerbocker in 1962[35]. It was adopted after extensive testing on dogs showed it to be effective and particularly safe (though it is not clear whether it was actually compared with other waveforms), and they found it to be clinically effective. Schuder *et al.* in 1964 compared[36] one, two and three phase square-wave pulses in dogs and showed that near threshold current the monophasic pulse was effective within a much narrower range of durations than the others. Their later studies on epicardial electrodes in calves[37] suggested bidirectional pulses were more effective and safer. Meanwhile, Negovsky *et al.*[38] in 1980 reported their considerable clinical experience using diphasic pulses with a maximum total energy of only 200 J achieving a high (80–100%) success rate. Jones and Jones[39,40], working with a myocardial tissue culture, showed a reduced depression of rhythmicity and contraction when diphasic sinusoidal or asymmetrical bidirectional square-wave pulses were used in which the reverse component was 5–20% of the initial pulses current (similar to the Lown waveform), but they did not assess the therapeutic ratio for symmetrical pulses.

A third pulse waveform, which avoids the need for a bulky inductor, is the truncated exponential pulse (loosely described as trapezoidal), generated by discharging a capacitor through a resistor for a limited duration. To achieve a reasonably square pulse of similar duration the product of capacitance and resistance must be much higher than that where inductance is included. Although this pulse has a theoretical advantage in minimizing energy dissipation in the heart[41], Geddes, Niebauer et al., working with isolated perfused dog hearts in a saline tank, found no significant difference in therapeutic ratio for square, truncated exponential or damped sinusoidal pulses nor for single, double or symmetrical bidirectional square pulses[42].

Clearly the value of non-human models in this context is very limited as both geometry and electrophysiology are crucial determinants. Research in this important area has been sadly lacking but there is likely to be a resurgence of interest related to implantable devices where threshold is critically important. Investigation of the use of multiple shocks using different combinations of three electrodes has not been applied to external defibrillation.

Output energy

Although a maximum energy of 400 J (stored) has been widely adopted, Tacker et al. (1974) suggested that this was inadequate, especially for heavy patients[43]. This was partly based on animal work which seemed to indicate that there was a general dose per kg; this was extrapolated to humans without reference to relative heart size and chest geometry. The other basis was a retrospective analysis of defibrillation attempts in which there was a substantial failure rate, worst (50%) for patients over 80 kg. In response to this, high output defibrillators were developed by several manufacturers. Pantridge, on the other hand, reported[44] a very high success rate (80 out of 82) using one or two low energy shocks (200 J stored). A multitude of papers appeared over the next 4 years supporting high or low energy defibrillation, and these were reviewed in 1980 by Crampton[45] who concluded that:

(1) the patients' clinical condition mainly determines the outcome;
(2) body weight does not affect the defibrillation success rate;
(3) there was no evidence for extra efficacy of shocks greater than 400 J, or in most cases 200 J.

Subsequent prospective human studies[46,47] have confirmed these views.

The pulse generator

The basic circuit of the damped sinusoidal pulse generator consists of a capacitor in series with an inductor. Either a charging circuit or the electrode paddles are connected via switches.

Typical values chosen are capacitance: 30–45 μF, inductance: 20–50 mH, charge voltage (max) 4–5 kV, total internal resistance 5–12 Ω. The charging voltage is achieved by an oscillator driving a step-up transformer. The charging level is monitored by a voltmeter across the capacitor (with a non-linear scale) calibrated in energy (Joules) delivered into a 50 Ω load. Control of charging is either manual, charging continuously while a switch is held on, or automatic, charging up to an operator-determined level. The charge stored should be maintained for a period within close limits or automatically topped-up – this is especially required for devices using a compact type of capacitor in which the dielectric (K-film) slowly absorbs the stored charge.

Unused charge is dumped by connecting an internal load of about 10 kΩ across the capacitor. This is done either by the operator or automatically when the device is switched off and whenever a shock is delivered (as dielectric charge may otherwise regenerate a dangerous voltage across the capacitor). Charge dumping should also be performed automatically when a lower energy setting is selected, though this is not done in some devices. Dumping the charge through an external load of less than 50 Ω, especially by shorting the electrode paddles together, can damage the K-film type capacitor because of the large reverse polarity voltage of the very under-damped discharge.

The high voltage components should be well isolated from the case and other parts of the circuit and preferably embedded in a suitable insulating material. Standards for isolation, circuit performance, mechanical strength and other parameters have been proposed in the UK[48,49] and USA[50] and generally adopted.

Electrode paddles

The construction of the paddles should ensure that the operator is able to apply the electrodes with adequate force without coming into contact with them either directly or via conductive gel. In some older types force on the handle towards the body closes electrical contacts against a stiff spring ensuring adequate skin pressure; unfortunately this has not been generally adopted, probably in the interests of compactness. A 'fire' button should be incorporated in both paddles and preferably a 'charge' button in one. Sometimes a 'ready' indicator is included.

A flat paddle, shaped like a hand mirror and having no buttons, should be available for anterior–posterior shocks. Alternatively, large disposable self-adhesive pre-gelled electrodes may be used.

ECG monitoring

Almost all modern defibrillators incorporate an ECG monitor. This records either from a separate cable with standard ECG electrodes or, for emergency use, directly from the paddle electrodes. The input is disconnected when a shock is delivered, but even so it must be well protected against high voltages that may remain transiently on the electrodes. The signal is severely filtered to minimize interference and base-line drift and is therefore significantly distorted, QRS amplitude and ST shift being uninterpretable. Where ECG print-out is available there should be an 'unfiltered' option for this reason.

Synchronization

The timing signal is derived from the ECG monitor, triggered by the rectified differentiated QRS complex so that trigger level and signal polarity do not require adjustment. Correct synchronization should be indicated by a marker on the ECG or audibly. It is recommended[48] that synchronized mode is indicated by a warning light or tone as its unintended use in emergency resuscitation of VF has been a common operator cause of defibrillation failure. It is preferable that reversion to asynchronous mode occurs automatically on start-up and possibly also after synchronous shocks are delivered (in case VF results).

These and other technical features of defibrillator design have been discussed by O'Dowd[51].

Ventricular defibrillation

Consciousness is lost within 10–20 seconds on the onset of VF, but this period may be apparently longer when preceded by a period of rapid VT, as often happens. It is very upsetting to a patient to be defibrillated while awake and this is quite possible with alert coronary care staff. A few soothing words while preparations are calmly made will generally suffice to allow the 'cardiac anaesthetic' to take effect. Failing this intravenous diazepam immediately after the defibrillation may erase the unpleasant memory.

Outside this brief period defibrillation should be performed as early as possible. The rhythm should be apparent from the monitor connected to the paddle electrodes; if it is unclear in the cardiac arrest situation the first shock should be delivered anyway ('blind defibrillation') while arrangements for better ECG monitoring are made. External cardiac massage should be performed while setting-up and charging the defibrillator if the arrest has been longer than 30 seconds, and continued between attempts and after successful defibrillation until a good pulse returns. Attention to the airway and ventilation can be left until after the first shock unless a primary respiratory cause is suspected (see Chapter 23). The procedure proposed by the Resuscitation Council of

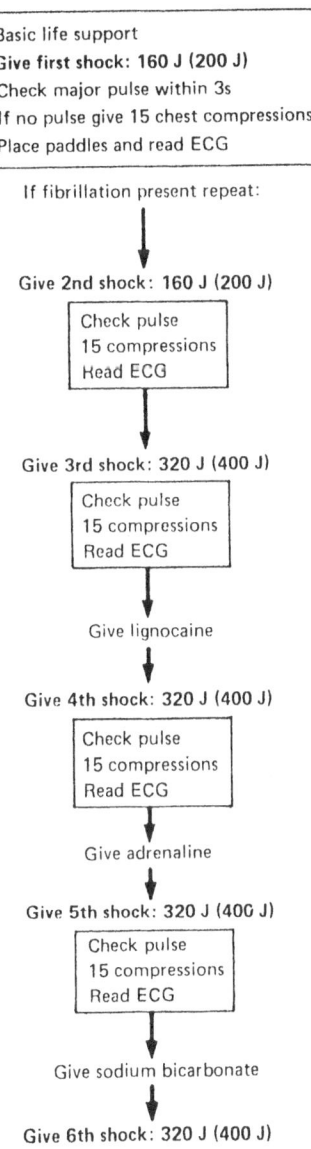

1 Basic life support
2 **Give first shock: 160 J (200 J)**
3 Check major pulse within 3s
4 If no pulse give 15 chest compressions
5 Place paddles and read ECG

If fibrillation present repeat:

Give 2nd shock: 160 J (200 J)

Check pulse
15 compressions
Read ECG

Give 3rd shock: 320 J (400 J)

Check pulse
15 compressions
Read ECG

Give lignocaine

Give 4th shock: 320 J (400 J)

Check pulse
15 compressions
Read ECG

Give adrenaline

Give 5th shock: 320 J (400 J)

Check pulse
15 compressions
Read ECG

Give sodium bicarbonate

Give 6th shock: 320 J (400 J)

Figure 16.4   Resuscitation from cardiac arrest. From Chamberlain, 1986[52], reproduced with permission

the UK is summarized in Figure 16.4 (from Chamberlain, 1986[52]) and is similar to that recommended by the American Heart Association[53]. Before antiarrhythmic agents are used (which could prolong electromechanical dissociation) a period of 1–2 minutes of intensive CPR followed by another shock has sometimes been found to be successful by the author. The use of lignocaine can be used which is traditional and based mainly on its efficacy against ventricular extrasystoles; it may well be that intravenous amiodarone, bretylium or flecainide will prove more helpful.

Cardioversion

Emergency cardioversion for acute onset arrhythmias with haemo-dynamic deterioration, especially in the context of myocardial infarc-tion, requires only a brief partial but amnesic intravenous anaesthetic, though, if immediately available, full anaesthesia with endotracheal intubation is preferable when the patient's fasting status is in doubt. For elective cardioversion a proper anaesthetic is probably safer.

The energy required for conversion of AF is similar to that for VF but in an elective procedure smaller shocks may be tried first. The anterior–posterior paddle configuration may be preferable as discussed above.

Other tachycardias – atrial flutter, SVT and VT – generally respond to much lower energy shocks of 10–50 J although higher energies may be required (or may still be ineffective) for automatic arrhythmias.

Paediatric defibrillation

Because of the relatively greater size of the heart compared to the chest in children, the electrode paddles should be the largest that can be applied leaving an adequate gap. Adult paddles are suitable for most children over 3 years of age though smaller paddles should be available for babies.

An energy 'dose' related to body-weight, 2 J/kg, has been widely adopted, but there is little data to support this. An alternative is to start with a very low energy shock of 5 J, doubling with rapidly successive shocks until successful.

AVOIDANCE OF COMPLICATIONS

Resnekov and McDonald in 1967[54] reported a complication rate of nearly 15% in 220 patients treated with cardioversion. Apart from systemic emboli (two patients) most of these could be attributed in retrospect to the underlying disease, the precardioversion arrhythmia or the additional non-electrical treatment. In addition, despite the dis-continuation of digoxin for 24 hours prior to the procedure, transient rhythm disturbance occurred in over 50%.

Emboli

Atrial fibrillation causes loss of atrial contraction and may result in thrombus formation within the atria. Reversion to sinus rhythm, however caused, is associated with a small but significant risk of systemic embolization. Elective cardioversion allows the institution of anti-coagulation and this has been shown, prospectively, to reduce the incidence of emboli[55]. As there may be a delay before effective atrial systole returns (Stewart, R. 1987; personal communication) anti-coagulation should be continued at least for a few days.

Arrhythmias

The significant postshock arrhythmias are sinus arrest or prolonged severe bradycardia and VT or VF. For bradycardias intravenous atropine should be given, and the possible need for pacing should be considered in cases of 'lone AF' without obvious structural disease as this may be a manifestation of sinus node disease. To avoid ventricular arrhythmias electrolyte (especially potassium) disturbance, metabolic (especially thyroid) abnormalities and drug toxicity should be excluded or corrected before elective cardioversion, and synchronization used whenever possible.

Digoxin, especially, has been associated with shock-induced refractory VF since the early report of three cases by Rabbino et al.[56] in 1964. Kleiger and Lown[57] within 2 years published a study of 107 cardioversions from AF. They found signs of digitalis toxicity in the preshock ECG as well as a high digoxin dose were associated with electrically induced ventricular arrhythmias. They also noted that in cases reported elsewhere serious complications followed shocks of 200 J or more, and suggested the use of a very low energy shock, starting with 25 J. This practice has since been widely adopted for all digitalized patients. Their use of antiarrhythmic drugs to suppress ectopic beats, however, has not been shown to be of any prophylactic benefit in this (or any other) context. A recent study by Mann et al.[58] claimed to show that cardioversion of digitalized patients is 'safe' if the serum drug level is in the therapeutic range (<2 mg/ml). Although this is an attractive hypothesis, their evidence is far from compelling, being based on only 19 cases. With the generally lower doses of digoxin used in recent years and a greater awareness of the problem, toxicity is becoming much less frequent. This may lead to complacency and it is essential that the possibility be consciously considered in every case.

Tissue injury

Myocardial damage by the shock itself has been shown to occur in cell cultures[39,40] and dogs[59,60] at an energy level of five times that required for defibrillation[59]. Although the findings of elevated serum creatinine kinase (CK) following cardioversion raised fears of myocardial injury, it was shown that the myocardial CK (CKMB) rose very little, indicating that skeletal muscle was the main source[60]. Changes in the ECG, especially ST-segment shift, are commonly seen and, though generally attributed to injury may reflect alterations in coronary flow caused by stimulation of the intrinsic nerves[22] or their direct adrenergic, cholinergic or peptidergic effects on the myocardium. Hypotension[61], cardiac enlargement and pulmonary oedema[56] may be seen transiently especially after high energies are used, but the mechanism has not been delineated. Positive radionuclide scans following defibrillation have been reported[62-64], but again the nature of the abnormalities is not clear, nor to what extent the shock itself is responsible. Overall there is no compelling evidence that permanent myocardial damage is a significant clinical problem though transient injury or functional depression may occur for a variety of reasons.

Other structures may be affected by shock, especially the skin and skeletal muscle as discussed above. DC shock may be delivered safely in pregnancy[65,66], though a fetal arrhythmia could theoretically be induced.

Pacemakers

In patients with implanted pacemakers defibrillation shocks may cause malfunction or complete failure[67,69] of the pulse generator, despite protection of the circuits by zener diodes; these problems are more likely to occur with unipolar systems and the risk is minimized by:

(1) Avoiding placing either defibrillator paddle near the pacemaker pocket or the right ventricular apex;
(2) Keeping the fields orthogonal, by making the line between the paddles perpendicular to the line between the pocket and the lead tip (Figure 16.5).

Loss of pacing capture is sometimes seen for a few seconds after

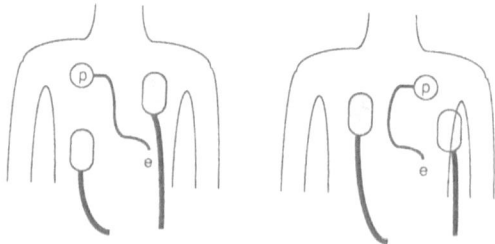

Figure 16.5 Defibrillation of a patient who has an implanted pacemaker. The paddles must be kept as far as possible from the pulse generator **p** and the pacing electrode **e** in the heart. They should be positioned so that a line between them is orientated at right-angles to a line between **p** and **e**

delivery of a large shock, and probably represents transient myocardial depression.

The increasing programmability of modern pacemakers widens the range of possible subtle malfunctions which may be produced by corruption of memory, and in entirely 'software based' devices there could be complete loss of function. It is, therefore, advisable to identify the pacemaker and have the appropriate programmer immediately to hand. The pacemaker function and programming should be checked after the procedure.

Alternatives

Adverse effects should, of course, be considered in the context of the alternative treatments (including no treatment). For VF there is no alternative while for cardioversion the use of intravenous drugs results both in more severe vascular, inotropic and arrhythmic problems and in a variety of other specific drug side effects. With oral drugs the haemodynamic effects are less, but so is efficacy, and specific side effects are common. Additionally, the timing of anticoagulant treatment is more difficult though no less important.

AUTOMATIC DEFIBRILLATOR

A serious limitation to the success of out-of-hospital resuscitation is the lack of personnel adequately trained in arrhythmia detection to make safe use of a defibrillator, even if it were available. In 1972 Friedberg[70] suggested that the widespread community use of automatic defibrillators could ovecome this problem, but it was not until 10 years later that Chamberlain's team reported its first clinical use by ambulance staff[71].

The device they used, the first version of the automatic external defibrillator-pacemaker, AEDP 'Heart Aid' (Cardiac Research Corporation, Secaucus, NJ 07094, USA) uses both ECG and respiration to identify cardiac arrest with VF[28]. It uses as one electrode a stainless steel plate built into a plastic airway making contact with the back of the tongue, and as the other, a self-adhesive stannous chloride pad applied to the epigastrium. The interelectrode impedance is monitored and shocks inhibited if it is greater than 200Ω or if a breath is detected by a transducer in the airway. VF is detected by comparison of two analog derivations of the ECG which are highly correlated during regular rhythm, but not with the disorganized ECG of VF. When both ECG and apnoeic criteria have been met for 12 seconds, a 200 J shock is delivered without further intervention from the operator. Asystole is also detected and results in external pacing at 80 bpm. Continued VF or asystole is treated even if breathing is detected. Reliability of VF detection in successive models in field or laboratory testing was quite good[71], poor[72] and good[73-75], later designs using digital methods for VF detection.

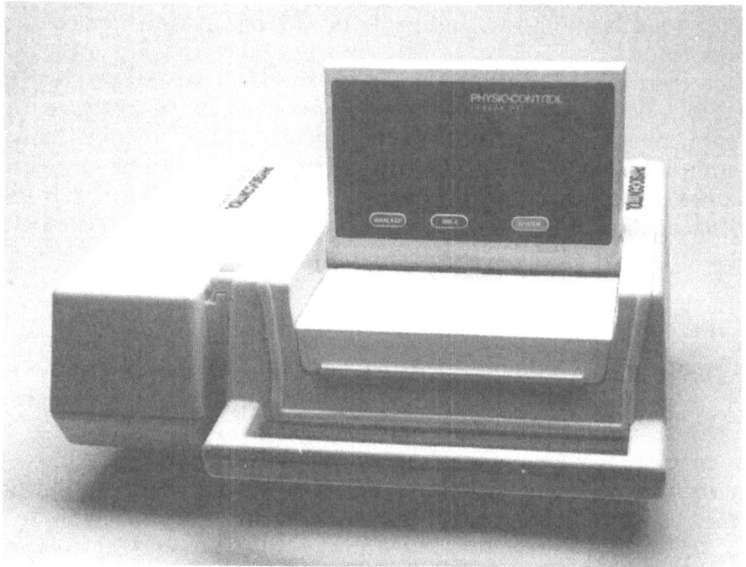

Figure 16.6   A semi-automatic portable defibrillator

An alternative to the fully automatic system is one in which VF detection is indicated on ECG monitoring alone, and the operator makes the final decision to defibrillate based on this and observation of the patient. Such devices (e.g. 'Lifepak 100' and 'Lifepak 200', Physio-Control, Redmond, Washington 98052, USA) are described as 'semi-automatic'. Both types have been successful in large scale practice used by emergency medical technicians[76,77].

THE FUTURE

The adequate resuscitation training of ambulance staff in the UK is belatedly being undertaken, and this will lead to the much greater out-of-hospital use of defibrillators. Small automatic or semi-automatic devices may be issued to be used in the home for high-risk patients, at least until internal devices can be implanted without thoracotomy.

An alternative method for inducing the necessary current by magnetic induction may be made possible by the new ceramic superconductors. This or an improvement in the pulse waveform may result in shocks producing much less stimulation of nerves or skeletal muscle, and hence obviating the need for anaesthesia.

References

1. McWilliam, J. A. (1889). Cardiac failure and sudden death. *Br. Med. J.*, 1, 6–8
2. Hawes, H. (1774). Electricity restored vitality. *Trans. R. Humane Soc.*, 1, 51
3. (a) Abildgaard, P. C. (1775). Tentamina electrica in animalibus instituta. *Soc. Med. Havniensis Collectanea*, 2, 157–61
   (b) Driscol, T. E., Ratnoff, O. R. and Nygaard, O. F. (1975). The remarkable Dr. Abildgaard and countershock. *Ann. Intern. Med.*, 83, 878–82
4. Erichsen, J. E. (1842). The influence of the coronary circulation on the action of the heart. *London Med. Gazette*, 2, 561–4
5. Hoffa, M. and Ludwig, C. (1850). Einige neue Versuche uber Herzewegung. *Z. Rationale Med.*, 9, 107
6. Prevost, J. L. and Battelli, F. (1900). Quelques effets des decharges electriques sur le coeur des mammiferes. *J. Physiol. Pathol. Gen.* (Paris) 2, 40–52
7. Hooker, D. R , Kouwenhoven, W. B. and Langworth, O. R. (1933). The effect of alternating current on the heart. *Am. J. Physiol.*, 103, 444–54
8. Wiggers, C. J. (1936). Cardiac massage followed by countershock in revival of mammalian ventricular fibrillation due to coronary occlusion. *Am. J. Physiol.*, 116, 161–2
9. Beck, C. S. and Mautz, F. R. (1937). The control of the heart beat by the surgeon with special reference to ventricular fibrillation occurring during operation. *Ann. Surg.*, 106, 525–37
10. Beck, C. S. (1941). Resuscitation for cardiac standstill and ventricular fibrillation occurring during operation. *Am. J. Surg.*, 54, 273–9
11. Beck, C. S., Pritchard, W. H. and Feil, H. S. (1947). Ventricular fibrillation of long duration abolished by electric shock. *J. Am. Med. Assoc.*, 135, 985–6
12. Zoll, P. M., Linenthal, A. J., Gibson, W., Paul, M. H. and Norman, L. R. (1956). Termination of ventricular fibrillation in man by externally applied electric countershock. *N. Engl. J. Med.*, 254, 727–32
13. Kouwenhoven, W. B., Jude, J. R. and Knickerbocker, G. G. (1960). Closed-chest cardiac massage. *J. Am. Med. Assoc.*, 173, 1064–7
14. Lown, B., Amarasingham, R. and Neuman, J. (1962). New method for terminating cardiac arrhythmias – use of synchronized capacitor discharge. *J. Am. Med. Assoc.*, 182, 548–55
15. Julian, D. G. (1961). Treatment of cardiac arrest in acute myocardial ischaemia and infarction. *Lancet*, 2, 840–4
16. Pantridge, J. F. and Geddes, J. S. (1967). A mobile coronary care unit in the management of myocardial infarction. *Lancet*, 2, 271–3
17. McWilliam, J. A. (1887). Fibrillary contraction of the heart. *J. Physiol.*, 8, 296–310
18. Garrey, W. E. (1914). The nature of fibrillary contraction of the heart. *Am. J. Physiol.*, 33, 397–413
19. Zipes, D. P., Fischer, J., King, R. M., Nicoll, A. and Jolly, W. W. (1975). Termination of ventricular fibrillation in dogs by depolarizing a critical amount of myocardium. *Am. J. Cardiol.*, 36, 37–44
20. Peleska, B. (1966). Optimal parameters of electrical impulses for defibrillation by condenser discharges. *Circ. Res.*, 18, 10–17
21. Hoffman de Visme, G. and Furness, A. (1983). Electrical waveforms for cardiac defibrillation which dissipate least heat in the cardiac circuit. *Med. Biol. Eng. Comp.*, 21, 259–63
22. Cobb, F. R., Wallace, A. G. and Wagner, G. S. (1968). Cardiac inotropic and coronary vascular responses to countershock: evidence for excitation of intracardiac nerves. *Circ. Res.*, 23, 731–42
23. Roberts, D. E., Hersh, L. T. and Scher, A. M. (1979). Influence of cardiac fiber orientation on waveform voltage, conduction velocity and tissue resistivity in the dog. *Circ. Res.*, 44, 701–12
24. Karber, R. E., Jensen, S. R., Grayzel, J., Kennedy, J., and Hoyt, R. (1981). Elective cardioversion: influence of paddle-electrode location and size on success rates and energy requirements. *N. Engl. J. Med.*, 305, 658–62

25. Lown, B., Kleiger, R. and Wolff, G. (1964). The technique of cardioversion. *Am. Heart J.*, **67**, 282–4
26. Morris, J. J. Jr., Kong, Y., North, W. C. and Mcintosh, H. D. (1964). Experience with 'cardioversion' of atrial fibrillation and flutter. *Am. J. Cardiol.*, **14**, 94–100
27. Resnekov, L. and McDonald, L. (1968). Appraisal of electroconversion in treatment of cardiac dysrhythmias. *Br. Heart J.*, **30**, 786–811
28. Drack, A. W., Welborn, W. S., Rullman, R. G. *et al.* (1979). An automatic cardiac resuscitator for emergency treatment of cardiac arrest. *Med. Instr.*, **13**, 78–82
29. Kerber, R. E., Grayzel, J., Hoyt, R., Marcus, M. and Kennedy, J. (1981). Transthoracic resistance in human defibrillation: influence of body weight, chest size, serial shocks, paddle size and paddle contact pressure. *Circulation*, **63**, 676–82
30. Wojtczak, J. (1979). Contractures and increase in internal longitudinal resistance of cow ventricular muscle induced by hypoxia. *Circ. Res.*, **44**, 88–95
31. Kerber, R. E., Kouba, C., Martins, J. *et al.* (1934). Advance prediction of transthoracic impedance in human defibrillation and cardioversion: importance of impedance in determining the success of low-energy shocks. *Circulation*, **70**, 303–8
32. Gurvich, N. L. and Yuniev, G. S. (1947). Restoration of heart rhythm during fibrillation by a condenser discharge. *Am. Rev. Soviet Med.*, **4**, 252–6
33. MacKay, R. S. and Leeds, S. E. (1953). Physiological effects of condenser discharges with application to tissue stimulation and ventricular defibrillation. *J. Appl. Physiol.*, **6**, 67–75
34. Edmark, K. W. (1963). Simultaneous voltage and current waveforms generated during internal and external direct current pulse defibrillation. *Surgical Forum*, **14**, 262–4
35. Jude, J. R., Kouwenhoven, W. B. and Knickerbocker, G. G. (1962). An experimental and clinical study of a portable external cardiac defibrillator. *Surgical Forum*, **13**, 185–7
36. Schuder, J. C., Stoeckle, H. and Dolan, A. M. (1964). Transthoracic ventricular defibrillation with square-wave stimuli: one-half cycle, one cycle and multicycle waveforms. *Circ. Res.*, **15**, 258–64
37. Schuder, J. C., Gold, J. H., Stoeckle, H. *et al.* (1981). Defibrillation in the calf with bidirectional trepezoidal wave shocks applied via chronically implanted pericardial electrodes. *Trans. Am. Soc. Artif. Intern. Organs.*, **27**, 467–70
38. Negovsky, V. A., Smeridov, A. A., Tabak, V. Y., Venin, I. V. and Bogushevich, M. S. (1980). Criteria of efficiency and safety of the defibrillating impulse. *Resuscitation*, **8**, 53–87
39. Jones, J. L. and Jones, R. E. (1983). Improved defibrillator waveform safety factor with biphasic waveforms. *Am. J. Physiol.*, **245**, H60–H65
40. Jones, J. L. and Jones R. E. (1984). Decreased defibrillator-induced dysfunction with biphasic rectangular waveforms. *Am. J. Physiol.*, **247**, H792–H796
41. Geddes, L. A., Niebauer, M. J., Babbs, C. F. and Bourland, J. D. (1985). Fundamental criteria underlying the efficacy and safety of defibrillating current waveforms. *Med. Biol. Eng. Comput.*, **23**, 122–30
42. Niebauer, M. J., Babbs, C. F., Geddes, L. A. and Bourland, J. D. (1984). Efficacy and safety of the reciprocal pulse defibrillator current waveform. *Med. Biol. Eng. Comput.*, **22**, 28–31
43. Tacker, W. A., Galioto, F. M., Giuliani, E., Geddes, L. A. and McNamara, D. G. (1974). Energy dosage for human transchest electrical defibrillation. *N. Engl. J. Med.*, **290**, 214–15
44. Pantridge, J. F., Adgey, A. A. J., Webb, S. W. and Anderson, J. (1975). Electrical requirements for ventricular defibrillation. *Br. Med. J.*, **2**, 313–15
45. Crampton, R. (1980). Accepted, controversial and speculative aspects of ventricular defibrillation. *Prog. Cardiovasc. Dis.*, **3**, 167–86
46. Kerber, R. E., Jensen, S. R., Gascho, J. A. *et al.* (1983). Determinants of defibrillation: prospective analysis of 183 patients. *Am. J. Cardiol.*, **52**, 739–45
47. Weaver, W. D., Cobb, L. A., Copass, M. K. and Hallstrom, A. P. (1982). Ventricular

defibrillation – a comparative trial using 175–J and 320–J shocks. *N. Engl. J. Med.*, 307, 1101–6

48. British Standards Institution. (1980). Draft standard specification for the safety of cardiac defibrillator monitors, IEC 62D-8. Document 80/25763 DC. (London: BSI)
49. British Standards Institution. (1982). Draft – amendments to document 62D-8. Document 82/23869. (London: BSI)
50. Association for the advancement of medical instrumentation. (1980). Standard for cardiac defibrillator devices (proposed). (Arlington, VA, USA: AAMI)
51. O'Dowd, W. J. (1983). Defibrillator design and development – a review. *J. Med. Eng. Technol.*, 7, 5–15
52. Chamberlain, D. (1986). ABC of resuscitation: ventricular fibrillation. *Br. Med. J.*, 292, 1068–70
53. Standards and guidelines for cardiopulmonary resuscitation (CPR) and emergency cardiac care (ECC). (1986). *J. Am. Med. Assoc.*, 255, 2905–89
54. Resnekov, J. and McDonald, I. (1967). Complications in 220 patients with cardiac dysrhythmias treated by phased direct current shock, and indications for electroconversion. *Br. Heart J.*, 29, 926–36
55. Bjerkelund, C. J. and Orning, O. M. (1969). The efficacy of anticoagulant therapy in preventing embolism related to DC electrical conversion of atrial fibrillation. *Am. J. Cardiol.*, 23, 208–16
56. Rabbino, M. D., Likoff, W. and Dreifus, L. S. (1964). Complications and limitations of direct current countershock. *J. Am. Med. Assoc.*, 190, 417–20
57. Kleiger, R. and Lown B. (1966). Cardioversion and digitalis: II Clinical studies. *Circulation*, 33, 878–87
58. Mann, D. L., Maisel, A. S., Atwood, J. E., Engler, R. L. and LeWinter, M. M. (1985). Absence of cardioversion-induced ventricular arrhythmias in patients with therapeutic digoxin levels. *J. Am. Coll. Cardiol.*, 5, 882–8
59. Babbs, C. F., Tacker, W. A., Van Vleet, J. F., Bourland, J. D. and Geddes, L. A. (1980). Therapeutic indices for transchest defibrillator shocks: effective, damaging, and lethal electrical doses. *Am. Heart J.*, 99, 734–8
60. Ehsani, A., Ewy, G. A. and Sobel, B. E. (1976). Effects of electrical countershock on serum creatinine phosphokinase (CPK) isoenzyme activity. *Am. J. Cardiol.*, 37, 12–18
61. Pansegrau, D. G. and Abboud, F. M. (1970). Hemodynamic effects of ventricular defibrillation. *J. Clin. Invest.*, 49, 282–97
62. Di Cola, V. C., Freedman, G. S., Downing S. E. *et al.* (1979). Myocardial uptake of technetium-99m stannous pyrophosphate following direct current transthoracic countershock. *Circulation*, 54, 980–9
63. Sonnenblick, M., Gelmont, D., Karen, A. *et al.* (1977). Positive radionuclide myocardial infarction pattern after ventricular fibrillation and direct current countershock. *Chest*, 71, 673–4
64. Davison, R., Spies, S. M., Przyblek, J. *et al.* Technetium-99m stannous pyrophosphate myocardial scintigraphy after cardiopulmonary resuscitation with cardioversion. *Circulation*, 60, 292–6
65. Vogel, J. H. K., Pryor, R. and Blount, S. G. (1965). Direct current defibrillation during pregnancy. *J. Am. Med. Assoc.*, 193, 970–1
66. Schroeder, J. S. and Harrison, D. C. (1971). Repeated cardioversion during pregnancy. *Am. J. Cardiol.*, 27, 445–6
67. Das, G. and Eaton, J. (1981). Pacemaker malfunction following transthoracic countershock. *Pacing Clin. Electrophysiol.*, 4, 487–90
68. Gould, L., Patel, S., Gomes, G. I. *et al.* (1981). Pacemaker failure following external defibrillation. *Pacing Clin. Electrophysiol.*, 4, 575–7
69. Levine, P. A., Barold, S. S., Fletcher, R. D. *et al.* (1983). Adverse acute and chronic effects of electrical defibrillation and cardioversion on implanted unipolar cardiac pacing systems. *J. Am. Coll. Cardiol.*, 1, 1413–22
70. Friedberg, C. K. (1972). Introduction to symposium on myocardial infarction. *Circulation*, 45, 179–88

71. Jaggarao, N. S. V., Heber, M., Grainger, R. *et al.* (1982). Use of an automated external defibrillator pacemaker by ambulance staff. *Lancet*, **2**, 73–5
72. Heber, M. (1983). Out-of-hospital resuscitation using the 'Heart Aid', an automated external defibrillator–pacemaker. *Int. J. Cardiol.*, **3**, 456–8
73. Rosenthal, E., Carroll, D., Vincent, R. and Chamberlain, D. A. (1984). Automated external defibrillation; laboratory evaluation. *Int. J. Cardiol.*, **5**, 441–7
74. Cummins, R. O., Eisenberg, M., Bergner, L. and Murray, J. A. (1984). Sensitivity, accuracy, and safety of an automatic external defibrillator: report of a field evaluation. *Lancet*, **2**, 318–20
75. Stults, K. R., Brown, D. D. and Kerber, R. E. (1986). Efficacy of an automated external defibrillator in the management of out-of-hospital cardiac arrest: validation of the diagnostic algorithm and initial clinical experience in a rural environment. *Circulation*, **73**, 701–9
76. Weaver, W. D., Copass, M. K., Hill, D. L. *et al.* (1986). Cardiac arrest treated with a new automatic external defibrillator by out-of-hospital first responders. *Am. J. Cardiol.*, **57**, 1017–21
77. Cummins, R. O., Eisenberg, M. S., Litwin, P. E. *et al.* (1987). Automatic external defibrillators used by emergency medical technicians. *J. Am. Med. Assoc.*, **257**, 1605–10

17
Drugs used for the treatment of tachycardias

R. S. BEXTON

There is no one antiarrhythmic agent which is a panacea for all cardiac arrhythmias. There are probably now over 40 agents available for the treatment of cardiac rhythm disturbances, and the selection of the correct and most appropriate drug for any given arrhythmia is dependent upon a knowledge of the basic and clinical electrophysiological properties of that drug, a knowledge of the site and mechanism of the arrhythmia and perhaps most importantly clinical experience. Mechanisms of arrhythmias are discussed elsewhere in this book (see Chapter 1), but it is perhaps relevant to mention the possible mechanisms of action of antiarrhythmic drugs. The antiarrhythmic action of a drug may be due to the abolition of a re-entry circuit by increasing the refractory period and/or conduction velocity of one part of that circuit, the conversion of unidirectional block within a re-entry circuit to bidirectional block, the suppression of enhanced automaticity or triggered activity of an ectopic pacemaker or it may be due to synchronization of an electrophysiologically inhomogeneous myocardial substrate of an arrhythmia. Very occasionally the antiarrhythmic action of a drug may be due to the suppression of the pathophysiological event underlying the arrhythmia, e.g. calcium channel blocking drugs in the arrhythmias of Prinzmetal angina and β-blocking drugs in exercise-induced arrhythmias. Prior to considering specific clinical situations it is pertinent to discuss the electrophysiological properties of the various antiarrhythmic agents.

CLASSIFICATION OF ANTIARRHYTHMIC AGENTS

Many classifications of antiarrhythmic agents have been described, but there are perhaps three major classifications which exemplify the possible approaches to this difficult problem.

Table 17.1 Basic electrophysiological classification of antiarrhythmic drugs (from reference 1)

Class 1	Class 2	Class 3	Class 4	Class 5
A	Propranol	Amiodarone	Verapamil	Alinidine
Quinidine	Oxprenolol	Bretylium	Diltiazem	
Procainamide	Alprenolol	Sotalol		
Disopyramide	Practolol	Bethanidine		
B	Pindolol	Meobentine		
Diphenylhydantoin	Sotalol	Clofilium		
Mexiletine				
Lignocaine				
C				
Flecainide				
Lorcainide				
Encainide				

Basic electrophysiological classification

This classification, commonly called the Vaughan Williams classification[1-3], is based upon the effect of the antiarrhythmic agent on the action potential of isolated tissue models *in vitro*. The action of commonly used antiarrhythmic agents can be divided into four reasonably distinct groups (Table 17.1), based on the observation that virtually all the drugs have one major electrophysiological effect on the myocardial cell, although obviously there is overlap between groups in their subsidiary pharmacological characteristics. Recently a fifth class of antiarrhythmic action has been described[4], although this has no relevance to this chapter.

Class 1 agents are the 'membrane stabilizing', local anaesthetic drugs. Their dominant electrophysiological property is to block the fast inward sodium current during depolarization of the cardiac membrane, thus reducing membrane responsiveness. They decrease conduction velocity, increase the threshold for excitability and prolong the effective refractory period of cardiac muscle. These drugs also depress diastolic depolarization, thus reducing spontaneous automaticity. By depressing Phase 4 depolarization the drugs of this class may control arrhythmias which are due to enhanced automaticity, and by altering the refractory period they are likely to be effective in re-entrant arrhythmias. This class is further subdivided into three groups based on their effect on action potential duration: 1A consists of drugs which lengthen the duration of the action potential, 1B of drugs which shorten it and 1C consists of drugs which have no effect on the duration of the action potential.

Class 2 include the sympathetic nervous inhibitors – drugs which block the effects of catecholamines on the action potential. The majority of the members of this class are the β-blocking drugs. They have no direct electrophysiological effects at clinically relevant concentrations, but block the effect of catecholamines on the outward potassium current

Table 17.2   Clinical electrophysiological classification of antiarrhythmic drugs

Class 1 (AV node)	Class 2 (H–P system)	Class 3 (Both)
Propranolol Verapamil Digoxin	a { Disopyramide Quinidine Ajmaline Flecainide b { Lignocaine Mexiletine Diphenylhydantoin Bretylium	Amiodarone Aprindine

AV = Atrioventricular, H–P = His–Purkinje

thus depressing Phase 4 depolarization leading to a reduction in automaticity. They may also block the effect of catecholamines on the slow inward calcium current thus abolishing slow responses.

Class 3 is a relatively small group of drugs whose only electrophysiological action is prolongation of action potential duration with consequent lengthening of the effective refractory period.

Class 4 drugs antagonize transmembrane calcium fluxes, thus blocking the slow inward current of the action potential. The tissue of the sinoatrial and atrioventricular nodes depends primarily on slow response action potentials which rely on this slow inward current that flows through the calcium channels, and hence these agents are particularly useful and effective in arrhythmias involving nodal tissue.

This basic electrophysiological classification has proved invaluable for the classification of new drugs. Although it is obviously a non-clinical classification, with the increasing knowledge of the electrophysiological mechanisms of arrhythmias it is perhaps becoming of greater clinical relevance. Its disadvantages are that it does not include several important antiarrhythmic drugs such as digoxin, and it ignores the indirect and extracardiac actions of drugs.

Clinical electrophysiological classification

This newer classification[5] divides antiarrhythmic agents into three classes dependent upon their major action delineated during clinical electrophysiological studies (Table 17.2). Drugs are classified according to whether their predominant action is upon the atrioventricular node (Class 1), the His–Purkinje system (Class 2) or both (Class 3). Class 2 is further subdivided into those drugs which primarily affect His–Purkinje conduction (2a) and those whose major effect is on refractoriness (2b). This classification is obviously more clinically orientated than the Vaughan Williams classification, but it does have the major disadvantage of ignoring the sinus node and atrium.

Table 17.3 Clinical classification of antiarrhythmic drugs

Sinus node	*Atrium*	*AV Node*
Beta-blockers	Procainamide	Beta-blockers
Digoxin	Quinidine	Digoxin
Verapamil	Disopyramide	Verapamil
Reserpine	Amiodarone	Flecainide
	Flecainide	
Anomalous	*Ventricle*	
pathway	Procainamide	
Procainamide	Quinidine	
Quinidine	Disopyramide	
Disopyramide	Amiodarone	
Amiodarone	Lignocaine	
Flecainide	Mexiletine	
	Bretylium	
	Phenytoin	
	Flecainide	

AV = Atrioventricular

Clinical classification

Finally, antiarrhythmic drugs may be classified based upon the results of clinical studies and one's own clinical experience (Table 17.3). This is obviously the least scientific of all these classifications, but is perhaps the most clinically useful. As indicated in the introduction if the site and mechanism of the arrhythmia is known then knowledge of the basic and clinical electrophysiological properties of an antiarrhythmic agent and its major sites of clinical action, based on the above three classifications, should allow a reasoned approach towards the correct agent.

DRUG TREATMENT OF TACHYCARDIAS

The aims of drug treatment for tachycardias may be threefold: conversion, prophylaxis or rate control. Before considering the commoner tachyarrhythmias, it should be stressed that a careful search for any arrhythmia precipitating factors should be made, and if possible corrected, prior to the initiation of antiarrhythmic therapy. These precipitating factors include biochemical disturbances, hormonal imbalances such as thyrotoxicosis or phaeochromocytoma, infection, anaemia, hypotension, heart failure, drug overdose or intoxication particularly with antiarrhythmic agents, myocardial ischaemia including Prinzmetal angina, bradycardia and specific conditions such as the long QT syndrome.

Atrial fibrillation, flutter and tachycardia

The treatment of these three arrhythmias is essentially similar and, therefore, they may be considered together. Each may present as either an acute, paroxysmal or established arrhythmia. The aim of treatment in the acute form is conversion and possibly subsequent prophylaxis, in the paroxysmal form it is prophylaxis and in the established arrhythmia the aim is usually rate control.

Acute onset atrial fibrillation or flutter with a fast ventricular response may present as acute collapse and, therefore, require immediate external DC cardioversion. If the arrhythmia is well tolerated then elective conversion, by electrical or pharmacological means, may be planned. If elective DC cardioversion, perhaps the most successful form of treatment, is considered it has been suggested that 3–4 weeks of effective anticoagulant therapy may reduce the risk of systemic embolization at the time of conversion[6]. Pharmacological agents most effective in the conversion of such arrhythmias are those which prolong action potential duration, i.e. Vaughan Williams Class 1A and 3. The drugs most commonly used are disopyramide, procainamide, quinidine, amiodarone and more recently flecainide. In acute onset atrial arrhythmias, intravenous disopyramide has been reported to be successful in converting between 29%[7] and 62%[8] of arrhythmias. When the arrhythmias have been present for more than 7 days the success rate is, however, considerably diminished[8,9]. Similar results have been obtained with oral disopyramide[10,11], and again conversion rates were highest in recent onset arrhythmias. In general the drug is more successful in those patients with atrial fibrillation when compared with atrial flutter and tachycardia.

Similar results have previously been reported with procainamide[12-14], administered both orally and intravenously, and with quinidine[15]. As with disopyramide these drugs are considerably more effective in recent onset arrhythmias. Results with intravenous procainamide indicate conversion rates varying from 60%[12] to 90%[13] in atrial fibrillation which has been present for less than 24 hours, but from 0%[12] to 33%[13] in atrial fibrillation of longer duration. Conversion rates with the oral preparation are of a similar magnitude[14]. It should be remembered that these Class 1A drugs, particularly disopyramide and quinidine, with their anticholinergic effects, may lead to an increase in the ventricular response to these arrhythmias when a degree of atrioventricular block is present. The drugs will decrease the atrial rate but enhance atrioventricular nodal conduction thus reducing concealed conduction and resulting in conduction of a greater proportion of atrial beats. This is most commonly seen with atrial flutter with 2:1 atrioventricular block[16]. Pretreatment with an atrioventricular blocking drug such as digoxin, verapamil or a β-blocker will prevent this phenomenon.

Two relatively new agents which have proved encouraging in the treatment of atrial tachyarrhythmias are amiodarone and flecainide. Although the numbers of studies are relatively small, amiodarone has been shown to be extremely effective in the restoration of sinus rhythm when administered either orally or intravenously. Santos et al.[17] reported the successful reversion from stable atrial fibrillation to sinus rhythm in

86% of cases given oral amiodarone. In 50% of patients reversion occurred between the third and fifth day and 72% of those who converted were still in sinus rhythm one year later. The results of this study would imply that amiodarone is considerably more effective than any other conventional antiarrhythmic agent in the treatment of chronic stable atrial fibrillation. However, there have been no further large series to confirm these impressive results. A more recent, smaller study using intravenous amiodarone[18] has reported an overall conversion rate of 73% in patients with recent onset atrial fibrillation with a fast ventricular rate, and perhaps most clinically relevant was the fact that the ventricular rate slowed in all cases, including the non-converters. Another Class III agent, sotalol, has also been shown to be effective in a variety of supraventricular arrhythmias, including atrial fibrillation and flutter[19].

The new Class 1C antiarrhythmic agent flecainide has also recently been reported as highly effective in the treatment of a variety of atrial tachyarrhythmias[20,21], including atrial tachycardia[22]. The success of these newer agents, amiodarone and flecainide, has rekindled interest in the chemical conversion of atrial tachyarrhythmias, although as with the older established antiarrhythmics they are generally more effective in atrial fibrillation than in other forms of atrial arrhythmias.

Once sinus rhythm has been restored by either electrical or pharmacological means, a decision has to be made as to whether long term prophylaxis is to be administered, with the possibility of unwanted effects from antiarrhythmic agents, to prevent a recurrence of the arrhythmia. A reasonable strategy, at the present time, would seem to be not to employ a long term prophylactic drug after the first cardioversion. If the arrhythmia recurs, then following a second cardioversion a trial of prophylaxis would be appropriate. This strategy may avoid the administration of potentially dangerous therapy to a subgroup of patients who do not require such therapy. The maintenance of sinus rhythm following cardioversion is dependent on a number of factors including left atrial size[23], patient age[23] and the aetiology of the arrhythmia[24]. However, in general the relapse rate within the first year is between 50% and 80% of untreated patients[25], but if sinus rhythm is maintained for more than 2 years further relapse is unlikely. Quinidine[26-28], procainamide[28] and disopyramide[29] have all been demonstrated to be significantly more effective than placebo in maintaining sinus rhythm. A recent uncontrolled study[30] also suggests that amiodarone may be useful in this clinical situation.

In paroxysmal atrial tachyarrhythmias, particularly atrial fibrillation, the basic aim of treatment is prophylaxis. Studies with Holter monitoring have suggested that the autonomic nervous system may play an important role in the initiation of these arrhythmias[31]. These studies have indicated that paroxysmal atrial fibrillation may be the common result of two opposite mechanisms related to either increased vagal or sympathetic drive. The arrhythmias of vagal origin tend to occur at night, at rest or in the digestive period and are not helped, and indeed may even be exacerbated, by drugs such as digoxin and β-blockers[31]. One would expect the Class 1A drugs, with their parasympathetic activity, to be particularly effective in this type of arrhythmia, but clinical reports do not support this. The only drug which has been shown to be effective is amiodarone[30,32,33]. The arrhythmias of sympathetic origin occur mainly during the day, on exercise, with emotional stress and are often preceded by an increase in sinus rate. These arrhythmias are generally responsive to β-blockade and digoxin, with or without the addition of a membrane stabilizing drug[31]. Amiodarone would also appear to be successful in this group. These studies suggest that Holter monitoring should be extremely useful in determining the initiating factors in paroxysmal atrial tachyarrhythmias and thus allow consideration of the most appropriate therapeutic strategy.

In established, chronic atrial fibrillation the basic aim of treatment is control of the ventricular rate. Before initiation of treatment the route of atrioventricular conduction must be determined. In the majority of cases this will be the atrioventricular node and the His–Purkinje system. In these patients rate control can be achieved rapidly with verapamil[34] and long term with digoxin[35]. If rate control is inadequate with digoxin alone, verapamil[36] or propranolol[37] may be added with a particularly beneficial effect on exercise related tachycardia. If these established agents, alone or in combination, do not provide adequate control then amiodarone may prove effective[30]. If the route of atrioventricular conduction is an accessory pathway as in the Wolff–Parkinson–White syndrome, then the aim of therapy is to primarily slow conduction within this pathway (see below) as well as the atrioventricular node.

Junctional tachycardias

This group primarily includes paroxysmal re-entrant tachycardias due to either functional duality of atrioventricular nodal conduction (dual AH pathways) or to the presence of an accessory atrioventricular connection (pathway) as in the Wolff–Parkinson–White or Lown–Ganong–Levine syndromes. Much rarer are the accelerated junctional rhythms and automatic junctional tachycardias which primarily occur in the setting of heart disease and are often transient. The two basic strategies in these paroxysmal re-entrant arrhythmias are conversion of an acute arrhythmia and prophylaxis against further recurrences.

Drug treatment of the acute arrhythmia is usually extremely effective and resort to direct current cardioversion is rarely required. As the vast majority of these re-entrant tachycardias utilize the atrioventricular node as part of their tachycardia circuit, initial treatment should be aimed at the atrioventricular node. Verapamil, given as a rapid intravenous bolus, is currently the agent of choice, and is effective in the majority of cases[38,39]. Intravenous propranolol may also be used but has proved less successful[40]. More recently the potent atrioventricular nodal blocking drugs adenosine-5 triphosphate and adenosine[41] have been shown to be highly effective with success rates of 90% (comparable to verapamil) and with conversion often occurring within 30 seconds. However, these latter two drugs may cause heart block and bradycardia, and their short half-lives may allow relatively early recurrence of the arrhythmia. Digoxin is sometimes used, particularly in children, but is much slower and less effective[42], and there is some evidence that digoxin may improve conduction in anomalous pathways and hence may be extremely hazardous if atrial fibrillation supervenes. Other agents which have been shown to be highly efficacious by a direct effect on the atrioventricular node include flecainide[20,43], and more recently Yeh *et al.*[44] have investigated the use of combined oral diltiazem and propranolol in the termination of junctional tachycardias. These drugs terminated nearly all arrhythmias, and this approach may be of interest in those patients whose attacks are too infrequent to warrant continuous drug prophylaxis.

When the tachycardia is known to involve an anomalous pathway the treatment may also be directed at this pathway. Intravenous disopyramide[45], flecainide[20,43], amiodarone[46], procainamide[47], quinidine[47] and ajmaline[47] have all been shown to significantly effect refractoriness and conduction within anomalous pathways, and thus to be of use in the termination of re-entrant arrhythmias involving such a mechanism. Prophylaxis against paroxysmal re-entrant junctional tachycardias may be aimed at preventing the premature beats which initiate the tachycardia, at equalizing the recovery times of both pathways so that unidirectional block in one pathway cannot occur, at total blockade of one of the pathways or at prolongation of the refractory period of a localized part of the circuit so preventing impulse circulation. In clinical practice, as with the conversion of these arrhythmias, prophylactic therapy may be directed at either the atrioventricular node or the anomalous pathway if it is present. Verapamil[48] and diltiazem[49] have both been shown to be effective via their action on the atrioventricular node. Of the agents known to influence accessory pathway conduction and refractoriness (see above), only amiodarone has been extensively studied in terms of prophylaxis and has been found to be highly effective with reported suppression rates of up to 100%[32]. However, the newer agents such as flecainide have electrophysiological properties[43,50] which suggest they should be equally efficacious.

Ventricular arrhythmias

The decision to be made with ventricular arrhythmias is perhaps not which antiarrhythmic agent to use but which patient to treat. Arrhythmias following myocardial infarction are dealt with elsewhere in this book and I shall contain this discussion to chronic ventricular arrhythmias. For the sake of simplicity these can be divided into three groups: ventricular premature beats, ventricular tachycardia and ventricular fibrillation.

The decision as to which patient to treat is perhaps most difficult with the theoretically most benign of these three groups, i.e. ventricular premature beats. Patients with no underlying heart disease but with frequent ventricular premature beats, couplets or short runs of non-sustained ventricular tachycardia are probably at little risk from these arrhythmias[51]. However, these patients may be severely disturbed by palpitations and thus require treatment. If the symptoms do not subside with reassurance and reduction of potential arrhythmogenic factors (e.g. caffeine, nicotine) then antiarrhythmic therapy may be indicated. In this subgroup of patients, with minimal risk of sudden death, it is essential that a therapy is not introduced that will place the patient at risk for sudden death from a proarrhythmic effect of the drug administered. In such patients a 50% reduction in ventricular premature beats is often enough to abolish symptoms, and occasionally patients may become asymptomatic with no reduction in the number of ventricular premature beats. This may occur if the ventricular premature beats occur later in the cardiac cycle or if the postectopic enhancement of contractility is attenuated with treatment such as β-blockers.

Several population studies over the past 15–20 years[52–54] have demonstrated that ventricular ectopic activity is an index of risk for sudden cardiac death and that the more frequent and complex the ectopy, the greater the risk. The risk is greater still if the ectopy is combined with documented structural heart disease. However, it is not clear from these studies whether ventricular ectopy is purely a 'marker' of underlying heart disease and hence increased risk and thus whether treatment of the ectopy alone will be beneficial. Interestingly, a more recent study[51] in a population of patients with documented minimal or no underlying heart disease and ventricular ectopy has shown them to have an excellent prognosis.

The treatment of ventricular ectopy following a myocardial infarction is perhaps a clearer issue. It has been shown that patients with ventricular premature beats (documented and quantified during the second or third week following infarction) are at increased risk of sudden death[55,56] or death from cardiac origin[57] and that patients with complex forms of ventricular arrhythmias, particularly repetitive forms, are at a greater risk of sudden death compared with patients with simple forms[58]. It would, therefore, appear logical to treat frequent ventricular premature beats following a recent myocardial infarction although it has not been demonstrated that antiarrhythmic therapy reduces mortality in these patients[59]. The beneficial effect of antiarrhythmic therapy has been clearly demonstrated in patients with complex forms of ventricular arrhythmias postinfarction[60]. It would, therefore, appear that ventricular premature beats should be treated in the following groups of patients: (1) patients with distressingly symptomatic ventricular premature beats whether or not they have underlying heart disease, (2) patients with frequent or complex ventricular arrhythmias who have recently sustained a myocardial infarction, and (3) possibly patients with underlying structural heart disease who have complex ventricular ectopy, although the rationale for treatment in this last group has not really been clearly established. Certainly the goal of therapy in these latter two groups should be the prevention of more complex ventricular arrhythmias rather than merely the suppression of ventricular premature beats, although these may be the trigger of more complex arrhythmias. Ideally antiarrhythmic therapy should result in at least a 75% (ideally up to 90%) reduction in the frequency of ventricular premature beats and a total abolition of sustained and non-sustained ventricular tachycardia.

Probably nearly all antiarrhythmic agents have been used for the suppression of ventricular premature beats at some time. In those patients with 'normal' hearts and symptomatic ventricular ectopy, β-blocking drugs should be tried. These agents may provide mild sedation as well as a decrease in sympathetic tone. The Class 1 agents quinidine[61], procainamide[62], disopyramide[63], mexiletine[64], flecainide[65] and tocainide[66] have all been demonstrated to be highly effective in suppressing chronic ventricular premature beats. These studies have all shown a similar potency for the above agents with the possible exception that flecainide appeared more effective when compared with quinidine[65], the 'gold standard' agent of Class 1. Similarly, amiodarone has recently been shown to be more effective than Class 1 agents in patients with complex ventricular ectopy[67].

There is considerably less debate concerning the need for treatment of recurrent sustained ventricular tachycardia. Recurrent ventricular tachycardia which is symptomatic or which is in the setting of underlying structural heart disease requires antiarrhythmic therapy. Asymptomatic sustained ventricular tachycardia in the presence of a normal heart, a relatively rare phenomenon, should probably also be treated (and most clinicians would find it difficult not to), although the need for such treatment has not been demonstrated. All the antiarrhythmic agents known to be effective in suppressing ventricular premature beats have also been demonstrated to be effective in ventricular tachycardia to some extent or other. However, by general consensus, amiodarone is the most effective agent in the prophylaxis of refractory and recurrent ventricular tachycardia. A recent study by Prystowsky et al.[68] has demonstrated long term control of malignant ventricular arrhythmias by oral amiodarone in a large group of patients.

The ability to reproduce arrhythmias, with the use of programmed electrical stimulation, in patients with malignant ventricular arrhythmias or a history of 'failed' of sudden death has improved the evaluation of drug therapy. Patients whose inducible arrhythmia has become non-inducible when retested on an oral antiarrhythmic have a better prognosis compared to patients whose arrhythmia is still inducible[69]. Depending on a number of factors, such as the antiarrhythmic agent under test, the stimulation protocol used, the definition of success and failure etc., the positive predictive value of the technique (i.e. the percentage of non-inducible patients after treatment who do not have a spontaneous recurrence of arrhythmia on treatment) is 90–95%, and the negative predictive value (i.e. the percentage of patients still inducible after treatment who do have a spontaneous recurrence of arrhythmia on treatment) is 40–85%[70]. There have been several reports of the poor predictive value of serial testing with amiodarone. However, patients in whom amiodarone is effective, as assessed by programmed stimulation, have a better outcome than patients in whom it is ineffective[71]. Despite a wealth of literature on the subject, there is still debate as to the precise worth of this technique, although it would appear to be an enormous advance on empirical treatment of life-threatening arrhythmias. Ambulatory electrocardiographic monitoring and exercise stress testing have also been used successfully for the evaluation of drug efficacy in certain clinical situations[60]. Serum drug level determination may also be useful. Myerburg et al.[72] found that maintaining therapeutic plasma drug levels protected against sudden death, but interestingly there was no relationship between drug levels and the degree of suppression of arrhythmias.

Perhaps the easiest ventricular arrhythmia to treat is the most serious, ventricular fibrillation. The treatment of choice is electrical defibrillation. Patients who do not initially respond to defibrillation may benefit from the administration of intravenous bretylium. This is the only antiarrhythmic agent known to cause 'chemical defibrillation'[73] and may also facilitate successful electrical cardioversion. Very 'fine' ventricular fibrillation may be unresponsive to defibrillation, and in such circumstances isoprenaline may be helpful. The prophylaxis of recurrent ventricular fibrillation, recurrent failed sudden death, is dependent upon programmed stimulation guided therapy as discussed above.

When choosing an antiarrhythmic agent for a particular arrhythmia in a particular patient, the possible side effects should always be considered. Many antiarrhythmic agents are negatively inotropic, particularly in the presence of underlying structural heart disease. Many are proarrhythmic and may cause life-threatening ventricular arrhythmias as a direct result of the treatment administered. It is, therefore, important to ascertain the benefits to be gained by treating the patient, and to balance these against the possible disadvantages of the therapy before initiating a potentially toxic medication.

References

1. Vaughan Williams, E. M. (1970). Classification of antiarrhythmic drugs. In Sandoe, E., Flensted-Jensen, E. and Olesen, K. H. (eds.) *Symposium on Cardiac Arrhythmias*. pp. 449–492 (Sodertalje, Sweden: Astra AB)
2. Singh, B. N. and Vaughan Williams, E. M. (1972). A fourth class of antiarrhythmic action? Effect of verapamil on ouabain toxicity, on atrial and ventricular intracellular potentials and on other features of cardiac function. *Cardiovasc. Res.*, 6, 109–14
3. Singh, B. N. and Hauswirth, O. (1974). Comparative mechanism of action of antiarrhythmic drugs. *Am. Heart J.*, 87, 367–82
4. Millar, J. S. and Vaughan Williams, E. M. (1981). Anion antagonism – A fifth class of antiarrhythmic action? *Lancet*, I, 1291–2

5. Touboul, P. and Morena, H. (1979). Electrophysiological effects of antiarrhythmic drugs. In Puech, P. and Siama, R. (eds.) *The Cardiac Arrhythmias by the Arrhythmia Working Group of the French Cardiac Society*. pp. 245–51. (Paris: Corbiere and Roussel)

6. Bjerkelund, C. J. and Orning, O. M. (1969). The efficacy of anticoagulant therapy in preventing embolism related to D.C. electrical conversion of atrial fibrillation. *Am. J. Cardiol.*, **23**, 208–16

7. Deano, D. A., Wu, D., Mautner, R. K., Sherman, R. H., Ehsani, A. E. and Rosen, K. M. (1977). The antiarrhythmic efficacy of intravenous therapy with disopyramide phosphate. *Chest*, **71**, 597–606

8. Luoma, P. V., Kujala, P. A., Juustila, H. J. and Takkunen, J. T. (1978). Efficacy of intravenous disopyramide in the termination of supraventricular arrhythmias. *J. Clin. Pharm.*, **18**, 293–301

9. Mizgala, H. F. and Huvelle, P. R. (1976). Acute termination of cardiac arrhythmias with intravenous disopyramide. *J. Int. Med. Res.*, **4**, 82–5

10. Beck, O. A., Gunther, R. and Hochrein, H. M. (1982). Conversion of chronic atrial fibrillation and flutter with disopyramide and a verapamil–quinidine combination: A comparative study. *Dtsch. Med. Wochenschr.*, **107**, 1419–23

11. Rulliere, R., Vial, F. and Pornin, M. (1976). La reduction des fibrillations auriculaires par le disopyramide: 70 tentatives. *N. Presse Med.*, **5**, 581–2

12. Halpern, S. V., Ellrodt, G., Singh, B. N. and Mandel, W. J. (1980). Efficacy of intravenous procainanide infusion in converting atrial fibrillation to sinus rhythm: Relation to left atrial size. *Br. Heart J.*, **44**, 589–95

13. Fenster, P. E., Comess, K. A., Marsh, R., Katzenberg, C. and Hager, W. D. (1983). Conversion of atrial fibrillation to sinus rhythm by acute intravenous procainamide infusion. *Am. Heart J.*, **106**, 501–4

14. Miller, G., Weinberg, S. L. and Pick, A. (1952). The effect of procaine amide in clinical auricular fibrillation and flutter. *Circulation*, **6**, 41–50

15. Storstein, L. (1983). Chronic treatment of supraventricular arrhythmias. In Van Durme, J. P., Bogaert, M. G., Julian, D. G. and Kulbertus, H. E. (eds.) *Chronic Antiarrhythmic Therapy*. pp. 200–206. (Molndal, Sweden: A. B. Hassle)

16. Robertson, C. E. and Miller, H. C. (1980). Extreme tachycardia complicating the use of disopyramide in atrial flutter. *Br. Heart J.*, **44**, 602–3

17. Santos, A. L., Aleixo, A. M., Landeiro, J. and Luis, A. S. (1979). Conversion of atrial fibrillation to sinus rhythm with amiodarone. *Acta Med. Portuguesa*, **1**, 15–23

18. Strasberg, B., Arditti, A., Sclarovsky, S., Lewin, R. F., Buimovici, B. and Agmon, J. (1985). Efficacy of intravenous amiodarone in the management of paroxysmal or new atrial fibrillation with fast ventricular response. *Int. J. Cardiol.*, **7**, 47–55

19. Teo, K. K., Harte, M. and Horgan, J. M. (1985). Sotalol infusion in the treatment of supraventricular tachyarrhythmias. *Chest*, **87**, 113–18

20. Nathan, A. W., Hellestrand, K. J., Bexton, R. S. and Camm, A. J. (1984). Clinical use of intravenous flecainide for acute atrial, junctional and ventricular tachycardias (Abstract). *J. Am. Coll. Cardiol.*, **3**, 557

21. Goy, J-J., Grbic, M., Hurni, M., Finci, L., Maendly, R., Duc, J. and Sigwart, U. (1985). Conversion of supraventricular arrhythmias to sinus rhythm using flecainide. *Eur. Heart J.*, **6**, 518–24

22. Creamer, J. E., Nathan, A. W. and Camm, A. J. (1985). Successful termination of atrial tachycardias with flecainide acetate. *Br. Heart J.*, **53**, 164–6

23. Henry, W. L., Morganroth, J., Pearlman, A. S., Clark, C. E., Redwood, D. R., Itscoitz, S. B. and Epstein, S. E. (1976). Relation between echocardiographically determined left atrial size and atrial fibrillation. *Circulation*, **53**, 273–9

24. Ewy, G. A., Ulfers, L., Hager, W. D., Rosenfeld, A. R., Roeske, W. R. and Goldman, S. (1980). Response of atrial fibrillation to therapy; role of etiology and left atrial diameter. *J. Electrocardiol.*, **13**, 119–23

25. Radford, M. D. and Evans, D. W. (1968). Long-term results of DC reversion of atrial fibrillation. *Br. Heart J.*, **30**, 91–6

26. Hartel, G., Louhija, A., Konttinen, A. and Halonen, P. I. (1970). Value of quinidine

in maintenance of sinus rhythm after electric conversion of atrial fibrillation. *Br. Heart J.*, **32**, 57–60

27. Hillestad, L., Bjerkelund, C., Dale, J., Maltau, J. and Storstein, O. (1971). Quinidine in the maintenance of sinus rhythm after electroconversion of chronic atrial fibrillation. *Br. Heart J.*, **33**, 518–21

28. Szekeley, P., Sideris, D. A. and Batson, G. A. (1970). Maintenance of sinus rhythm after atrial defibrillation. *Br. Heart J.*, **32**, 741–6

29. Hartel, G., Louhija, A. and Konttinen, A. (1974). Disopyramide on the prevention of recurrence of atrial fibrillation after electroconversion. *Clin. Pharmacol. Ther.*, **15**, 551–5

30. Blomstrom, P., Edvardsson, N. and Olsson, S. B. (1984). Amiodarone in atrial fibrillation. *Acta Med. Scand.*, **216**, 517–24

31. Coumel, P., Leclerq, J-F. and Attuel, P. (1982). Paroxysmal atrial fibrillation. In Kulbertus, H. E., Olsson, S. B. and Schlepper, M. (eds.) *Atrial Fibrillation.* pp. 158–75. (Molndal, Sweden: A. B. Hassle)

32. Rosenbaum, M. B., Chiale, P. A., Halpern, M. S., Nau, G. J., Przybylski, J., Levi, R. J., Lazzari, J. O. and Elizari, M. V. (1976). Clinical efficacy of amiodarone as an antiarrhythmic agent. *Am. J. Cardiol.*, **38**, 934–44

33. Rowland, E. and Krikler, D. M. (1980). Electrophysiological assessment of amiodarone in the treatment of resistant supraventricular arrhythmias. *Br. Heart J.*, **44**, 82–90

34. Aronow, W. S., Landa, D., Plasencia, G., Wong, R., Karlsberg, R. P. and Ferlinz, J. (1979). Verapamil in atrial fibrillation and atrial flutter. *Clin. Pharmacol. Ther.*, **26**, 578–83

35. Storstein, L. (1982). Role of digitalis in ventricular rate control in atrial fibrillation. In Kulbertus, H. E., Olsson, S. B. and Schlepper, M. (eds.), *Atrial Fibrillation.* pp. 285–292. (Molndal, Sweden: A. B. Hassle)

36. Klein, H. O., Pauzner, H., Di Segni, E., David, D. and Kaplinsky, E. (1979). The beneficial effects of verapamil in chronic atrial fibrillation. *Arch. Intern. Med.*, **139**, 747–9

37. Klein, H. O. and Kaplinsky, E. (1982). Verapamil and digoxin: Their respective effects on atrial fibrillation and their interaction. *Am. J. Cardiol.*, **50**, 894–902

38. Sung, R. J., Elser, B. and McAllister, R. G. (1980). Intravenous verapamil for termination of re-entrant supraventricular tachycardias. *Ann. Intern. Med.*, **93**, 682–9

39. Klein, G. J., Gulamhusein, S., Prystowsky, E. N., Carruthers, S. G., Donner, A. P. and Ko, P. T. (1982). Comparison of the electrophysiologic effects of intravenous and oral verapamil in patients with paroxysmal supraventricular tachycardia. *Am. J. Cardiol.*, **49**, 117–24

40. Wu, D., Denes, P., Dhingra, R., Khan, A. and Rosen, K. M. (1974). The effects of propranolol on induction of A–V nodal reentrant paroxysmal tachycardia. *Circulation*, **50**, 665–77

41. Belhassen, B. and Pelleg, A. (1984). Acute management of paroxysmal supraventricular tachycardia: Verapamil, adenosine triphosphate or adenosine?. *Am. J. Cardiol.*, **54**, 225–7

42. Greco, R., Musto, B., Arienzo, V., Alborino, A., Garofalo, S. and Marsico, F. (1982). Treatment of paroxysmal supraventricular tachycardia in infancy with digitalis, adenosine 5-triphosphate and verapamil: A comparative study. *Circulation*, **66**, 504–8

43. Hellestrand, K. J., Nathan, A. W., Bexton, R. S., Spurrell, R. A. J. and Camm, A. L. (1983). Cardiac electrophysiologic effects of flecainide acetate for paroxysmal reentrant junctional tachycardias. *Am. J. Cardiol.*, **51**, 770–6

44. Yeh, S-J., Lin, F-C., Chou, Y-Y., Hung, J-S. and Wu, D. (1985). Termination of paroxysmal supraventricular tachycardia with a single oral dose of diltiazem and propranolol. *Circulation*, **71**, 104–9

45. Camm, A. J., Ward, D. and Spurrell, R. A. J. (1979). The effect of intravenous disopyramide phosphate on recurrent paroxysmal tachycardias. *Br. J. Clin. Pharmacol.*, **8**, 441–9

46. Wellens, H. J. J., Lie, K. I., Bar, F. W., Wesdorp, J. C., Dohmen, H. J., Duren, D. R. and Durrer, D. (1976). Effect of amiodarone in the Wolff–Parkinson–White syndrome. *Am. J. Cardiol.*, **38**, 189–94

47. Wellens, H. J. J. and Durrer, D. (1974). Effect of procainamide, quinidine and ajmaline in the Wolff–Parkinson–White syndrome. *Circulation*, **50**, 114–20

48. Tonkin, A. M., Aylward, P. E., Joel, S. E. and Heddle, W. F. (1980). Verapamil in prophylaxis of paroxysmal atrioventricular nodal reentrant tachycardia. *J. Cardiovasc. Pharmacol.*, **2**, 473–86

49. Yeh, S-J., Fu, M., Lin, F-C., Lu, Y-S., Hung, J-S. and Wu, D. (1985). Serial electrophysiologic studies of the effect of oral diltiazem on paroxysmal supraventricular tachycardia. *Chest*, **87**, 639–43

50. Bexton, R. S., Hellestrand, K. J., Nathan, A. W., Spurrell, R. A. J. and Camm, A. J. (1983). A comparison of the antiarrhythmic effects on AV junctional re-entrant tachycardia of oral and intravenous flecainide acetate. *Eur. Heart J.*, **4**, 92–102

51. Kennedy, H. L., Whitlock, J. A., Sprague, M. K., Kennedy, L. J., Buckingham, T. A. and Goldberg, R. J. (1985). Long-term follow-up of asymptomatic healthy subjects with frequent and complex ventricular ectopy. *N. Engl. J. Med.*, **312**, 193–7

52. Chiang, B. N., Perlman, L. V., Ostranger, L. D. and Epstein, F. H. (1969). Relationship of premature systoles to coronary heart disease and sudden death in the Tecumseh epidemiologic study. *Ann. Intern. Med.*, **70**, 1159–66

53. Fisher, F. D. and Tyroler, H. A. (1973). Relationship between ventricular premature contractions on routine electrocardiography and subsequent sudden death from coronary heart disease. *Circulation*, **47**, 712–19

54. Hinkle, L. E., Carver, S. T. and Stevens, M. (1969). The frequency of asymptomatic disturbances of cardiac rhythm and conduction in middle-aged men. *Am. J. Cardiol.*, **24**, 629–50

55. Kotler, M. N., Tabatznik, B., Mower, M. M. and Tominaga, S. (1973). Prognostic significance of ventricular ectopic beats with respect to sudden death in the late postinfarction period. *Circulation*, **47**, 959–66

56. Vismara, L. A., Amsterdam, E. A. and Mason, D. T. (1975). Relation of ventricular arrhythmias in the late hospital phase of acute myocardial infarction to sudden death after hospital discharge. *Am. J. Med.*, **59**, 6–12

57. Moss, A. J., Davis, H. T., DeCamilla, J. and Bayer, L. W. (1979). Ventricular ectopic beats and their relation to sudden and nonsudden death after myocardial infarction. *Circulation*, **60**, 998–1003

58. Ruberman, W., Weinblatt, E., Goldberg, J. D., Frank, C. W., Chaudhary, B. S. and Shapiro, S. (1981). Ventricular premature complexes and sudden death after myocardial infarction. *Circulation*, **64**, 297–305

59. Bigger, J. T., Weld, F. M. and Rolnitzky, L. M. (1982). Which postinfarction ventricular arrhythmias should be treated? *Am. Heart J.*, **103**, 660–4

60. Graboys, T. B., Lown, B., Podrid, P. J. and DeSilva, R. (1982). Long-term survival of patients with malignant ventricular arrhythmias treated with antiarrhythmic drugs. *Am. J. Cardiol.*, **50**, 437–43

61. Morganroth, J. and Hunter, H. (1985). Comparative efficacy and safety of short-acting and sustained release quinidine in the treatment of patients with ventricular arrhythmias. *Am. Heart J.*, **110**, 1176–81

62. Bigger, J. T. and Heissenbuttel, R. H. (1969). The use of procaine amide and lidocaine in the treatment of cardiac arrhythmias. *Prog. Cardiovasc. Dis.*, **11**, 515–34

63. Vismara, L. A., Mason, D. T. and Amsterdam, E. A. (1974). Disopyramide phosphate: Clinical efficacy of a new oral antiarrhythmic drug. *Clin. Pharm. Ther.*, **16**, 330–5

64. Talbot, R. G., Julian, D. G. and Prescott, L. F. (1976). Long-term treatment of ventricular arrhythmias with oral mexiletine. *Am. Heart J.*, **91**, 58–65

65. Flecainide Quinidine Research Group (1983). Flecainide versus quinidine for treatment of chronic ventricular arrhythmias. A multicenter clinical trial. *Circulation*, **67**, 1117–23

66. Morganroth, J., Nestico, P. F. and Horowitz, L. N. (1985). A review of the uses and limitations of tocainide – a class IB antiarrhythmic agent. *Am. Heart J.*, **110**, 856–63

67. Schmidt, G., Goedel-Meinen, L., Jahns, G., Linne, R., Schaudig, U., Kein, G., Baedeker, W. and Wirtzfeld, A. (1985). Long-term efficacy of class I antiarrhythmic agents and amiodarone in patients with malignant ventricular arrhythmias. *Drugs*, **29** (Suppl 3), 37–46

68. Prystowsky, E. N., Heger, J. J., Miles, W. M. and Zipes, D. P. (1985). Amiodarone treatment in patients with ventricular arrhythmias. *Drugs*, **29** (Suppl 3), 47–52

69. Mason, J. W. and Winkle, R. A. (1980). Accuracy of ventricular tachycardia-induction study for predicting long-term efficacy and inefficacy of antiarrhythmic drugs. *N. Engl. J. Med.*, **303**, 1073–7

70. Ruskin, J. N., Schoenfeld, M. H. and Garan, H. (1983). Role of electrophysiologic techniques in the selection of antiarrhythmic drug regimens for ventricular arrhythmias. *Am. J. Cardiol.*, **52**, 41C–46C

71. Horowitz, L. N., Greenspan, A. M., Spielman, S. R., Webb, C. R., Morganroth, J., Rotmensch, H., Sokoloff, N. M., Rae, A. P., Segal, B. L. and Kay, H. R. (1985). Usefulness of electrophysiologic testing in evaluation of amiodarone therapy for sustained ventricular tachyarrhythmias associated with coronary heart disease. *Am. J. Cardiol.*, **55**, 367–71

72. Myerburg, R. J., Kesler, K. M., Kiem, I., Pefkaros, K. C., Conde, C. A., Cooper, D. and Castellanos, A. (1981). Relationship between plasma levels of procainamide, suppression of premature ventricular complexes and prevention of recurrent ventricular tachycardias. *Circulation*, **64**, 280–90

73. Sanna, G. and Arcidiacono, R. (1973). Chemical ventricular defibrillation of the human heart with bretylium tosylate. *Am. J. Cardiol.*, **32**, 982–7

18
The arrhythmogenic effects of antiarrhythmic drugs. Types, mechanisms and predisposing factors

C. J. GARRATT and A. J. CAMM

It has been suggested that antiarrhythmic drugs may contribute directly to 5% of cases of out-of-hospital cardiac arrest.[1] Certainly, nearly all antiarrhythmic agents have been shown to induce or exacerbate ventricular arrhythmias in some patients. Such arrhythmogenic or pro-arrhythmic effects are more common in patients with severe ventricular disease or a history of life-threatening arrhythmias[2]. However, in individual cases there are few specific features predictive of such susceptibility. The following account is an attempt to review the types and mechanisms of antiarrhythmic drug-induced ventricular tachyarrhythmias, and to assess the possibility of predicting which patients are at risk. Antiarrhythmic drug-induced supraventricular tachycardias (such as those associated with digoxin toxicity) and bradyarrhythmias will not be discussed.

CLASSIFICATION OF ARRHYTHMOGENIC EFFECTS OF ANTIARRHYTHMIC DRUGS

Induction of polymorphic ventricular tachycardia associated with abnormal ventricular repolarization (torsade de pointes)

Delayed repolarization and specifically QT prolongation were first implicated in the origin of ventricular tachycardia with the discovery of the congenital long QT syndromes. Since that time a variety of acquired causes of QT prolongation associated with polymorphic ventricular tachycardia have been established (Table 18.1). Antiarrhythmic agents belonging to class 1a in the Vaughan Williams classification are the most common drug-related causes[3] (Figure 18.1). Class 3 agents (sotalol[4] and

Table 18.1 Causes of the acquired long QT syndrome

Common:	antiarrhythmic agents; Vaughan Williams classes 1a and 3
	bradycardia; usually sinus bradycardia or atrioventricular conduction block
	hypokalaemia
	psychotropic drugs: tricyclic antidepressants and phenothiazines
Less Common:	hypomagnesaemia
	hypocalcaemia
	myocardial infarction
	mitral valve prolapse
	cerebrovascular accidents

amiodarone[5]) have also been implicated. The polymorphic ventricular tachycardia induced under these circumstances is termed '*torsade de pointes*'. This arrhythmia has several specific characteristics[3].

It is an irregular, wide complex arrhythmia in which the QRS complexes appear to twist around a baseline. The tachycardia is usually self-terminating, but often degenerates into ventricular fibrillation. The arrhythmia is often recurrent and repetitive. The onset is preceded by ventricular beats exhibiting a long–short cycle length. A typical sequence is as follows: the first complex is a ventricular premature beat, followed by a compensatory pause (long cycle length) and a subsequent sinus beat; a second ventricular premature beat then occurs on the T wave of the sinus beat (short cycle length) and precipitates the polymorphic ventricular tachycardia[3] (Figure 18.2).

The most effective treatment is overdrive atrial or ventricular pacing. There are several reports of successful treatment with isoprenaline although in some cases it has been found to be unreliable[3]. In individual cases Vaughan Williams class 1b drugs have been effective (lignocaine[6], tocainide[6] and mexiletine[7]).

Exacerbation of monomorphic ventricular arrhythmias

This form of proarrhythmic event differs from the induction of *torsade de pointes* in that it involves an arrhythmia already present before therapy is commenced (Figure 18.3). The arrhythmia in question is monomorphic rather than polymorphic. Using serial Holter monitoring studies a worsening of arrhythmia was observed in 11% of drug tests in patients being treated for ventricular tachyarrhythmias[8]. Under conditions of electrophysiological study, conversion of induced, non-sustained ventricular tachycardia to sustained ventricular tachycardia has occurred in 5–13% of patients undergoing antiarrhythmic drug testing[9,10]. All drug classes are involved in this type of proarrhythmic effect: in the study by Rinkenberger and co-workers[10] sustained ventricular tachycardia occurred during drug testing with disopyramide (two patients), quinidine (two patients), amiodarone (four patients) and

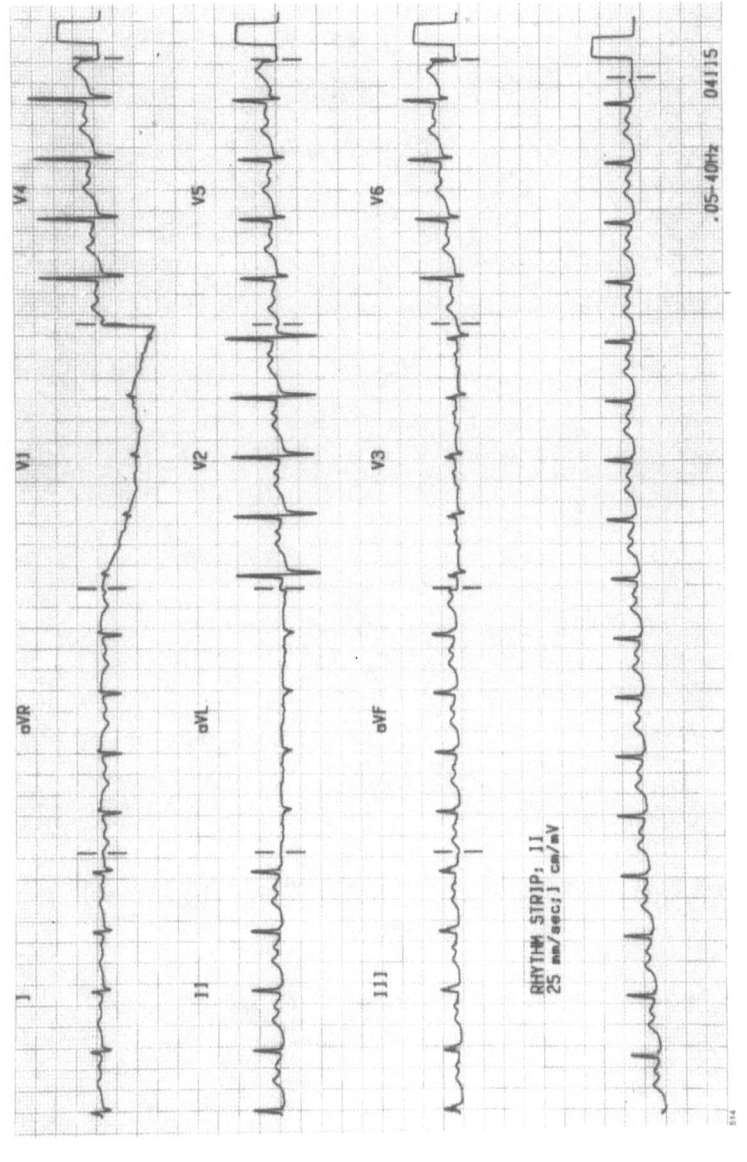

Figure 18.1 The 12-lead ECG (in sinus rhythm) of a 65-year-old man on quinidine therapy who had been admitted with a self-terminating episode of polymorphic ventricular tachycardia

303

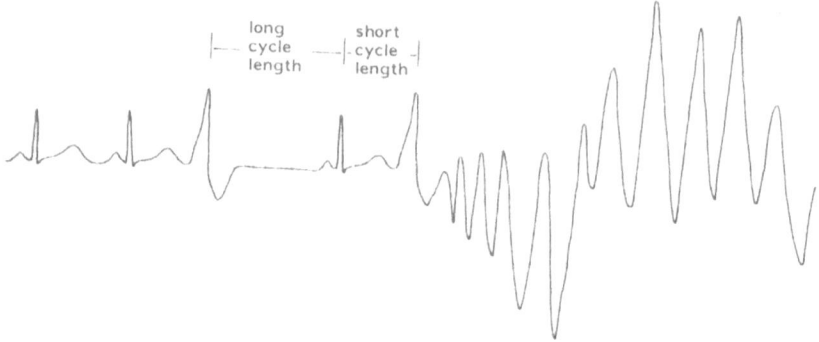

Figure 18.2 An illustration of the long–short cycle length sequence preceding *torsade de pointes*.

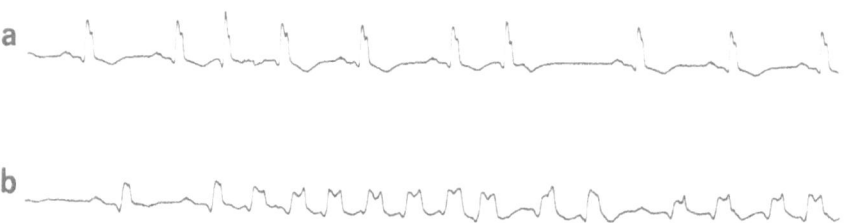

Figure 18.3 Uniform ventricular tachycardia which occurred more frequently after treatment with a class 1c drug.

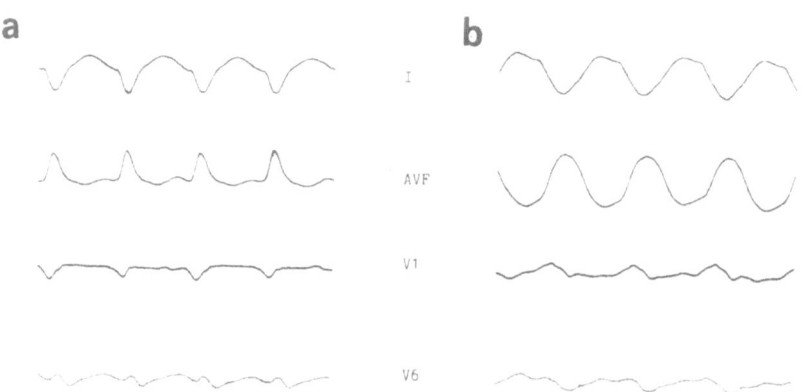

Figure 18.4 Spontaneous uniform ventriculur tachycardia: **a:** before treatment; **b:** after treatment with a class 1c drug.

encainide (seven patients). In all patients only non-sustained ventricular tachycardia could be initiated in the control studies. In some cases, particularly during treatment with agents of class 1c, a monomorphic tachycardia may be so sustained as to become incessant[11].

Induction of 'sinusoidal' ventricular tachycardia

This form of ventricular tachyarrhythmia is characterized by a sinusoidal appearance with marked QRS widening[11], and is, therefore, different in morphology from the spontaneous ventricular arrhythmias in the drug-free state (Figure 18.4). There is no associated QT prolongation. A striking characteristic of the arrhythmia is that it is often resistant to electrical cardioversion, and sudden cardiac death, even in hospital, is common. This proarrhythmic effect is primarily associated with anti-arrhythmic drugs of class 1c. Drugs demonstrated to have this effect include flecainide[2], propafenone[12] and encainide[13].

MECHANISMS OF PROARRHYTHMIC EFFECTS

It has already been stated that *torsade de pointes* is usually precipitated by a premature ventricular complex occurring to the T wave of the previous sinus beat. If it is assumed that the onset of premature ventricular complexes corresponds to the recovery of excitability in some portion of the ventricle, while the end of the QT interval corresponds to a similar instant in some other portion of the ventricle[14], then it is clear that some asynchrony of repolarization exists at the onset of *torsade de pointes*.

The role of asynchrony of repolarization in the genesis of *torsade de pointes* has been studied by Bonatti and co-workers[15]. They recorded right ventricular monophasic action potentials (MAPs) in patients with the long QT syndrome of different aetiologies and with a documented history of *torsade de pointes*. The aetiologies were hypokalaemia (two cases), hypocalcaemia (two cases), bradycardia (two cases), prenylamine treatment (one case), amiodarone treatment (one case), idiopathic non-familial (one case) and idiopathic familial (one case). In each of the 10 cases studied, MAPs recorded in several areas of the right ventricle showed large differences in duration, ranging from 100 to 270 milliseconds. In the normal right ventricle MAPs did not vary by more than 40 milliseconds in the same patient. In areas where the MAP was prolonged this was seen to be due to 'humps' occurring on the falling phase of repolarization. Several spontaneous episodes of *torsade de pointes* occurred during the recordings; they were precipitated by extrasystoles occurring during the course of 'humps' of MAPs, i.e. during the phase of delayed repolarization. Bonatti interpreted these studies as suggesting that the humps arose from 'focal re-excitations' that delay normal repolarization of the cardiac potential. He considered that focal re-excitations are responsible not only for isolated ventricular extrasystoles but also for *torsade de pointes*.

Camm and Ward[16] and later, Brugada and Wellens[17] proposed an alternative mechanism for *torsade de pointes*. They conjectured that the asynchrony of repolarization may result in electrotonic depolarization of the normal myocardium by a form of local re-entry. If another structure (or more than two) were being depolarized by the same mechanism, an arrhythmia similar in morphology to *torsade de pointes* would occur. However, clinical electrophysiological studies on patients with the familial or idiopathic long QT syndrome do not provide support for a re-entrant mechanism. The ability to initiate an arrhythmia reproducibly by programmed electrical stimulation has been believed to be a hallmark of re-entrant arrhythmias[18]. Programmed right and left ventricular stimulation with up to three extrastimuli before and during isoprenaline treatment resulted in non-sustained polymorphic tachycardia in only six out of 15 cases of familial or idiopathic long QT syndrome[19]. The induced arrhythmias appeared to differ from the spontaneous episodes in rate as well as morphology of the QRS complexes. None of the induced episodes had the typical *torsade de pointes* configuration.

There is evidence that the ionic basis for the humps and prolongation of repolarization is a defect in potassium conductance. Brachmann and co-workers[20] have shown that caesium infusion in dogs can provide a model for *torsade de pointes* induction, in that it can produce bradycardia-dependent ventricular ectopy and, in some cases, multiform ventricular tachycardia. Microelectrode studies in canine endocardial preparations[20] revealed that caesium infusion resulted in early afterdepolarizations which interrupted phase 3 of Purkinje fibre action potentials. Caesium is known to delay repolarization by blocking potassium currents. It has been proposed that certain individuals are especially sensitive to the effects of certain antiarrhythmic agents to block outward potassium current, and as a result these individuals are susceptible to the generation of *torsade de pointes*.

There is overwhelming evidence that the basis for sustained, monomorphic ventricular tachycardia is macro- or micro- re-entry[21]. Initiation and maintenance of re-entrant arrhythmias are dependent on a critical balance between refractoriness and conduction slowing in the re-entrant circuit. Any antiarrhythmic agent which affects both properties has the potential to alter the balance between these factors such that the arrhythmia is more easily initiated or maintained. In patients with drug-exacerbated monomorphic ventricular tachycardia Rinkenberger and co-workers[10] showed that the drugs associated with sustained ventricular tachycardia increased the mean tachycardia cycle length by 112 milliseconds but increased the median ventricular effective refractory period by only 30 milliseconds. If the refractory period of the individual elements in the re-entrant loop was similarly only minimally increased then fibres in the re-entrant pathway would have more time to repolarize in advance of the returning wavefront and thus perpetuate the re-entrant circuit. This cannot be the mechanism in all cases of drug-exacerbated monomorphic ventricular tachycardia however, as in some patients the tachycardia may become accelerated as well as more sustained[22]. It is possible that small changes in refractoriness and conduction lead to the use of new, previously latent pathways for re-entrant excitation.

The mechanism of the sinusoidal tachycardia associated with class 1c agents is unstudied and unknown, but presumably is related to the marked conduction slowing that is the major feature of these drugs.

PREDISPOSING FACTORS

Regardless of the microelectrophysiological correlates of the arrhythmias associated with the acquired long QT syndromes, a QT interval beyond which the risk of *torsade de pointes* rises abruptly has not been established. Measurement of antiarrhythmic drug levels has been shown to be similarly unhelpful. Kay and co-workers[3] reviewed the circumstances surrounding the development of *torsade de pointes* in 32 patients receiving antiarrhythmic medication (quinidine, disopyramide, procainamide or amiodarone). In 22 of 26 patients in whom the drug levels were measured, the levels were found to be within the therapeutic range.

The fact that an antiarrhythmic agent has been administered to an individual patient for a considerable period of time does not exclude the possibility of the development of *torsade de pointes*. Bauman and co-workers[23] reported the development of *torsade de pointes* in 31 patients receiving quinidine. Although 74% of these had been receiving quinidine for less than 1 week, the range in time delay from initiation of therapy to *torsade* was up to 3 years. Interestingly, in this study two-thirds of the patients had long QT intervals whilst not taking quinidine. The study by Kay and co-workers[3] revealed that 20 of the 32 patients with *torsade* had baseline prolongation of the QT interval (before antiarrhythmic therapy) or co-existent hypokalaemia or hypomagnesaemia. There is a strong suggestion, therefore, that the presence of a long QT interval prior to antiarrhythmic therapy is a good predictor of the development of *torsade de pointes*, and may be a contraindication to therapy with class 1a agents.

There are theoretical reasons for supposing that an indicator of marked asynchrony of repolarization or the presence of early after-depolarizations would be a very useful predictor of the occurrence of polymorphic ventricular tachycardia. No such tests are currently routinely available.

Podrid and co-workers[24] compared 51 patients who had monomorphic ventricular arrhythmias which were aggravated by antiarrhythmic agents with 102 patients in whom no aggravation occurred. The only useful predictive features were the presence of left ventricular dysfunction and a history of life-threatening arrhythmias. Arrhythmia aggravation was not associated with abnormalities on the baseline electrocardiogram or drug-induced changes on the electrocardiogram.

Grouped data from several flecainide and encainide clinical studies[25] clearly identified structural heart disease, previous sustained ventricular tachycardia and rapid escalation of drug dosage as the risk factors for serious proarrhythmic events and death. QRS and QT duration are of no value in predicting patients at risk. Of the serious proarrhythmic effects that do occur with class 1c agents, 75% are apparent within the first 2 weeks of therapy[2].

SUMMARY AND CONCLUSIONS

There are three major groups of proarrhythmic effects of antiarrhythmic therapy. These correspond to some extent to the Vaughan Williams class of drug involved (Tables 18.2 and 18.3). Possible mechanisms of these arrhythmogenic effects have been discussed.

Several recommendations can be made regarding the initiation of antiarrhythmic drug therapy. Before starting treatment, close attention should be paid to the presence of baseline QT prolongation and to

Table 18.2 Vaughan Williams classification of antiarrhythmic drugs

Class		Effect on action potential	Examples
1		Reduction of rate of rise of phase 0:	
	a	+ prolongation	quinidine, disopyramide, procainamide
	b	+ shortening	lignocaine, mexiletine, tocainide
	c	+ no effect on duration	flecainide, propafenone, encainide
2		Reduction of rate of rise of phase 4	β-blockers
3		Prolongation	amiodarone, sotalol, bretylium
4		Depression of phase 2–3	verapamil, diltiazem

Table 18.3 Classification of proarrhythmic events

Proarrhythmic event	Drug class	Predisposing factors
Polymorphic ventricular tachycardia	1a and 3	Pre-existing QT prolongation coexistent hypokalaemia
Monomorphic ventricular tachycardia	all classes, particularly 1c	history of life-threatening arrhythmias poor left ventricular function high drug levels
'Sinusoidal' ventricular tachycardia	1c	history of life-threatening arrhythmias poor left ventricular function high drug levels

coexistent metabolic abnormalities, particularly when treatment with drugs of classes 1a or 3 are being considered.

Previous antiarrhythmic agents must be discontinued for several half-lives before a new antiarrhythmic agent is introduced. Drug combinations should be avoided if possible.

Patients with a history of life-threatening arrhythmias or poor left ventricular function should be admitted to hospital for initiation of therapy. Quantitative Holter monitoring, or in some cases electrophysiological studies, should be performed prior to and early after the start of treatment. Drug levels should be measured after initiation of therapy and after any dose increase. This is particularly important with patients with poor left ventricular function to whom a drug of class 1c is being administered.

References

1. Ruskin, J. N., McGovern, B., Garan, H., DiMarco, J. P. and Kelly, E. (1983). Antiarrhythmic drugs: A possible cause of out-of-hospital cardiac arrest. *N. Engl. J. Med.*, 309, 1302–6
2. Morganroth, J. and Horowitz, L. N. (1984). Flecainide: Its proarrhythmic effect and expected changes on the surface electrocardiogram. *Am. J. Cardiol.*, 53, 89B–94B
3. Kay, G. N., Plumb, V. J., Arciniegas, J. G., Henthorn, R. W. and Waldo, A. L. (1983). Torsade de pointes: the long–short initiating sequence and other clinical features: observations in 32 patients. *J. Am. Coll. Cardiol.*, 2, 806–17
4. McKibbin, J. K., Pocock, W. A., Barlow, J. B., Millar, R. N. S. and Obel, I. W. P. (1984). Sotalol, hypokalaemia, syncope and torsade de pointes. *Br. Heart J.*, 51, 157–62
5. Sclarovsky, S., Lewin, R. F., Kracoff, O., Strasberg, B., Arditti, A. and Agmon, J. (1983). Amiodarone-induced polymorphous ventricular tachycardia. *Am. Heart J.*, 105, 6–12
6. Bansal, A. M., Kugler, J. D., Pinsky, W. W., Norberg, W. J. and Frank, W. E. (1986). Torsades de pointes: Successful acute control by lidocaine and chronic control by tocainide in 2 patients. *Am. Heart J.*, 112, 618–21
7. Shah, A. and Schwartz, H. (1984). Mexiletine for treatment of torsade de pointes. *Am. Heart J.*, 107, 589–91
8. Velebit, V., Podrid, P., Lown, B., Cohen, B. H. and Graboys, T. B. (1982). Aggravation and provocation of ventricular arrythmias by antiarrhythmic drugs. *Circulation*, 65, 886–94
9. Buxton, A. E., Waxman, H. L., Marchlinski, F. E. and Josephson, M. E. (1984). Electropharmacology of nonsustained ventricular tachycardia: effects of class 1 antiarrhythmic agents, verapamil and propranolol. *Am. J. Cardiol.*, 53, 738–44
10. Rinkenberger, R. L., Prystowsky, E. N., Jackman, W. M., Naccarelli, G. V., Heger, J. J. and Zipes, D. P. (1982). Drug conversion of nonsustained ventricular tachycardia to sustained ventricular tachycardia during serial electrophysiologic studies: identification of drugs that exacerbate tachycardia and potential mechanisms. *Am. Heart J.*, 103, 177–84
11. Bigger, J. T. and Sahar, D. I. (1987). Clinical types of proarrhythmic response to antiarrhythmic drugs. *Am. J. Cardiol.*, 59, 32E–37E
12. Buss, J., Neuss, H., Bilgin, Y. and Schlepper, M. (1985). Malignant ventricular tachyarrhythmias in association with propafenone treatment. *Eur. Heart J.*, 6, 424–8
13. Winkle, R. A., Mason, J. W., Griffin, J. C. and Ross, D. (1981). Malignant ventricular tachyarrhythmias associated with the use of encainide. *Am. Heart J.*, 102, 857–64

14. Surawicz, B. and Knoebel, S. B. (1984). Long QT: good, bad or indifferent? *J. Am. Coll. Cardiol.*, **4**, 398–413
15. Bonatti, V., Rolli, A. and Botti, G. (1983). Recording of monophasic action potentials of the right ventricle in long QT syndromes complicated by severe ventricular arrhythmias. *Eur. Heart J.*, **4**, 168–79
16. Camm, A. J. and Ward, D. E. (1979). Clinical cardiac electrophysiology, Part 2. *Hospital Update*, **5**, 403–10
17. Brugada, P. and Wellens, H. J. J. (1985). Early afterdepolarisations: Role in conduction block, "prolonged repolarisation-dependent re-excitation", and tachyarrhythmias in the human heart. *Pacing Clin. Electrophysiol.*, **8**, 889–96
18. Wellens, H. J. J. (1978). Value and limitations of programmed electrical stimulation in ventricular tachycardia. *Circulation*, **57**, 845–53
19. Bhandari, A. K., Shapiro, W. A., Morady, F., Shen, E. N., Mason, J. and Scheinman, M. M. (1985). Electrophysiologic testing in patients with the long QT syndrome. *Circulation*, **71**, 63–71
20. Brachmann, J., Scherlag, B. J., Rosenshtraukh, L. V. and Lazzara, R. (1983). Bradycardia-dependent triggered activity: relevance to drug-induced multiform ventricular tachycardia. *Circulation*, **68**, 846–56
21. Josephson, M. E., Almendral, J. M., Buxton, A. E. and Marchlinski, F. E. (1987). Mechanisms of ventricular tachycardia. *Circulation*, **75**, (Suppl. III), 41–7
22. Torres, V., Flowers, D. and Somberg, J. C. (1985). The arrhythmogenicity of antiarrhythmic agents. *Am. Heart J.*, **109**, 1090–7
23. Bauman, J. L., Bauernfiend, R. A., Hoff, J. V., Strasberg, B., Swiryn, S. and Rosen, K. M. (1984). Torsade de pointes due to quinidine: Observations in 31 patients. *Am. Heart J.*, **107**, 425–30
24. Podrid, P. J., Lampert, S., Graboys, T. B., Blatt, C. M. and Lown, B. (1987). Aggravation of arrhythmia by antiarrhythmic drugs: Incidence and predictors. *Am. J. Cardiol.*, **59**, 38E–44E
25. Morganroth, J. (1987). Risk factors for the development of proarrhythmic events. *Am. J. Cardiol.*, **59**, 32E–37E

19
Digitalis and arrhythmias

R. HAYWARD

INTRODUCTION

Digitalis electrophysiology is straightforward by comparison with the impenetrable controversy which surrounds its use in chronic heart failure. In the following account, inotropic effects are mentioned only *en passant*, and the term digitalis is used to describe all glycoside-like compounds, whether or not derived from digitalis plants. Cardiac glycosides elude attempts to locate their electrophysiological actions within standard antiarrhythmic drug classifications. Effects differ in various parts of the heart, and interactions with the autonomic nervous system contribute substantially to the overall response.

CELLULAR ACTIONS

The principal site of digitalis activity is the myocardial cell membrane (sarcolemma); the glycoside molecule is not required to penetrate the cell. Even when firmly bound to a non-membrane permeable protein, digoxin remains able to stimulate contractility of cultured heart cells, and removal of digoxin from sarcolemmal binding sites by digoxin-specific antibody quickly reverses its effects. There is no lag as would be expected if the drug had to diffuse out of the cell. Unlike novel positive inotropic drugs, e.g. sulmazole and DPI 201–106[1], digitalis has no direct effect on contractile proteins.

Cardiac glycosides bind avidly to specific sites on the sarcolemma. The precise location is now known to be part of the sodium pump enzyme complex, termed Na^+-K^+-ATPase (sodium and potassium dependent adenosine triphosphatase). Na^+-K^+-ATPase binding accounts for most myocardial glycoside uptake, though some is non-specifically adsorbed onto cell membrane lipid. Loose uptake onto lipid probably accounts for the fast initial uptake of lipid soluble glycoside by the heart, which precedes any contractile response[2]. Binding of digitalis to the ATPase complex almost always inhibits the action of the sodium pump[3,4]. Inhibition is partial. In animal studies sodium expulsion is sufficiently inhibited by digitalis to allow the intracellular concentration of available sodium (termed a^iNa) to rise from approximately 6 mmol/1 to 7 mmol/l. As a result, contractile force approximately doubles[5].

Though intracellular calcium ion availability directly controls myocardial contractile force, a^iNa is also important[6]. A digitalis-induced increase in a^iNa enhances contractility via the membrane-located sodium–calcium counter transport system. It uses as a source of energy the passive entry of Na ions into the cell down the transmembrane gradient (extracellular sodium 140 mmol/l, intracellular 10 mmol/l), to expel calcium against its massive concentration gradient (extracellular 2.5 mmol/l, intracellular 10^{-4} mmol/l in diastole). By reducing the transmembrane sodium gradient, digitalis reduces sodium–calcium exchange, intracellular calcium tends to accumulate, and more is available to promote contractile element activation. Microelectrode studies in animals have validated this mechanism[5].

Extrapolating *in vitro* experimental data to man is complicated by a major dose-response difference. Therapeutic digitalis concentrations in man are approximately 10^{-9} mol/l (specifically 1–2 nmol/l or 0.8–1.6 ng/ml), while sodium pump inhibition is not readily demonstrable until 10^{-8} or even 10^{-7} molar concentrations are reached. Relative *in vitro* insensitivity is probably an artefact of tissue isolation techniques[7]. There is little doubt that significant sodium pump inhibition is present in patients on digitalis, but proof is elusive. Subtoxic digoxin administration in dogs caused a 25% inhibition of the sodium pump (measured by endomyocardial biopsy) at a time when left ventricular contractility as assessed by peak dP/dt was enhanced by 20%[8].

Though important, sodium pump inhibition is not the only mechanism of digitalis inotropy. In some studies, sodium pump stimulation can be detected with very low digitalis concentrations[9], despite onset of contractile stimulation[10,11].

Digitalis influences contractility by four additional actions:

(1) By inhibiting Na^+–K^+-ATPase activity on membranes of sympathetic nerve terminals in ventricular myocardium, neuronal reuptake of released noradrenaline diminishes and levels adjacent to myocardial β-receptors increase.

(2) Mainly in the atria, but also in the ventricles, increased vagal tone enhances acetylcholine liberation, though the effect on contractility would be negative.

(3) A secondary result of digitalis binding to sarcolemmal Na^+–K^+-ATPase is to increase the calcium storing capacity of nearby phospholipids. By this means, more calcium is held in the glycocalyx and on the sarcolemmal surface, ready to move into the cell during depolarization[4].

(4) Digitalis probably displaces an endogenous material from sarcolemmal ATPase. This material exerts a potent inhibitor action;

displacement by digitalis causes 'disinhibition', expressed as slight stimulation[9]. Evidence for the existence of an endogenous compound which has digitalis-like properties is now very strong.

ENDOGENOUS DIGITALIS

The reason for digitalis receptors in mammalian cells has been a mystery. The answer is probably that they are the site of action of one or more endogenous compounds whose physiological role is to regulate the sodium pump[12].

Digitalis-like immunoactivity (DLIA) is present in serum from patients with chronic renal failure[13], premature babies, neonates and some patients with paroxysmal atrial tachycardia[14]. The rat adrenal cortex secretes a compound (not ACTH) which is inotropic and reacts in digoxin assays[15]. Toads secrete cardioactive digitalis-like bufagins[16] which are used in Chinese folk-remedies.

Endogenous DLIA may be related to the so-called natriuretic hormone, found in patients with uraemia and volume overload[17]. By inhibiting the sodium pump in arteriolar smooth muscle cells and elevating intracellular calcium, arteriolar tone is enhanced. Hypertensive patients' serum contains a Na^+-K^+-ATPase inhibitor, and widespread depression of sodium pump activity is characteristic of hypertension[17]. There are probably a number of DLIA compounds (alternative isonyms include endoxin, endodigin and cardiodigin) produced by diverse tissues including the atrial myocardium, and with differing activity profiles. Exogenous digitalis displaces them from receptors and is a less potent Na^+-K^+-ATPase inhibitor. DLIA is not the same as atrial natriuretic peptide.

DIGITALIS RECEPTORS

Cardiac receptors take up digitalis with avidity. Myocardial glycoside concentrations (g/g) are 15–35 times those in plasma (g/ml). With therapeutic plasma concentrations approximately half the available heart receptor sites are occupied[18]. Receptor density is greatest in the left ventricle (1.5×10^{14} receptor sites/g tissue). The right ventricle carries 0.9×10^{14} and atrial myocardium 0.6×10^{14} sites/g tissue. Some animals have two classes of digitalis receptor. They have relatively few high affinity receptors (800 sites/cell), which bind digitalis in low concentrations ($10^{-8}-10^{-9}$ mol/l), and mediate subtle contractile enhancement with minimal sodium pump inhibition. More numerous are low-affinity receptors (10^6/cell). These take up digitalis when levels are high ($10^{-6}-10^{-7}$ mol/l), and mediate a further increment in contractility due to substantial sodium pump inhibition, plus emergence of toxic rhythm disturbances. The goal of tailoring a novel glycoside which would bind only to the 'safe' high affinity receptor seems remote, but recent studies have discerned two receptor populations in man[19].

CELLULAR ELECTROPHYSIOLOGY

Electrophysiological changes in cardiac cells exposed to therapeutic concentrations of digitalis are subtle. Most data come from a classic cross-perfusion study in dogs[20]. Alterations in the surface ECG of a dog receiving cumulative doses of ouabain were correlated with transmembrane action potentials recorded simultaneously via microelectrodes in His–Purkinje (HP) fibres of a second dog perfused with blood from the first. The earliest effect on the ECG was ST segment depression and altered T-wave shape, correlating in the second dog with an approximate 10% (significant) lengthening of HP fibre action potential. Increased action potential duration reflected a prolonged plateau phase (phase 2) and delayed onset of repolarization (phase 3), implying that slow calcium current influx might be enhanced. Resting membrane potential was unaffected, indicating that sodium pump inhibition had not yet commenced. Alterations in sarcolemmal function probably include increased resistance to transmembrane potassium flux (decreased potassium conductance) and reduced background potassium efflux. Enhanced inward calcium current (I_{Ca}) may also contribute[21].

Though action potential prolongation is usually considered an antiarrhythmic effect (Vaughan Williams class III), it is doubtful if the initial result of digitalis administration is protective. Lack of antiarrhythmic activity may stem from non-uniform dispersal of action potential prolongation throughout the cardiac chambers[22]. Action potential prolongation takes place in atrial and ventricular myocardium and in HP fibres. Action potential amplitude, rate of rise of upstroke (phase 0 V_{max}) and conduction velocity are initially unaffected.

The response is biphasic. In the canine study[20], attainment of toxic ouabain concentrations caused action potential abbreviation due to accelerated repolarization. In other studies action potentials begin to shorten simply with more prolonged sub-toxic exposure. Onset of toxicity is presaged by junctional and ultimately ventricular arrhythmias. Features of fulminant digitalis toxicity are loss of resting membrane potential due to progressive paralysis of the sarcolemmal sodium pump, with reduced action potential amplitude. Repolarization is accelerated and action potentials shortened, an effect of the lowered transmembrane potassium gradient which enhances sarcolemmal potassium permeability. At this stage, phase 0 V_{max} is reduced and conduction velocity is correspondingly slowed. In clinical toxicity these potent proarrhythmic effects are further exacerbated by enhanced sympathetic drive[23].

The digitalis-toxic abnormalities described above relate to systolic electrical function. Toxic phenomena also emerge during diastole. The rate of spontaneous diastolic depolarization (phase 4 slope) is increased in HP fibres and cells of the AV node, but not in atrial or ventricular working myocardium. Consequently the automaticity of these potential pacemaker foci is increased, favouring emergence of accelerated junc-

Table 19.1   Digitalis toxic arrhythmias

---

(1) *Ectopic tachycardias*
     (a) Automatic (highly characteristic)
          Non-paroxysmal junctional tachycardia
          Junctional escape rhythm
          Ventricular tachycardia: bidirectional (alternating BBB pattern)
                                   parasystolic
          Fascicular tachycardia
     (b) Re-entrant (less characteristic)
          Atrial flutter and fibrillation
          Ventricular premature beats
          Ventricular tachycardia, flutter and fibrillation
     (c) Uncertain mechanism (highly characteristic)
          Paroxysmal atrial tachycardia plus AV block ('PAT with block')

(2) *Pacemaker depression* (relatively uncommon)
     Sinus bradycardia, sinus arrest.

(3) *Depressed conduction* (common)
     AV block: e.g. AF with complete AV block, 1st or 2nd degree block
     Exit block in atrial or junctional tachycardia
     (Acquired bundle branch block is rare)

(4) *Ectopic rhythms with depressed conduction*
     Atrial or junctional tachycardia with AV block

(5) *AV dissociation*
     Accelerated junctional or ventricular rhythm ± sinus bradycardia

(6) *'Triggered' automatic arrhythmias*
     Junctional tachycardia following an atrial premature beat
     Ventricular tachycardia following supraventricular tachycardia

---

tional and fascicular rhythms. The diastolic membrane potential begins spontaneously to oscillate. Oscillations are termed delayed after-depolarizations, and may exceed the threshold potential, causing repetitive firing[24]. Intracellular calcium ion accumulation is responsible, itself the result of sodium accumulation and reduced sodium-calcium exchange. The level of a^{i}Ca increases on the cell membrane interior, and sarcoplasmic reticular calcium uptake is intermittently unable to compensate, so that a^{i}Ca fluctuates. The conductivity of a recently identified sarcolemmal sodium channel depends upon adjacent a^{i}Ca. Accordingly, the effect of diastolic oscillations of a^{i}Ca is to promote surges of transient inward sodium current which are expressed electrically as diastolic afterdepolarizations. The clinical importance of this mechanism is unknown. Certain digoxin-toxic arrhythmias are triggered by shortened cycle length (Table 19.1). Afterdepolarizations behave similarly. Some investigators now consider the afterdepolarization mechanism more clinically important than enhanced phase 4 automaticity[23]. Paradoxically, hypoxia seems to oppose afterdepolarizations, probably by modifying sarcoplasmic calcium release[25].

Table 19.2 Summary of therapeutic electrophysiological actions of digitalis

Structure	Direct effect	Indirect effect	Net result
Sinoatrial node	variable depression	slight vagal slowing	slower sinus rate and conduction velocity
Atrium	ERP prolonged	bisphasic, but ERP reduced	ERP reduced, CV enhanced
Atrioventricular junction	slight slowing	major ERP prolongation, conduction slowed	important gains in ERP and conduction time
Accessory pathways	ERP probably reduced	probably vagal ERP reduction but undefined	varies; ERP may shorten dangerously
His–Purkinje system	ERP slightly increased, conduction unchanged	minimal effect with non-toxic exposure	slight ERP prolongation
Ventricular myocardium	slight ERP prolongation	vagal ERP reduction in upper regions	variable; ERP reduced slightly

CV: Conduction velocity
ERP: Effective refractory period

ELECTROPHYSIOLOGICAL ACTIONS ON SELECTED CARDIAC TISSUES

The therapeutic electrophysiological effects of digitalis are summarized in Table 19.2, and explained below.

Atrial myocardium

The direct actions of digitalis on atrial myocardium are swamped by potent indirect effects mediated via the vagal nerves[26]. In denervated preparations, digitalis initially increases atrial effective refractoriness and prolongs action potential duration[22], though even this direct action may involve release of locally stored acetylcholine. Indirect effects are those of vagal hypertonia and enhanced acetylcholine liberation. Sarcolemmal permeability to potassium is potentiated, the atrial cell is hyperpolarized and action potential amplitude is increased. Phase 0 V_{max} and conduction velocity are accelerated[27]. The combination of reduced refractoriness and enhanced conduction equates with a proarrhythmic effect in the atria.

Sinoatrial node

Direct actions on the sinoatrial node are minimal relative to indirect, neurally mediated effects. After pharmacological blockade of autonomic innervation (propranolol 0.2 mg/kg plus atropine 0.04 mg/kg), digoxin caused no change in sinus cycle length, sinus node recovery time or sinoatrial conduction time. But with intact autonomic innervation, sinus cycle length was significantly prolonged[28]. Important indirect effects include vagal (parasympathetic) and sympathetic influences. Phase 0 upstroke in sinoatrial and atrioventricular node cells is dominated by slow calcium currents; fast sodium channels do not mediate depolarization in these special areas. Acetylcholine liberated by vagal nerve endings in and around the sinus node depresses slow calcium flux, depressing the action potential upstroke velocity and slowing conduction. Further sinus node depressant actions include a diminished phase 4 slope, and thus a reduced discharge rate. Sinus node responsiveness to catecholamines is also impaired, consistent with a slight β-blocking action[23].

Atrioventricular node

Due to the dependence on slow calcium currents of AV nodal n-cells, the indirect vagal effects mediated by acetylcholine predominate over direct digitalis actions, causing slowed conduction and increased refractoriness[26]. Direct actions are complementary, but minimal or undetectable after elimination of autonomic influences[28]. Toxic glycoside concentrations, however, cause the slope of phase 4 to increase in cells of the AV node, favouring the emergence of junctional tachycardia[23].

His–Purkinje fibres

Sensitivity to digitalis is greater in His–Purkinje fibres than in working myocardium. In dogs, action potential duration increased by approximately 10% during non-toxic exposure to ouabain[20]. There was a non-significant trend towards reduced action potential amplitude and V_{max} at this time, coinciding with ST segment and T-wave changes. Predictably on this evidence, refractory periods increased by approximately 5% in intact canine His–Purkinje tissue after therapeutic doses of ouabain[29].

Conduction velocity was unchanged, so that from these data, digitalis is most unlikely to engender bundle branch block other than following very early premature beats of junctional origin, these being more liable to elicit aberrant conduction. Onset of bundle branch block has been ascribed to digitalis toxicity[30]. Glycoside administration with pre-existing bundle branch disease has been deprecated, and likened to the situation with first or second degree atrioventricular block, in which digitalis is relatively contraindicated, although no ill-effect may be detectable[31].

Toxic levels precipitate an increase in phase 4 slope, not seen in ventricular myocardial cells. Spontaneous afterdepolarizations (described above), emerge in both specialized conducting tissue and working myocardial cells[25]. Depending on their timing, premature impulses can elicit fascicular re-entry and reflection by falling close to diastolic depolarizations[23]. Longitudinal dissociation develops, whereby the sequence of proximal then distal Purkinje system activation is reversed. Action potential amplitude, duration and resting membrane potential all decline. His–Purkinje fibres provide the principal anatomical substrate for toxic ventricular tachyarrhythmias.

Ventricular myocardium

Therapeutic glycoside exposure slightly increases action potential duration of ventricular myocardium, but higher doses accelerate repolarization[23]. Effects on the intact human ventricle are modest; refractoriness decreased by approximately 10% after ouabain and reduction was most pronounced under the influence of overdrive pacing[32].

Working myocardial cells lack intrinsic automaticity and phase 4 is isoelectric; spontaneous diastolic depolarization does not develop in these cells with digoxin toxicity. In the base of the right ventricle, parasympathetic innervation contributes a small acetylcholine-mediated reduction in effective refractoriness[33]. Vagal nerve supply is less dense elsewhere in the ventricles but has been identified around the bundle branches[34]. Unless toxicity has supervened, sympathetically-mediated actions are subtle but probably contribute to reduced refractoriness.

Bypass pathways

Effects of digitalis on accessory atrioventricular pathways in man have been variable, but definite facilitation has been observed. Thus in 21 patients with Wolff–Parkinson–White syndrome studied by Sellers and co-workers[35], the shortest R–R interval during induced periods of atrial fibrillation was reduced in six but increased in seven patients. The decrement in R–R interval ranged from 15 to 77 ms after digoxin, although increments of similar size occurred in seven patients, implying a safe response to digitalization. Onset of ventricular fibrillation was linked with digitalis administration in nine subjects. Bombardment by increasingly frequent transmission of impulses from the fibrillating atria probably provoked fibrillation in the ventricles.

Digitalis is, therefore, contraindicated in WPW syndromes unless proven safe by electrophysiological study. Precipitation of VF seems highly likely if the shortest control R–R interval in atrial fibrillation, closely correlated with the anterograde bypass tract refractory period, is less than 220 ms[35].

INTERACTIONS WITH THE CENTRAL NERVOUS SYSTEM

Parasympathetic system

The dominance of parasympathetic effects on supraventricular structures is achieved by digitalis actions at multiple levels in the vagal control system[36,37]. Carotid, aortic and cardiopulmonary baroreceptors supplying afferent innervation are sensitized. In heart failure, left atrial baroreceptor activity is depressed relative to the raised atrial pressure.

Sensitization by digitalis means that baroreceptor activity is elevated to more appropriate levels, and previously excessive constriction of resistance and capacitance vessels is reduced. Parasympathetic drive to the heart is enhanced, with familiar effects on intracardiac conduction described above, by three means:

(1) Central vagal nuclei are stimulated and vagal efferent traffic is increased.
(2) Sensitivity of supraventricular cholinergic receptor sites is enhanced.
(3) Acetylcholine is released from local stores in the myocardium.

Accordingly digitalis is a potent vagotonic drug. Indeed its most useful roles in arrhythmia control are achieved by enhanced vagotonia.

Sympathetic system

Low-dose digitalis exposure causes a subtle increase in local catecholamine concentrations within the ventricular myocardium, as described above. Both the positive inotropic effect and the pro-arrhythmic potential of these drugs are thereby enhanced. Sympathetic interactions assume major importance with digitalis toxicity, and summate with direct toxic effects on cardiac cells (above). Indirect sympathetic effects are more potent than direct toxic actions; in the cat, spinal cord transection trebles the concentration of digitalis needed to induce toxicity. Animal studies have identified a specific region of the medulla oblongata as responsible for both arrhythmias and widespread vasoconstriction seen in digitalis toxicity[38].

Termed the 'area postrema', this site on the floor of the fourth ventricle is one of a small number of CNS structures that is not protected by the lipid-selective blood–brain barrier. As in the posterior pituitary and the pineal body, vascular anatomy is unusual in that a perivascular glial membrane is absent and vascular sinusoids are plentiful. All cardiac glycosides attain high concentrations here independent of their lipid-solubility. Attempts to design safer compounds by ensuring failure to penetrate the blood–brain barrier have, therefore, been frustrated. For example the experimental glycoside AS1-222 is highly polar and poorly lipid soluble. It is thus minimally taken up by the brain in general and achieves low CSF concentrations but is no less toxic[38].

Enhanced sympathetic drive to the peripheral and coronary vascular systems characterizes digitalis toxicity; the latter has been implicated in proarrhythmic activity because of its propensity to exacerbate ischaemia[39]. Digitalis vasoconstriction has proved sufficient to precipitate myocardial ischaemia[40] as well as mesenteric infarction and bowel necrosis[37].

By inhibiting Na^+-K^+-ATPase of vascular smooth muscle cells, arteriolar tone is increased. Vascular α-receptors are also stimulated. Glycoside penetration into sympathetic control centres provokes renal β_1-receptor stimulation, followed by renin release and increased angiotensin II constrictor activity. The direct arterioconstrictor effect of digitalis is ultimately mediated by increased intracellular calcium concentrations; predictably, therefore, it is reversed by calcium channel blockers such as verapamil[39].

CLINICAL ELECTROPHYSIOLOGY OF DIGITALIS

Atrial fibrillation

Control of the ventricular rate in atrial fibrillation is the prime indication for digitalis therapy. Because of its unusual profile, incorporating suppression of sinus and AV nodes and positive inotropism, it matches exquisitely the requirements for treating patients with atrial fibrillation and heart failure[41]. The atria behave as a syncytium, with no intervening electrical barriers. During fibrillation the depolarizing wavefront spreads through the atrial myocardium in a manner that is best described as random re-entry[42]. Some 500 impulses/minute, therefore, reach the upper approaches to the AV node at random if very brief intervals[43]. After digitalis administration both the median R–R interval and the minimum R–R interval encountered increase. Meijler[44] has found that the upper limit of R–R interval increases more than does the lower limit, so that the R-R interval scatter is greater after digitalis. There is debate as to whether the ventricular rate is truly irregular in atrial fibrillation, and whether the AV node imposes some mathematical order upon transmission of random impulses to the ventricles[43,45]. Certainly phenomena such as chaining, featuring a series of very similar R–R intervals, and alternans, in which a long interval is followed by a short one, are frequently seen, but digitalis does not promote regularity, even though the ventricular response is slowed. Slowing of the ventricular rate is achieved by two complementary actions:

(1) Increased refractoriness and slowed conduction through the AV node stems principally from enhanced vagal tone as described above. The ERP of the AV node is rarely prolonged to more than 600 ms after digitalis, inadequate to explain the appearance of R–R intervals of some 1500 ms.

(2) Concealed conduction is of more importance. Occurring within the AV node, concealed conduction increases after digoxin, causing extinction of the majority of wavefronts as they traverse

the upper portion of the node. Because of its capacity to reduce refractoriness and accelerate conduction in atrial myocardium, the atrial fibrillation frequency increases after digoxin and a greater number of impulses impinge on the node, resulting in increased nodal refractoriness and impulse extinction[44].

By virtue of these actions digitalis is effective in chronic atrial fibrillation. The resting ventricular rate is reduced and diastolic ventricular filling improves; benefit is particularly striking when diastolic filling is impaired as in mitral stenosis. With exertion the rate may climb excessively despite digitalization, probably because vagal drive is minimized during upright exercise[46]. Co-administration of a β-blocker or verapamil is then helpful. Up to 480 mg of verapamil may be needed and seems safe[47] despite the recognized digoxin–verapamil interaction which increases the serum digoxin concentration[48].

Paroxysmal atrial fibrillation

Shortening of the atrial refractory period and accelerated atrial conduction are proarrhythmic actions, even though AV nodal transmission is reduced as a consequence. The initial component of the biphasic early response includes transient prolongation of atrial action potential and refractory period[22]. Unfortunately because this effect is inhomogeneously dispersed in the atrium, little antiarrhythmic protection is demonstrable in the laboratory setting. Clinical experience is often diametrically opposite, however. For example, paroxysmal supraventricular tachyarrhythmias, including paroxysmal atrial fibrillation and flutter, are frequent after open heart surgery, and can be prevented by early postoperative digitalization[49]. Likewise, the incidence of supraventricular premature contractions in patients with mitral leaflet prolapse was significantly reduced on oral digoxin therapy[50].

Coumel[51] has been able to segregate patients with paroxysmal atrial fibrillation into two groups of unequal size. The majority, typically males aged 40–50 years, suffer increasingly frequent episodes of atrial fibrillation (often with periods of flutter) in which a vagal mechanism is strongly implicated. Attacks are not provoked by manoeuvres which involve sympathetic hyperactivity, i.e. exercise and emotion, but occur when vagal drive is enhanced, as during rest and sleep and after meals. Onset of the tachycardia may be heralded by prolongation of the sinus cycle length suggesting a surge of vagal activity. On this evidence, the potent supraventricular, vagotonic actions of digitalis should not be helpful, a prediction confirmed by Coumel and colleagues[51]. Quinidine and its local anaesthetic congeners are suitable, but amiodarone may be needed for adequate control; β-blockers share with digitalis an undesirable proarrhythmic propensity.

In contrast a smaller group of paroxysmal atrial fibrillators is regarded as having adrenergic atrial arrhythmias. Paroxysms are usually precipitated by exertion or emotion and are rare at rest. They are presaged

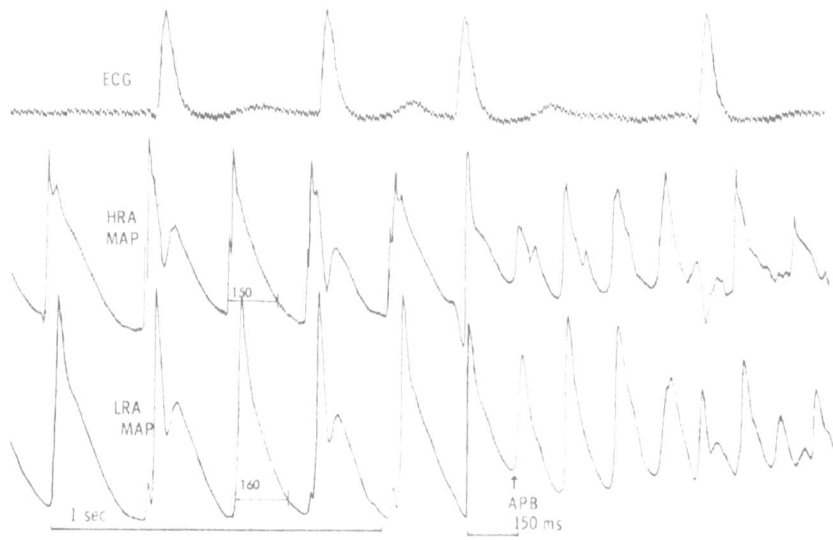

Figure 19.1 Intracardiac recording of two atrial monophasic action potentials plus surface ECG channel, showing spontaneous transition from atrial flutter, 300/minute, to atrial fibrillation, 40 minutes after methyldigoxin infusion. Fibrillation results from a sudden shortening of the atrial cycle length at point labelled APB, resulting in an action potential upstroke incident upon the repolarization wave of the preceding complex
(Reproduced by kind permission from *Cardiovascular Research*)

by sinus tachycardia, implying enhanced sympathetic drive, followed by salvoes of atrial ectopic beats, ectopic atrial tachycardia and ultimately atrial fibrillation with a ventricular rate of 120–150 beats/minute. Digitalis and β-blockers are helpful. For resistant cases, amiodarone, plus or minus quinidine or flecainide has been required. Propafenone, combining local anaesthetic, β-blocking and calcium antagonist activity, should be of value.

By employing a progressively more analytical approach to paroxysmal atrial fibrillation, the traditional first line role of digitalis may be eroded, with beneficial consequences to the patient. Rapid digitalization has been deployed in atrial fibrillation of recent onset; cardioversion was achieved with i.v. digoxin 1.5 mg over 12 h in 32 of 45 patients[52]. In this study tachycardia termination was not preceded by ventricular rate reduction, implying that if digoxin was causally involved, an effect on the atrium not the AV junction was responsible.

Atrial flutter

Classically, digitalis converts atrial flutter to fibrillation, and so transforms a drug-refractory arrhythmia into one which is relatively easily controlled. One method by which digitalis achieves this effect is illustrated in Figure 19.1. Monophasic action potentials measured from the

322

human right atrium show an accelerating atrial rate close to 300/minute, ultimately with a spontaneously very short coupling interval which initiates atrial fibrillation. This result was achieved 40 minutes after digitalis infusion, at a stage when the biphasic response referred to above is completed and both atrial action potentials and refractory periods are shortened. Figures 19.2 and 19.3 illustrate the control phase and the phase of action potential shortening, respectively. An alternative response is conversion to sinus rhythm. Animal data suggest that reversion to sinus rhythm is a direct action not involving the vagus, whereas conversion to fibrillation represents a vagally mediated decrease in atrial refractoriness.

Paroxysmal atrial tachycardia

On the basis of the atrial actions described, digitalis would be expected to be proarrhythmic in this context. Indeed paroxysmal atrial tachycardia with AV block is considered a classic digitalis toxic arrhythmia. The underlying mechanism is uncertain, but may be enhanced automaticity. In a previously digitalized patient, appearance of atrial tachycardia with block should be considered a sign of toxicity till proved otherwise. If the ventricular rate is not excessively fast, management comprises digoxin withdrawal and maintenance of a normal serum potassium.

Intrauterine arrhythmias

Tachyarrhythmias are now being diagnosed *in utero* using either echocardiography alone or combined with Doppler blood flow analysis (see Chapter 11). Once diagnosed, digoxin is usually the first drug tried. When given to pregnant women, digoxin successfully terminated fetal supraventricular tachycardia with associated heart failure in six cases[53]. Effects were slow after oral administration (3–35 days), against 24 hours for intravenous digoxin. Wolff–Parkinson–White syndrome was identified later in two of the three fetuses in which the response to digoxin was most prompt; these probably had reciprocating junctional tachycardia involving the AV node, and were accordingly relatively digoxin-sensitive, while others may have had less amenable atrial tachycardias[54].

A recent case report describes the successful control of paroxysmal supraventricular tachycardia in a fetus with multiple cardiac tumours, a condition in which drug resistance might have been anticipated[55]. Digoxin was unsuccessful in controlling one case of fetal atrial flutter[56], though it may not have been given an adequate trial.

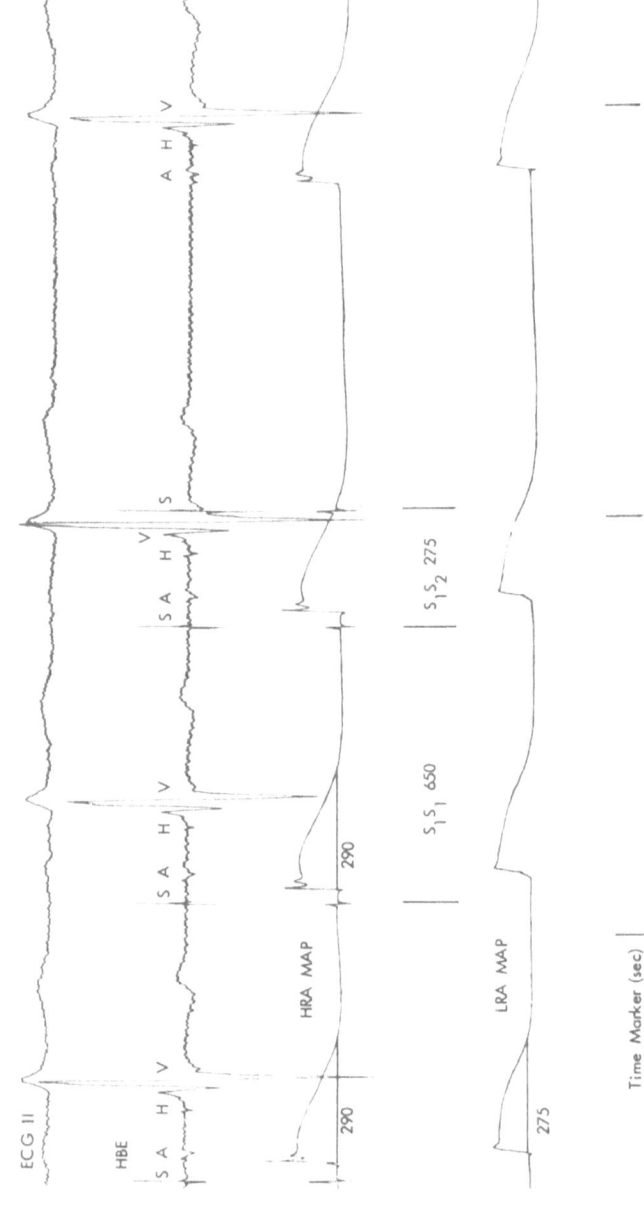

Figure 19.2 Intracardiac recordings of monophasic action potential from two positions in the human right atrium, recorded via bipolar electrodes (lower traces), plus His bundle electrogram and surface ECG channel. Prior to digitalis administration, showing atrial extrastimulus (S2) with a 275 ms coupling interval falling just within atrial effective refractory period (time intervals in ms)

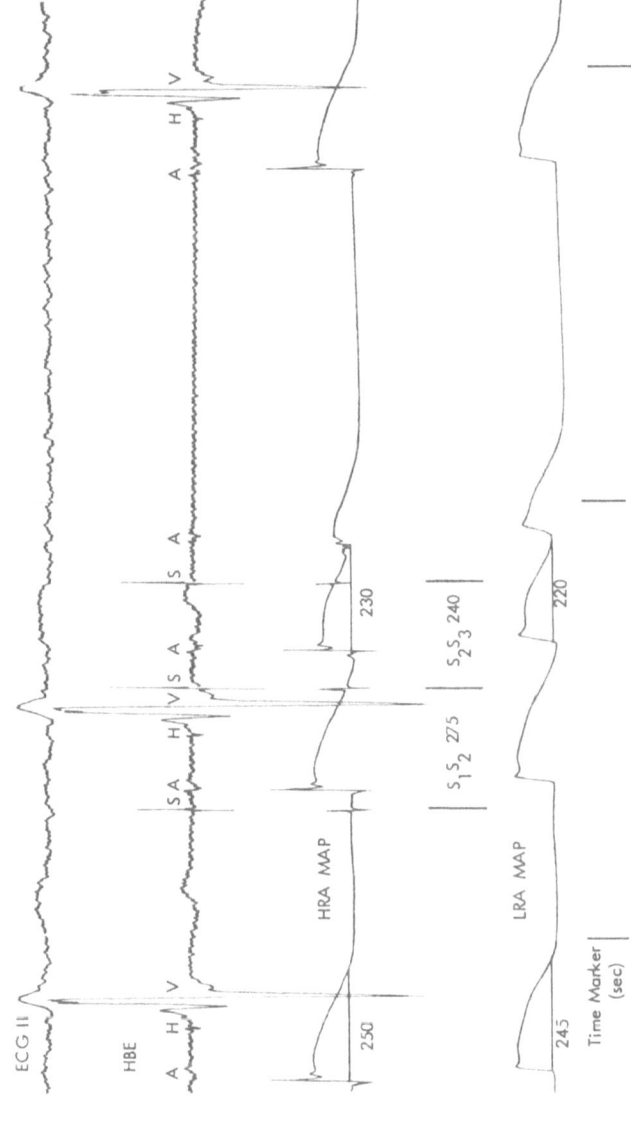

Figure 19.3 Intracardiac recording from same subject as in Fig 1 above, 40 minutes after infusion of methyldigoxin. Atrial action potentials now reduced, and with a 275 ms coupling interval, S2 now evokes an atrial depolarisation, consistent with reduced atrial effective refractoriness

325

Childhood arrhythmias

Amiodarone and Class I drugs such as disopyramide are increasingly used in supraventricular tachyarrhythmias of childhood. Digoxin remains popular with many clinicians who have become expert in handling it[57], and is well tolerated. For the same plasma digoxin concentration, myocardial levels are approximately twice as high in infants as in adults, probably due to relatively lower renal clearance combined with a greater myocardial binding capacity. Pre-term infants develop particularly high myocardial concentrations[58]. Binding avidity declines during early infancy, and the ability to clear digoxin via the kidneys rises during the first month.

Under the age of one month, the digitalizing dose is 2–4 doses of $10 \mu g \, kg^{-1}$ 6-hourly by mouth, with $10 \mu g \, kg^{-1} d^{-1}$ as maintenance. Full paediatric doses are appropriate after the first month, giving $20 \mu g \, kg^{-1} d^{-1}$. As with alternative antiarrhythmic drugs in children, this dose is several fold greater than that used in adults as a function of body weight; calculations based on surface area may be more realistic[59]. The range of therapeutic digoxin concentrations quoted in children is usually 1.3–3.9 mmol/l (1–3 ng/ml).

The role of digoxin in paediatric heart failure with normal rhythm has seemed secure in contrast with adult practice. Even here digoxin has been criticized as ineffective on the basis of studies in children with ventricular septal defects[60]. This may be a special situation in which cardiac contractile indices are already nearly maximal despite apparent heart failure; the margin available for a digoxin effect may be very small[61]. The place of digitalis looks secure as an antiarrhythmic agent in children despite in-roads made by novel agents.

Pre-excitation syndromes and junctional tachycardias

The potential dangers of giving digoxin to patients with Wolff–Parkinson–White (WPW) syndrome are well-known. As Sellers and colleagues[35] demonstrated, the shortest R–R interval between pre-excited complexes in atrial fibrillation, an important prognostic factor relating to vulnerability to ventricular fibrillation, is dangerously reduced by digoxin in approximately one third of patients. Shortening of the anterograde effective refractory period of the accessory pathway permits more rapid transmission of impulses from the fibrillating atria through to the ventricles, but it is not the sole mechanism. Probably just as important is the reduced opportunity for concealed conduction within the bypass tract which results from reduced refractoriness and accelerated conduction. By decreasing anterograde transmission via the AV node, the potential for concealed retrograde penetration into the accessory pathway, also important in modulating the ventricular rate in atrial fibrillation[62] likewise diminishes.

Digitalis, therefore, shares with verapamil and lignocaine an undesirable liability to increasing the ventricular rate in atrial fibrillation. Digoxin should not be given unless the response has been evaluated at electrophysiological study. This caveat extends to patients with WPW syndrome who seem solely to suffer from re-entry junctional tachycardia, since atrial fibrillation can ensue during such an attack.

Digitalis has been rarely used in combination to deal with re-entry junctional tachycardia in fully investigated WPW syndrome. Its effects on AV node conduction and refractoriness help prevent and terminate circus movement, but agents which impair the conducting properties of the accessory pathway, such as disopyramide, flecainide and other Class I drugs are preferred. Intracardiac electrophysiological study of patients with re-entry junctional tachycardia and concealed WPW syndrome suggest that digitalis can reduce vulnerability to tachycardia initiation by atrial premature beats, but in a minority of subjects, new echo zones were created indicating a proarrhythmic response[63].

Ventricular arrhythmias

Despite a secure role as an atrial antiarrhythmic agent, digitalis glycosides are considered proarrhythmic in the ventricles. Ventricular effective refractoriness is shortened by ouabain in man, and the electrocardiographic QT interval is reduced in parallel[32]. Major ventricular tachyarrhythmias are a cardinal feature of digitalis toxicity.

Despite these powerful considerations, the incidence of complex ventricular arrhythmias (ventricular tachycardia, couplets, bigeminy and multiform ectopics) did not increase in a heterogeneous group of patients, some with impaired left ventricular function, given oral digoxin by Gradman and co-workers[64]. Furthermore, the occurrence of ventricular ectopic beats declined during digoxin treatment relative to placebo. This effect was greatest in patients with normal left ventricular function, tending to contradict the hypothesis that any antiarrhythmic action in the ventricles is due to withdrawal of sympathetic hyperactivity as part of the response to improved myocardial function.

A decade has now passed since Lown and colleagues demonstrated complete abolition of ventricular ectopy by the short acting cardiac aglycone acetyl strophanthidin in 21% of 146 patients with frequent ventricular premature contractions[65]. A reduction in both the frequency and the degree of malignancy of ventricular premature contractions was achieved in a further 25%. Ectopic frequency, however, increased in 28% and was unchanged in 26%. Though approximately half these patients had impaired left ventricular function, again this was not predictive of a beneficial response. Lown and co-workers suggested that acetyl strophanthidin opposed ventricular ectopy by enhancing vagal drive and opposing sympathetic stimulation.

The same workers in Boston have subsequently evolved an advanced non-invasive protocol for the assessment of patients with malignant ventricular tachyarrhythmias and for an evaluation of their responsiveness to antiarrhythmic drug therapy[66]. The highly productive and individualistic philosophy adopted by this group eschews the use of intracardiac electrophysiology studies. An integral component of their protocol is the administration of intravenous acetyl strophanthidin. Suppression of ventricular ectopic activity during the brief and almost immediate (1–30 minute) time course is regarded as a favourable response, justifying long term oral digoxin therapy.

Results achieved by this group are impressive but the contribution made by digoxin is not clear. Frank toxicity and major arrhythmias can emerge during an acetyl strophanthidin challenge and it is not widely employed. At present the use of digoxin in ventricular arrhythmias cannot be commended, other than as adjunctive therapy for heart failure.

DIGITALIS AND MYOCARDIAL INFARCTION (MI)

Concerns about arrhythmogenic responses and about possibly increased infarct size have inhibited the use of digoxin in the coronary care situation. These concerns may have been exaggerated. For example in a careful short-term CCU study[67], patients with left ventricular failure due to extensive myocardial necrosis treated with digoxin showed no sign of increased infarct size or of worsened ventricular arrhythmias when compared with controls. Moreover, ejection fraction increased significantly during the study in digitalized patients, but declined in controls. Using the acetyl strophanthidin challenge test referred to above, Lown and colleagues showed that unlike the experimental animal, patients with acute MI are not more vulnerable to digitalis-induced arrhythmias[68]. Digitalis glycosides are effective against an unacceptably fast ventricular rate in atrial fibrillation complicating acute MI, but should not be used when high-grade AV block limits the ventricular rate to less than 110–120/minute[69]. Some authorities advocate the use of ouabain in the CCU environment, because of its rapid peak effect (30–45 minutes after infusing 0.25 mg slowly over 10 minutes). Any glycoside should be infused over not less than 10 minutes to avoid the potent arterioconstrictor effect of a bolus injection[37].

Major concern has recently arisen over the possibility that digitalis may increase long term mortality in post-MI survivors, at least in part due to a possible arrhythmogenic effect. Six large scale studies have addressed the issue[70-75]. In three of these[70,71,74], digoxin treatment appeared to confer an increase in mortality, i.e. digitalis was an independent risk factor for death post-infarction.

Particularly striking were the conclusions of Moss and colleagues[70], that the digoxin-related mortality clustered in a high-risk subset, those who had congestive failure while in the CCU, plus evidence on pre-discharge Holter recordings of 'complex' ventricular premature beats (multiform, repetitive, bigeminal or early). The mode of death in the digitalized group was sudden (within 1 hour of onset of agonal illness) in six of 21 cases, implying that proarrhythmic activity may have played a part. Results from the remaining three studies, however, tend to exculpate digitalis. The presence of worse left ventricular function and other factors in the patients given digoxin was sufficient to account for the excess mortality. Digoxin served, therefore, as a marker of a poor prognosis rather than its cause. The security of the statistical evidence against digoxin post-MI has been vigorously criticized[76]; by the same token evidence that it is safe is weak. Digoxin certainly does not improve long term survival. In the absence of digoxin-amenable arrhythmias, alternative strategies for heart failure are preferable.

DIGITALIS TOXICITY: RECOGNITION AND TREATMENT

Early studies identified toxicity in up to 35% of digitalized patients, though the prevalence is probably less now. Successful treatment depends on the early recognition of side effects. Symptoms accrue insidiously, and are listed below:
— Lassitude, nausea, anorexia, vomiting.
— Visual disturbance such as yellow-tinged vision (xanthopsia) or the perception of other colours (chromatopsia) and impaired recognition of colour.
— Headache, confusion, delirium, convulsions.
Tachyarrhythmias attributable to digitalis toxicity include ventricular premature beats, bigeminy and ventricular tachycardia[77]. Emergence of a regular ventricular rate in atrial fibrillation signifies the onset of accelerated junctional tachycardia. Paroxysmal atrial tachycardia with block is a classical digitalis toxic arrhythmia, also simultaneous atrial and junctional tachycardia with AV dissociation (double tachycardia). Bradycardia due to third degree AV block is common, often preceded by second degree block. Fisch and Knoebel have constructed a rational classification of digitalis toxic arrhythmias based upon underlying mechanisms[78], a summary of which appears in Table 19.1 The diagnosis is confirmed if the plasma digoxin concentration is in the toxic range (>2.6 nmol/l, 2.0 ng/ml), but lower concentrations are found in 10% of patients with toxicity[77]. Potentiating factors are old age (probably reflecting declining renal elimination), low potassium and/or magnesium concentrations[79], raised serum calcium, hypothyroidism, advanced lung disease, possibly myocardial ischaemia, and cardiac amyloidosis. The threat to life is substantial. Up to a two thirds mortality has been encountered in the past with suicidal digoxin overdosage, when serum concentrations may lie in the range 6–30 nmol/l. Accidental poisoning from tablets or bizarre sources such as herbal tea containing foxglove leaves[80], is less frequent. Treatment includes withdrawal of digitalis, correction of predisposing factors particularly hypokalaemia, use of atropine or of temporary pacing if unacceptable bradycardia is present, and control of tachyarrhythmias. Hyperkalaemia is a particularly bad sign and may emerge after some hours, reflecting general paralysis of Na^+-K^+-ATPase and loss of intracellular potassium. Correction of

hypokalaemia must be cautious for this reason, giving 20–40 mmol/hour by slow i.v. infusion. Oral administration of activated charcoal following gastric lavage reduces further absorption, and maintenance of urine flow is important.

Ventricular arrhythmias may respond to phenytoin 100 mg i.v., repeated at intervals, or to lignocaine. Phenytoin is favoured since it opposes digitalis binding and may improve AV conduction. If cardioversion is mandatory, very low energies should be used, starting at 10 joule, and progressing to 50, 100, 200 and so forth[81].

DIGOXIN-SPECIFIC ANTIBODIES

Ready access to Fab fragments of antidigoxin antibodies raised in sheep has dramatically reduced the lethality of severe digitalis toxicity[82].

This antibody has a very high affinity for digoxin in the serum and binds to it on a molecule for molecule basis, forming an inactive complex which is eliminated via the kidneys. The serum is rapidly cleared. Glycoside bound onto cardiac receptors, which exists in equilibrium with serum digoxin, migrates into the serum and is inactivated. Only the non-antigenic Fab fraction of sheep antibody is used; the antibody is first cleaved with papain and the antigenic Fc fragments are separated off. There have been no reports of anaphylaxis. Severe toxic manifestations are terminated within 30–60 minutes. The amount of Fab antibody needed is calculated on the basis of the estimated load of glycoside present in the body.

Ampoules of 40 mg are generally available from hospital pharmacies or regional poisons units; the average dose needed by patients encountered by Wenger and co-workers[82] was 520 mg, range 4 to 1600 mg. The digoxin concentrations with which they had to deal ranged from 2.4 to > 100 ng/ml, with an average of over 14. Hopefully digitalis toxicity will become increasingly rare, but the introduction of this remedy for toxicity with a dangerous drug in which the ratio between a therapeutic and a toxic dose has been estimated at 1:4 is most welcome. The essential principle may also be applicable to other toxic conditions.

DIGITALIS AND CARDIOVERSION

Supraventricular and ventricular arrhythmias can emerge following direct current cardioversion, usually because of injudiciously high energies or poor synchronization. Animal experiments confirm that prior digitalization enhances the arrhythmogenic effect of cardioversion[81]. For example the energy needed to precipitate ventricular tachycardia in dogs is reduced from 400 J to 0.2 J by near-toxic digitalization.

In clinical practice it is usual to stop digitalis for at least 24 hours. If this is not possible and there is no evidence of toxicity, cardioversion is probably safe, though the plasma concentration should be known to be sub-toxic, and the electrolytes normal[83].

DRUG INTERACTIONS AND DIGITALIS

Since the therapeutically important digoxin–quinidine interaction was appreciated, the effects of verapamil and many other antiarrhythmic and diverse drugs have come to light[48,84]. Quinidine, verapamil, and amiodarone increase plasma digoxin levels, whereas nifedipine probably does not and diltiazem may have a slight effect. Nicardipine and gallopamil do so weakly, while tiapamil substantially increases digoxin concentration[48]. Mechanisms are not fully established but verapamil decreases renal and non-renal clearance, and diminishes the volume of distribution. Quinidine increases digoxin absorption from the gut; quinine may have a lesser effect. Disopyramide, flecainide, procainamide, mexiletine and ethmozine are innocent in this regard. Hydralazine lowers digoxin levels by increasing renal tubular secretion. Captopril appears to elevate serum digoxin concentration by reducing renal clearance[85]. The increasing use of multiple drug regimens including antiarrhythmic agents and vasodilators particularly in cardiac failure must increase the risk of three-way interactions with digoxin. The above list does not accommodate the many interactions with non-cardiac drugs, listed in review articles[48,84].

References

1. Colucci, W. S., Wright, R. F. and Braunwald, E. (1983). New positive inotropic agents in the treatment of congestive heart failure. *N. Engl. J. Med.*, **314**, 349–58
2. Hayward, R., Greenwood, H., Stephens, J. and Hamer, J. (1983). Relationship between myocardial uptake and actions in heart failure of methyldigoxin. *Br. J. Clin. Pharmacol.*, **15**, 41–8
3. Katz, A. M. (1985). Effects of digitalis on cell biochemistry: sodium pump inhibition. *J. Am. Coll. Cardiol.*, **5**, 16A–21A
4. Schwartz, A. and Adams, R. J. (1980). Studies on the digitalis receptor. *Clin. Res.*, **46** (Suppl 1) I-154–I-160
5. Wasserstrom, J. A., Schwartz, D. J. and Fozzard, H. A. (1983). Relation between intracellular sodium and twitch tension in sheep cardiac Purkinje strands exposed to cardiac glycosides. *Circ. Res.*, **52**, 697–705
6. Lee, C. O. (1985). 200 years of digitalis. *Am. J. Physiol.*, **249**, C367–78
7. Poole-Wilson, P. A., Galindez, E. and Fry, C. H. (1979). Effect of ouabain in therapeutic concentrations on K exchange and contraction of human and rabbit myocardium. *Clin. Sci.*, **57**, 41520
8. Hougen, T. J., Lloyd, B. L. and Smith, T. W. (1979). Effects of inotropic and arrhythmogenic digoxin doses and of digoxin specific antibody on myocardial monovalent cation transport in the dog. *Circ. Res.*, **44**, 23–31
9. Godfraind, T., DePover, A., Hernandez, G. C. and Fagoo, M. (1982). Cardiodigin: endogenous digitalis-like material from mammalian heart. *Arch. Int. Pharmacodyn.*, **258**, 165–7
10. Noble, D. (1980). Mechanism of action of therapeutic levels of cardiac glycosides. *Cardiovasc. Res.*, **14**, 495–514
11. Bernabei, R. and Vassale, M. (1984). The inotropic effects of strophanthidin in Purkinje fibers and the sodium pump. *Circulation*, **69**, 618–31
12. Anon. (1983). Endogenous foxglove. *Lancet*, **2**, 1463–4
13. Graves, S. W., Brown, B. and Valdes, R. (1983). An endogenous digoxin-like substance in patients with renal impairment. *Ann. Intern. Med.*, **99**, 604–8

14. Kaye, G. C., Williams, A. and Camm, A. J. (1986). Digoxin-like immunoreactivity during atrial arrhythmias. *Lancet*, **1**, 689
15. Pudek, M. R., Seccombe, D. W., Whitfield, M. F. and Ling, E. (1983). Digoxin-like immunoreactivity in premature and full-term infants not receiving digoxin therapy. *N. Engl. J. Med.*, **308**, 904–5
16. Shimoni, Y, Gotsman, M., Deutsch, J., Kachalsky, S. and Licjtstein, D. (1982). Endogenous ouabain-like compound increases heart muscle contractility. *Nature*, **307**, 369–71
17. de Wardener, H. E. and Clarkson, E. M. (1982). The natriuretic hormone: recent developments. *Clin. Sci.*, **63**, 415–20
18. Erdmann, E. and Brown, L. (1983). Cardiac glycoside-receptor system. *Eur. Heart J.*, **4** (Suppl. A), 61–5
19. Godfraind, T. (1984). Subclassification of cardiac glycoside receptors. In Erdmann, E. (ed.) *Cardiac Glycoside Receptors and Positive Inotropy.* Suppl. to *Basic Researches in Cardiology*, **79**, 27–34. (Darmstadt: Steinkopf Verlag.)
20. Rosen, M. R., Gelband, H. and Hoffman, B. F. (1973). Correlation between effects of ouabain on the canine electrocardiogram and transmembrane potentials of isolated Purkinje fibers. *Circulation*, **47**, 65–72
21. Marban, E. and Tsien, R. W. (1982). Enhancement of calcium current during digitalis inotropy in mammalian heart: positive feed-back regulation by intracellular calcium? *J. Physiol.*, **329**, 589–614
22. Hayward, R., Hamer, J., Taggart, P. and Emanuel, R. (1983). Observations on the biphasic nature of digitalis electrophysiological actions in the human right atrium. *Cardiovasc. Res.*, **17**, 533–46
23. Rosen, M. R. (1985). Cellular electrophysiology of digitalis toxicity. *J. Am. Coll. Cardiol.*, **5**, 22A–34A
24. Smith, T. W., Antman, E. M., Friedman, P. L., Blatt, C. M. and Marsh, J. D. (1984). Digitalis glycosides: mechanisms and manifestations of toxicity. Part II. *Prog. Cardiovasc. Dis.*, **26**, 495–540
25. Di Gennaro, M., Vassale, M., Iacono, G., Pahor, M., Bernabei, R. and Carbonin, P. U. (1986). On the mechanisms by which hypoxia eliminates digitalis-induced tachyarrhythmias. *Eur. Heart J.*, **7**, 341–52
26. Goodman, D. J., Rossen, R. M., Cannom, D. S., Rider, A. K. and Harrison, D. C. (1975). Effect of digoxin on atrioventricular conduction. Studies in patients with and without cardiac autonomic innervation. *Circulation*, **151**, 251–6
27. Rosen, M. R., Wit, A. L. and Hoffman, B. F. (1975). Electrophysiology and pharmacology of cardiac arrhythmias. IV. Cardiac antiarrhythmic and toxic effects of digitalis. *Am. Heart. J.*, **89**, 391–9
28. Alboni, P., Shantha, N., Filippi, L., Pirani, R., Preziosis, S., Tomasi, A. M. and Masoni, A. (1984). Clinical effects of digoxin on sinus node and atrioventricular node function after pharmacologic autonomic blockade. *Am. Heart. J.*, **108**, 1255–61
29. Gomes, J. A. C., Damato, A. N., Bobb, G. A. and Lau, S. H. (1978). The effect of digitalis on refractoriness of the intact canine His–Purkinje system. *Circulation*, **58**, 284–94
30. Gould, L., Patel, C., Botzu, R., Judge, D. and Lee, J. (1986). Right bundle branch block: a rare manifestation of digitalis toxicity – case report. *Angiology*, **37**, 543–6
31. Spurrell, R. A. J., Harris, A. M. and Howard, M. R. (1971). Effect of digoxin on A–V conduction. *Br. Med. J.*, **3**, 563–4
32. Bissett, J. K., deSoyza, N. D. B., Kane, J. J., McConnell, J. R. and Doherty, J. E. (1978). Effect of digitalis on human ventricular refractoriness. *Cardiovasc. Res.*, **12**, 288–93
33. Edvardsson, N., Hirsch, I. and Olssen, S. B. (1984). Acute effects of lignocaine, procainamide, metoprolol, digoxin and atropine on human myocardial refractoriness. *Cardiovasc. Res.*, **18**, 463–70
34. Watanabe, A. M. (1985). Digitalis and the autonomic nervous system. *J. Am. Coll. Cardiol.*, **5**, 35A–42A

35. Sellers, T. D., Bashore, T. M. and Gallagher, J. J. (1977). Digitalis in the pre-excitation syndrome. *Circulation*, **56**, 260–7
36. Gillis, R. A. and Quest, J. A. (1979). The role of the nervous system in the cardiovascular effects of digitalis. *Pharmacol. Rev.*, **31**, 19–97
37. Longhurst, J. C. and Ross, J. Jr. (1985). Extracardiac and coronary vascular effects of digitalis. *J. Am. Coll. Cardiol.*, **5**, 99A–105A
38. Somberg, J. C. (1984). Localization of neurally mediated arrhythmogenic and coronary vasoconstrictor properties of digitalis. *Fed. Proc.*, **43**, 2963–5
39. Tanz, R. D. (1986). Possible contribution of digitalis-induced coronary constriction to toxicity. *Am. Heart. J.*, **111**, 812–17
40. DeMots, H., Rahimtoola, S. H., McAnulty, J. H. and Porter, G. A. (1978). Effects of ouabain on coronary and systemic vascular resistance and myocardial oxygen consumption in patients without heart failure. *Am. J. Cardiol.*, **41**, 88–93
41. Chamberlain, D. A. (1985). Digitalis: where are we now? *Br. Heart J.*, **54**, 227–33
42. Hoffman, B. F., Bigger, J. T. (1980). Digitalis and allied glycosides. In Gilman, A. G., Goodman, L. S. and Gilman, A. (eds.) *The Pharmacological Basis of Therapeutics*. 6th edn. pp. 729–60. (NY: Macmillan) 729–60
43. Meijler, F. L. (1986). Editorial: the pulse in atrial fibrillation. *Br. Heart. J.*, **56**, 1–3
44. Meijler, F. L. (1985). An 'account' of digitalis and atrial fibrillation. *J. Am. Coll. Cardiol.*, **5**, 60A–68A
45. Rawles, J. M. and Rowland, E. (1986). Is the pulse in atrial fibrillation irregularly irregular? *Br. Heart J.*, **56**, 4–11
46. Breasley, R. A., Smith, D. A. and McHaffie, D. J. (1985). Exercise heart rates at different serum digoxin concentrations in patients with atrial fibrillation. *Br. Med. J.*, **290**, 9–11
47. Panidis, I. P., Morganroth, J. and Baessler, C. (1983). Effectiveness and safety of oral verapamil to control exercise-induced tachycardia in patients with atrial fibrillation receiving digitalis. *Am. J. Cardiol.*, **52**, 1197–201
48. Marcus, F. I. (1985). Pharmacokinetic interactions between digoxin and other drugs. *J. Am. Coll. Cardiol.*, **5**, 82A–90A
49. Csicsko, J. F., Schatzlein, M. H. and King, R. D. (1981). Immediate postoperative digitalization in the prophylaxis of supraventricular arrhythmias following coronary artery bypass. *J. Thorac. Cardiovasc. Surg.*, **81**, 419–22
50. Saltissi, S., Crowther, A., Byrne, C., Clarke, S., Jenkins, B. S. and Webb Peploe, M. M. (1983). The effects of oral digoxin therapy in primary mitral leaflet prolapse. *Eur. Heart J.*, **4**, 828–37
51. Coumel, P., Escoubet, B. and Attuel, P. (1984). Beta-blocking therapy in atrial and ventricular tachyarrhythmias: experience with nadolol. *Am. Heart J.*, **108**, 1098–108
52. Weiner, P., Bassan, M. M., Jarchovsky, J., Iusim, S. and Plavnick, L. (1983). Clinical course of acute atrial fibrillation treated with rapid digitalization. *Am. Heart J.*, **105**, 223–7
53. Wiggins, J. W. Jr., Bowes, W., Hill, C., Clewell, W., Manco-Johnson, M., Manchester, D., Johnson, R., Appareti, K. and Wolfe, R. R. (1986). Echocardiographic diagnosis and intravenous digoxin management of fetal tacharrhythmias and congestive heart failure. *Am. J. Dis. Child.*, **140**, 202–4
54. Ward, D. E. (1987). Arrhythmias and electrophysiological studies in children. *Curr. Opin. Cardiol.*, **2**, 76–80
55. Birnbaum, S. E., McGahan, J. P., Janos, G. G. and Myers, M. (1985). Fetal tachycardia and intramyocardial tumors. *J. Am. Coll. Cardiol.*, **6**, 1358–61
56. Rey, E., Duperron, L., Gauthier, R., Lemay, M., Grignon, A. and Le Lorier, J. (1985). Transplacental treatment of tachycardia-induced fetal heart failure with verapamil and amiodarone: a case report. *Am. J. Obstet. Gynecol.*, **153**, 311–12
57. Coumel, P. (1985). Medical treatment of arrhythmias in children. How and when using old and new drugs. *G. Ital. Cardiol.*, **15**, 795–6
58. Hastreiter, A. R. and Van der Horst, R. L. (1983). Postmortem digoxin tissue concentration and oxygen content in infancy and childhood. *Am. J. Cardiol.*, **52**, 330–5

59. Garson, A. Jr. (1986). Dosing the new antiarrhythmic drugs in children: considerations in pediatric pharmacology. *Am. J. Cardiol.*, 57, 1405–7
60. Berman, W. Jr., Yabek, S. M., Dillon, T., Niland, C., Corlew, S. and Christensen, D. (1983). Effects of digoxin in infants with a congested circulatory state due to a ventricular septal defect. *N. Engl. J. Med.*, 308, 363–6
61. Alpert, B. S. and Barfield, J. A. (1985). Reappraisal of digitalis in infants with left-to-right shunts and heart failure. *J. Paediatr.*, 106, 66–8
62. Klein, G. T., Yee, R. and Sharma, A. D. (1984). Concealed conduction in accessory atrioventricular pathways: an important determinant of the expression of arrhythmias in patients with Wolff–Parkinson–White syndrome. *Circulation*, 70, 402–11
63. Wu, D., Wyndham, C., Amat-yLeon, F., Denes, P., Dhingra, R. C. and Rosen, K. M. (1975). The effects of ouabain on induction of atrioventricular nodal reentrant paroxysmal supraventricular tachycardia. *Circulation*, 52, 201–7
64. Gradman, A. H., Cunningham, M., Harbison, M. A., Berger, H. J. and Zaret, B. L. (1983). Effects of oral digoxin on ventricular ectopy and its relation to left ventricular function. *Am. J. Cardiol.*, 51, 765–82
65. Lown, B., Graboys, T. B., Podrid, P. J., Cohen, B. H., Stockman, M. B. and Gaughan, C. E. (1977). Effect of a digitalis drug on ventricular premature beats. *N. Engl. J. Med.*, 296, 301–6
66. Graboys, T. B., Lown, B., Podrid, P. J. and DeSilva, R. (1982). Long-term survival of patients with malignant ventricular arrhythmia treated with antiarrhythmic drugs. *Am. J. Cardiol.*, 50, 437–43
67. Morrison, J., Goromilas, J., Robbins, M., Oug, L., Eisenberg, S., Stechel, R., Zema, M., Reiser, P. and Scherr, L. (1980). Digitalis and myocardial infarction in man. *Circulation*, 62, 8–16
68. Lown, B., Klein, M. D., Barr, I., Hagemeijer, F., Kosowsky, B. D. and Garrison, H. (1972). Sensitivity to digitalis drugs in acute myocardial infarction. *Am. J. Cardiol.*, 30, 388–95
69. Marcus, F. I. (1980). Editorial: use of digitalis in acute myocardial infarction. *Circulation*, 62, 17–19
70. Moss, A. J., Davis, H. T., Conard, D. L., DeCamilla, J. J. and Odoroff, C. L. (1981). Digitalis-associated cardiac mortality after myocardial infarction. *Circulation*, 64, 1150–6
71. Moss, A. J., Davis, H. T., Odoroff, C. L. and Bigger, J. T. (1983). Digitalis-associated mortality in postinfarction patients. *Circulation*, 68. (Suppl. 3), III-368
72. Ryan, T. J., Bailey, K. R., McCabe, C. H., Luk, S., Fisher, L. D., Mock, M. B. and Killip, T. (1983). The effects of digitalis on survival in high-risk patients with coronary artery disease. *Circulation*, 67, 735–42
73. Madsen, E. B., Gilpin, E., Henning, H., Ahnve, S., LeWinter, M., Mazur, J., Shabetai, R., Collins, D. and Ross, J. Jr. (1984). Prognostic importance of digitalis after acute myocardial infarction. *J. Am. Coll. Cardiol.*, 3, 681–9
74. Bigger, J. T. Jr., Fleiss, J. L., Rolnitzky, L. M., Merab, J. P. and Ferrick, K. J. (1985). Effect of digitalis treatment on survival after acute myocardial infarction. *Am. J. Cardiol.*, 55, 623–30
75. Muller, J. E., Turi, Z. G., Stone, P. H., Rude, R. E., Raabe, D. S., Jaffe, A. S., Gold, H. K., Gustafson, W.K., Poole, E., Passamani, E., Smith, T. W., and Braunwald, E. (1986). Digoxin therapy and mortality after myocardial infarction. *N. Engl. J. Med.*, 314, 265–71
76. Yusuf, S., Wittes, J., Bailey, K. and Furberg, C. (1986). Digitalis – a new controversy regarding an old drug. *Circulation*, 73, 14–18
77. Haber, E. (1985). Antibodies and digitalis: the modern revolution in the use of an ancient drug. *J. Am. Col. Cardiol.*, 5, 111A–117A
78. Fisch, C. and Knoebel, S. B. (1985). Digitalis and cardiotoxicity. *J. Am. Coll. Cardiol.*, 5, 91A–98A
79. Whang, R., Oei, T. O. and Watanabe, A. (1985). Frequency of hypomagnesemia in hospitalized patients receiving digitalis. *Arch. Intern. Med.*, 145, 655–6

80. Bain, R. J. I. (1983). Accidental digitalis poisoning due to drinking herbal tea. *Br. Med. J.*, **290**, 1624
81. Lown, B. (1985). Cardioversion and the digitalized patient. *J. Am. Coll. Cardiol.*, **5**, 889–90
82. Wenger, T. L., Butler, V. P. Jr., Haber, E. and Smith, T. W. (1985). Treatment of 63 severely digitalis-toxic patients with digoxin-specific antibody fragments. *J. Am. Coll. Cardiol.*, **5**, 118A–123A
83. Mann, D. L., Maisel, A. S., Atwood, J. E., Engler, R. L. and LeWinter, M. M. (1985). Absence of cardioversion-induced ventricular arrhythmias in patients with therapeutic digoxin levels. *J. Am. Coll. Cardiol.*, **5**, 882–8
84. George, C. F. (1982). Interactions with digoxin: more problems. *Br. Med. J.*, **284**, 291–2
85. Cleland, J. G. F., Dargie, H. J., Pettigrew, A., Gillen, G. and Robertson, J. I. S. (1986). The effects of captopril on serum digoxin and urinary urea and digoxin clearances in patients with congestive heart failure. *Am. Heart J.*, **112**, 130–5

20
Implantable electrical devices for the treatment of tachyarrhythmias

D. B. O'KEEFFE

INTRODUCTION

The first occasion when it is likely that electricity was used to correct a cardiac arrhythmia was recorded in 1775, when Abilgaard[1] used a Leyden jar in an experiment on a chicken, and 'shocked it into lifelessness'. Application of a second shock revived the chicken which fled, bringing the experiment to a premature conclusion.

In investigating deaths due to electrocution, Prevost and Batelli[2] noted in 1899 that the electrical discharges which were capable of inducing ventricular fibrillation in dogs, were also able to terminate this arrhythmia.

It was in 1913 that Mines[3] in his seminal paper 'On dynamic equilibrium in the heart', pointed out the mechanism of reciprocating rhythm as a 'circulating excitation', and observed that

' ... The conditions (for circulating excitation) are easily upset by the occurrence of an extrasystole and they may be re-established by other extrasystoles. I venture to suggest that a circulating excitation of this type may be responsible for some cases of paroxysmal tachycardia as observed clinically.'

There followed several decades of intermittent experimentation before the first report[4], in 1947, of the use of electricity to reverse ventricular fibrillation in a human – the patient, a child who developed ventricular fibrillation during surgery, made a full recovery.

The work of Lown and others[5] in the early 1960s established the efficacy and safety of synchronized electrical cardioversion using a direct current shock applied externally to the chest. At the same time implantable pacemakers for the treatment of bradycardia were coming into widespread use, and in 1967 Durrer[6] and Coumel[7] independently reported on the use of programmed electrical stimulation of the heart in the study of tachycardias, and within a year the first report was published[8] documenting the use of a permanently implanted pacemaker

337

to terminate junctional tachycardias in a case of Wolff–Parkinson–White syndrome. The patient held a magnet over the pacemaker during tachycardia to give competitive asynchronous ventricular underdrive pacing which would regularly interrupt the arrhythmia, restoring sinus rhythm.

Amongst several subsequent reports of pacemaker termination of tachycardias by pacing, one[9] emphasized the ability of right ventricular pacing at slightly increased rates (88 and 86 bpm, respectively), to suppress the initiation of paroxysmal nodal and ventricular tachycardias, so acting in a prophylactic role.

From this initial work, and a perception that drug treatment for many tachycardias is beset by toxicity, lack of efficacy, compliance problems and arrhythmogenic effects, grew an appreciation that implantable electrical devices could offer a very satisfactory alternative form of treatment to at least some such patients. In the early stages the lack of purpose designed, readily adaptable implantable equipment imposed a severe limitation on what it was possible to achieve, and to some extent this remains true today. It became rapidly clear that careful individual assessment of the tachycardia in question, and a readiness to provide close and expert follow-up for such patients, are vital factors in achieving good results from this form of anti-arrythmic treatment.

The past decade has seen the rapid development of sophisticated implantable equipment, designed for the control of tachycardias. Pacemakers expressly aimed at the control of reciprocating tachycardias have become available and been assessed in clinical practice[10–12].

In 1980 Mirowski and his colleagues published their preliminary clinical experience[13] with a new device, the automatic implantable (cardioverter) defibrillator – usually now abbreviated to AICD – capable of automatically recognizing malignant ventricular tachyarrhythmias and responding with a direct current defibrillating shock, delivered directly to the myocardium using a combination of epicardial and endocardial electrodes. Subsequent experience[14] has suggested that the use of the AI(C)D in patients with refractory ventricular tachyarrhythmias may be associated with a substantial improvement in prognosis.

DEVICES DESIGNED TO SUPPRESS TACHYCARDIA

The rhythm of the heart tends to become unstable not only when unusually rapid rates are sustained for any length of time, but also with unusually slow rates. Either condition will predispose to the onset of malignant tachyarrhythmias and, for example, it has been long recognized that Stokes–Adams attacks in the setting of chronic complete atrioventricular block may be due to ventricular tachycardia as well as ventricular standstill (Figure 20.1). It is not surprising, therefore, that when permanent pacemaker treatment came into widespread use, reports began to appear confirming that pacing the heart at slightly more rapid rates than usual (80–110 bpm) had, in some patients, the

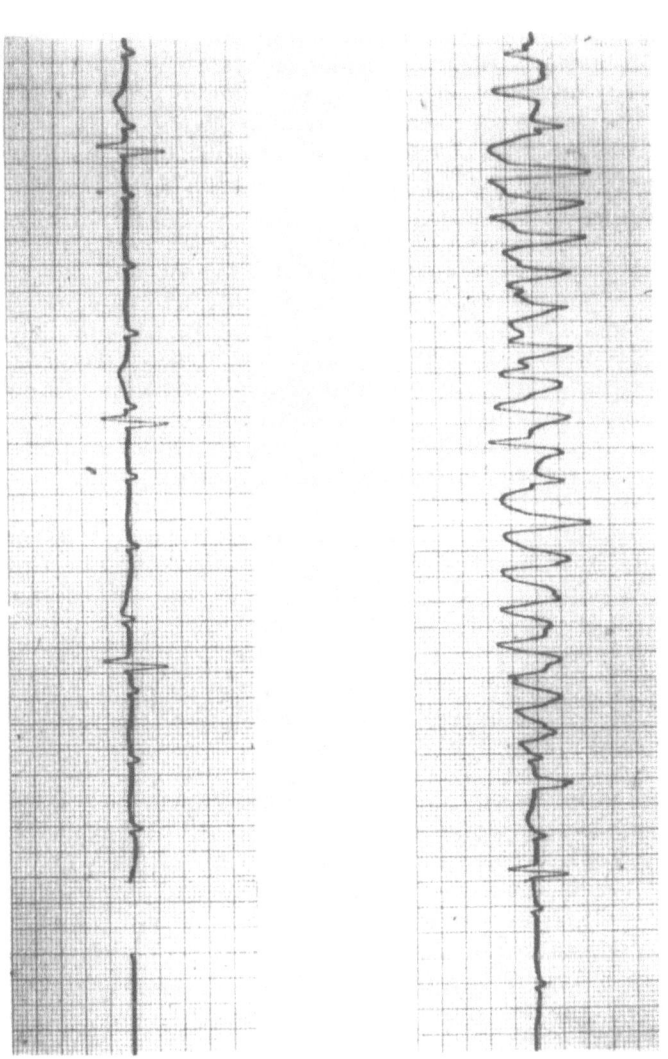

Figure 20.1 Complete atrioventricular block complicated by syncope due to paroxysms of the polymorphic ventricular tachycardia shown. Simple ventricular pacing (e.g. at 70 bpm) is usually sufficient, as in this case, to abolish the ventricular tachycardia.

effect of suppressing paroxysmal tachyarrhythmias[15-18]. This technique is known as overdrive suppression, and may be achieved by pacing in either the atrium or the ventricle.

Ventricular tachycardia

The classic indication for overdrive suppression, and the clinical situation in which the most predictable therapeutic effect may be anticipated, is *torsade de pointes* ventricular tachycardia – whether this is associated with the congenital long QT syndromes or other aetiologies[19]. In addition, overdrive suppression is undoubtedly effective in managing other forms of ventricular tachycardia, although its place in suppressing malignant arrhythmias in the setting of acute myocardial infarction has yet to be adequately defined.

In practice the response to overdrive suppression in a case of ventricular tachycardia may often be easily tested by inserting a temporary, transcutaneous pacing system and assessing the effect by ambulatory ECG monitoring. If paroxysms of ventricular tachycardia are sufficiently frequent then it will become clear within a few hours or days of testing whether implantation of a permanent system is worthwhile. Two points are of some importance in this context. First, both atrial and ventricular temporary electrodes should be inserted since an individual arrhythmia may respond to atrial, but not to ventricular overdrive pacing[20-25]. Atrial demand (AAI), ventricular demand (VVI) and ventricular inhibited atrioventricular (DVI) pacing at a variety of rates between 80 and 120 bpm should be tried for efficacy. Secondly, the effects of antiarrhythmic drugs may be additive with those of pacing[26], and the effect of the combination may prove successful where neither alone has a fully satisfactory suppressive effect. Pacing is sometimes useful in treating these cases, when drug dosage is limited by induced bradycardia[27,28] or arrhythmogenic effects, in that it may permit larger and possibly more effective doses of antiarrhythmic drugs to be employed, or to be employed without provoking drug-related tachyarrhythmias.

When ventricular tachycardia occurs only on widely separated occasions some difficulty will be encountered in assessing whether overdrive pacing is efficacious. Electrophysiological testing will only be helpful if a site in the heart can be found where single or double extrastimuli will reliably initiate the arrhythmia. If more complicated or prolonged sequences are required to start tachycardia the efficacy of overdrive pacing cannot be assessed in this way since the pacemaker is inevitably over-ridden by the initiation sequence. Difficulty is also encountered when single or double beat initiation is only intermittently effective.

In such cases some indication may be obtained from exercise testing as to whether a particular ventricular tachycardia is likely to respond well to overdrive pacing. If the rise in pulse rate with exertion tends to suppress ventricular arrhythmias (extrasystoles or more complex forms),

Table 20.1

Pacemaker (make/model)	Tachymode	Bradymode	Versatility	Availability	Implantability	Electrodes
Telectronics PASAR 4171	ES 1–7	SSI 60 ppm	scan	G	full	bipolar
Telectronics Optima MPT	dual demand	SSI prog.	dual demand	G	full	unipolar/ bipolar
Siemens-Elema 668	dual demand	SSI prog.	dual demand	G	full	unipolar/ bipolar
Siemens-Elema Tachylog	scan	SSI prog.	external prog.	R	full	bipolar
Siemens-Elema 704	short AV int.	DDD prog.	external prog.	G	full	unipolar
Medtronic Symbios 7007/7008	dual demand/ burst/ short AV int.	DDD prog.	external prog.	G	full	unipolar/ bipolar
Medtronic 5998 R/T	E	—	manual operation	G	partial	unipolar
Medtronic Spectrax 2331	E	SSI prog.	manual operation	G	partial	unipolar
Intermedics Intertach	ES	SSI prog.	external prog.	G	full	bipolar
CPI Ventak AICD	defib.	—	preset by maker	G	full	epicardial

ES: extrastimulus mode, G: general, E: externally determined, R = restricted; defib = defibrillator

it will be worth trying the effect of overdrive pacing, whereas if exertion provokes more frequent or more complex ventricular arrhythmias, overdrive pacing may prove disappointing.

In selecting an implantable device with which to treat a case of ventricular tachycardia responding to overdrive suppression, a wide variety of suitable equipment is freely available (Table 20.1). Only multiprogrammable pulse-generators with a wide range of rate, sensitivity and refractory period settings merit consideration. The optimal rate of overdrive may vary over time and need to be changed, the sensitivity setting in the ventricle will need to be carefully chosen to ensure accurate sensing of multiform complexes (so avoiding pacing during the vulnerable period of ectopic complexes) yet coarse enough to avoid T-wave sensing, since a short refractory period is desirable in order to ensure that early extrasystoles are also accurately sensed. Bipolar pacing systems are preferred in this context because:

(1) The chance of competitive pacing in interference mode is reduced.
(2) The risk of myopotential sensing and inappropriate pacer inhibition is reduced.

(3) In the case of atrial systems, bipolar electrodes can usually be relied upon to give accurate sensing of the lower amplitude signals without interference from far field ventricular signals or myopotentials.

When paroxysmal ventricular tachycardia is due to a re-entry mechanism, and the site of the circuit within the ventricle is accessible for a permanent electrode, then pre-excitation of the circuit by atrial triggered ventricular pacing, using a ventricular electrode placed as close as possible to the site of the origin of the tachycardia, may provide effective suppression of ventricular tachycardia by preventing initiation[29]. A variety of implantable bipolar DDD pacemakers (Intermedics Cosmos, Medtronic Symbios) are available and will perform this function satisfactorily. Important characteristics in this regard are programmable AV delay to a suitably low value ($\simeq 50$ ms) and $1:1$ AV tracking to high rate without increase in AV delay. Short AV delay 'pre-excitation' pacing has been more frequently used in the treatment of junctional tachycardias (see below).

Atrial tachycardias

Atrial tachycardias, including atrial flutter and fibrillation, tend to be more amenable to control or suppression by drug treatment, and less catastrophic in their clinical consequences than ventricular tachycardia. For these reasons the question of suppression by pacing arises less frequently. However, the combination of atrial tachycardias with sinus node disease (atrial tachy–brady syndrome) is a frequent indication for permanent pacemaker implantation, and when atrial demand pacing (AAI) is used in this clinical situation, the incidence of paroxysmal atrial tachyarrhythmia is substantially reduced[30]. Sometimes this effect may be due to the fact that pacing allows adequate drug therapy, whereas this may have been limited in the absence of pacemaker backup, by bradycardia[27]. The suppressive effect of AAI pacing is, however, evident in the absence of drug therapy. When ventricular demand (VVI) pacing is used for atrial tachy–brady syndrome it is possible that the same effect may be seen.

When selecting a pulse generator for the treatment of atrial tachy-brady syndrome there are, therefore, substantial advantages in choosing an atrial[31] demand system, provided that atrioventricular (AV) conduction disease can first be excluded[32]. This can easily be achieved by simple measurements (A–H and H–V times, atrioventricular Wenckebach point and response to carotid massage during atrial paced rhythm) using the permanent pacing electrode at the time of pacemaker implantation[33]. A multiprogrammable (rate, sensitivity and refractory period) bipolar generator is preferred, with parameters carefully programmed to ensure accurate sensing of the atrial electrogram, since competitive atrial pacing – in interference mode or due to undersensing – is likely to promote troublesome atrial tachyarrhythmias in these patients.

If AV conduction disease is present, an atrial inhibited ventricular inhibited atrioventricular (DDI) dual bipolar pacemaker (for example the Siemens-Pacesetter Advanced Function Pacemaker range) is the ideal choice. DVI (ventricular inhibited atrioventricular) pacemakers may suffer from the defect of atrial competitive pacing and are, therefore, not the ideal choice for this purpose. DDD ('physiological' atrioventricular) systems are to be avoided in this situation because they will transmit atrial tachyarrhythmias to the ventricle and are prone to support 'endless loop' tachycardias when retrograde VA conduction is intact, as is the case in up to 75% of these patients[34,35].

Junctional tachycardias

In 1967 Coumel and associates[36], noting that a delay in transmission of the cardiac impulse from atria to ventricles is usually a prerequisite for the initiation of reciprocating atrioventricular junctional tachycardia, described a method for preventing the onset of such junctional tachycardias by using continuous atrioventricular overdrive pacing with a short AV interval. In this way the delay in transmission between atria and ventricles is avoided, and the conditions for tachycardia cannot be met. Such pacemakers operating during both slow and fast heart rates, may also function as a termination system in the event of breakthrough tachycardia.

The effects of such AV pacing on the tachycardia initiation zone were examined by Akhtar[37] who confirmed Coumel's original suggestion that a collision of atrial and ventricular impulses within a re-entry circuit prevents the emergence of reciprocating tachycardia.

The advantages of a system which will reliably prevent the onset of paroxysmal tachycardia are obvious, and especially important if the tachycardia shows any tendency to become incessant[37] – as for example with the permanent junctional tachycardia of childhood. In these circumstances a perfectly working and effective termination antitachycardia pacemaker may yet leave the patient severely symptomatic because of repeated brief paroxysms of tachycardia in rapid succession. This problem is not uncommon in adult tachycardias although it often emerges only intermittently, and may, therefore, only become apparent after some length of follow-up with a permanent implanted tachycardia termination pacemaker.

Permanently implanted pacemakers of this short AV interval sequential type have been reported to give effective long term control[38], but are associated with some disadvantages. For instance the shortest atrial refractory periods available with regular (non-customized) units may be too long to sense and transmit the very early atrial extrasystoles which are frequently responsible for the initiation of paroxysmal junctional tachycardia[39]. On the other hand, a very short atrial refractory period carries with it the risks of rapid ventricular rate transmitted by the pacemaker during atrial tachycardia[40,41] – artificial pre-excitation may

343

Termination of SVT with a single premature stimulus

using the full 15 step scan

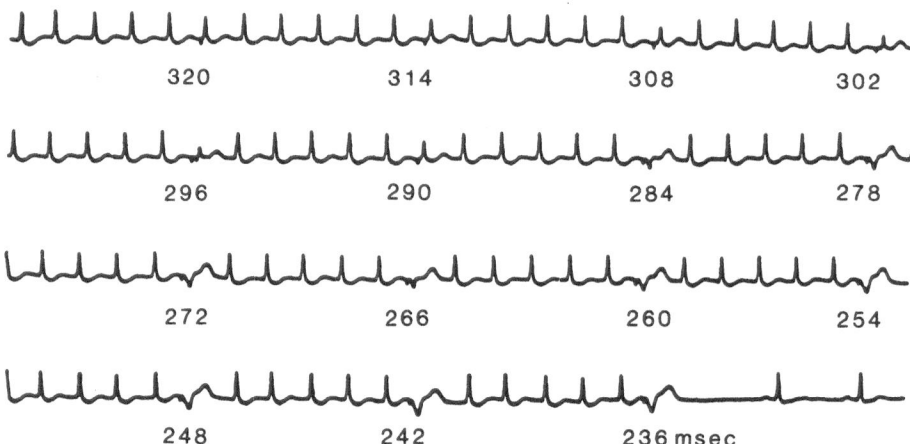

| 320 | 314 | 308 | 302 |

| 296 | 290 | 284 | 278 |

| 272 | 266 | 260 | 254 |

| 248 | 242 | 236 msec | |

Figure 20.2 Paroxysmal junctional tachycardia sensed by a PASAR 4152 anti-tachycardia pacemaker, which introduces increasingly premature extrastimuli, starting at 320 ms delay until the 15th attempt (236 ms delay) arrives within the termination zone and terminates tachycardia with restoration of sinus rhythm

carry the same risk during atrial fibrillation as Wolff–Parkinson–White syndrome – or early atrial extrasystoles may induce closely coupled ventricular stimulation, perhaps during the vulnerable period. Simultaneous or short-interval AV pacing may also have haemodynamic disadvantages because the atria contract against closed mitral and tricuspid valves[42].

Use of these techniques on a permanent basis, therefore, demands circumspection, very careful prior assessment and frequent skilled follow-up.

DEVICES DESIGNED TO SENSE AND TERMINATE TACHYCARDIAS

In 1967 it was shown that rapid atrial stimulation could be effective in terminating atrial flutter in humans[43], and in the same year Durrer and his colleagues[6] confirmed that critically timed atrial or ventricular extrasystoles would consistently terminate junctional tachycardia. These principles have been applied, with various embellishments, to the control of clinical tachycardias over the past 20 years. Initially a conventional demand pacemaker (atrial or ventricular) was employed, and at the onset of tachycardia an external magnet was applied to switch the pacemaker into fixed rate – competitive underdrive – mode[44]. This had the effect of introducing extrastimuli into the tachycardia cycle in the hope that, after a variable period of time, one would arrive within the termination window and interrupt tachycardia (Figure 20.2). Both

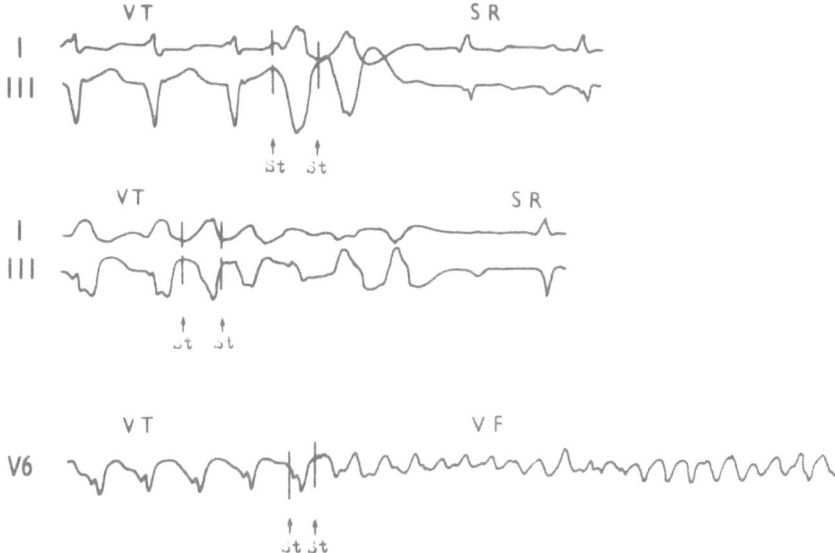

Figure 20.3 Termination of ventricular tachycardia by extrastimuli. Top – Double extrastimuli (St) give a clean termination with restoration of sinus rhythm. Middle – Double extrastimuli induce repetitive ventricular firing (3 beats) followed by restoration of sinus rhythm. Bottom – Double extrastimuli induce ventricular fibrillation

burst overdrive and extrastimulus modes in the atrium carry the risk of inducing atrial fibrillation.

While junctional tachycardias have proved most suitable for pacemaker treatment (Figure 20.2), the same principles have been applied to the treatment of ventricular tachycardia, in which they may sometimes be equally successful[45–48]. However, the catastrophic consequences of inducing malignant ventricular arrhythmias in the same way that atrial fibrillation can be induced, has so far inhibited the widespread use of these techniques for the control of ventricular arrhythmias (Figure 20.3). Latterly it has emerged that ventricular competitive pacing for junctional tachycardias, even in the absence of structural heart disease, may carry some risk, and is not now recommended out of hospital. Newer developments, for example antitachycardia pacemakers with defibrillation back-up, may in time change this situation.

Assessment for antitachycardia treatment

Pacemakers represent only one of a range of therapeutic options for the treatment of junctional tachycardia, and good results will only be obtained if careful attention is given to the choice of patients and initial assessment for antitachycardia pacing. Most cases of junctional tachycardia are amenable to atrial pacing, but not all are suitable for long term implantable antitachycardia pacing. Those who should be given consideration for this treatment include:

(1) Those with tachycardia causing substantial disability – it is not uncommon for junctional tachycardia to cause little disturbance, particularly in young people, and careful assessment of the possible risk of developing malignant arrhythmias followed by reassurance where appropriate, may be all that is necessary.

(2) Those cases where drug treatment is ineffectual or poorly tolerated – a substantial minority of patients affected by paroxysmal junctional tachycardia.

(3) Patients in whom junctional tachycardia coexists with sino-atrial disease or carotid hypersensitivity syndrome which may require permanent pacing in its own right. Here the choice of an anti-tachycardia unit with bradycardia standby mode can provide an elegant solution to both arrhythmias and may avoid the necessity of combining pacing with drug treatment.

(4) When attacks of junctional tachycardia occur only infrequently, but are associated with severe symptoms, some patients may prefer the solution provided by a permanent pacemaker to prolonged chronic drug therapy.

(5) Young women of child-bearing age represent a special case for consideration of antitachycardia pacing treatment since there are few antiarrhythmic drugs which are to be recommended for long term treatment in this patient group. The effects of these drugs on reproduction and the fetus are in most cases uncertain and in some cases known to be disastrous[49].

By the same token, a proportion of patients presenting with recurrent symptomatic junctional tachycardia will prove to be unsuitable for consideration of permanent pacemaker therapy, either because it may carry unacceptable risks or because other modalities of treatment will obtain superior results. Amongst these are:

(1) Patients with a rapidly conducting atrioventricular anomalous pathway who may be at risk if the pacemaker induces atrial fibrillation. The presence of any anomalous pathway, even if it appears to conduct slowly or only in the ventriculo–atrial (retrograde) direction, calls for a cautious approach, since behaviour of the refractory period in relation to sympathetic tone can be extremely variable.

(2) Cases in whom atrial fibrillation is easily induced and well sustained may be unsuitable for tachycardia conversion pacing, since this arrhythmia may be as troublesome or more troublesome than the junctional tachycardia which the pacemaker is designed to relieve.

(3) The easy or frequent occurrence of incessant tachycardia is a

relative contra-indication to tachycardia conversion pacing because in such patients (even with a perfectly functioning pacing system), the repetitive cycles of initiation and termination of tachycardia may leave patients little better off than they would be without a pacemaker.

(4) Previously relevant strictures regarding junctional tachycardias with a rate over 180 bpm or a very variable rate where there is substantial overlap between tachycardia rates and sinus rates, do not now constitute serious contra-indications to tachycardia conversion pacing. These considerations, however, will place constraints on the types of pacemaker which are suitable choices for the individual tachycardia being treated (see discussion below).

Some electrophysiological assessment is mandatory in each case of paroxysmal junctional tachycardia before embarking on permanent tachycardia conversion pacemaker treatment. However, the kind of exhaustive and exhausting study which is sometimes recommended in these cases produces largely academic information, and those pacing centres which cannot afford a large investment in operator time, training and sophisticated electrophysiological equipment need not be discouraged. This author favours a goal-directed approach designed with a minimum of invasive interference, to answer the questions of practical importance, which are:

(1) What is the diagnosis of the arrhythmia? Is more than one arrhythmia involved?

(2) Is antitachycardia pacing termination possible and reliable?

(3) Is antitachycardia pacing likely to be safe?

These questions can usually be satisfactorily answered by a scheme involving Holter monitoring, a resting EP study using two bipolar electrodes (in the right atrium and His positions) during which atrial fibrillation should be initiated, and attention directed to the ease and reliability of tachycardia termination and the sensing characteristics of the electrode during both tachycardia and sinus rhythm; the right atrial electrode should be left in place to test tachycardia termination and atrial fibrillation under controlled exercise conditions, and to allow a period of several days monitoring while a temporary external system is used to terminate spontaneous episodes of junctional tachycardia.

Choice of equipment

Since 1980 purpose designed, as opposed to customized, implantable antitachycardia pacemakers have become available, initially on an investigative basis and more recently on a general basis. Equipment design has been evolving rapidly and pacemakers which are non-programmable, lack a bradycardia back-up mode, can only be operated by an external unit or incorporate only single or double extrastimuli, can fairly be considered obsolete. Four units which meet these requirements are available in the United Kingdom at the time of writing and merit more detailed consideration (for full technical specifications the reader is referred to the manufacturer's literature – only the outstanding distinctions and limitations of each unit are discussed here):

Intermedics Cybertach 60

This is a purpose designed tachycardia conversion system designed automatically to identify tachycardia, on a high rate criterion alone, and to respond with an asynchronous rapid burst of pacing to give overdrive termination[50].

This unit features programmability of mode (so that it can be 'disarmed', to function in AAI mode only), tachycardia detection rate, burst rate and burst duration.

It lacks any facility for more sophisticated tachycardia recognition (e.g. using abrupt onset or rate stability criteria), the ability to deliver timed extrastimuli or to adapt to variations in tachycardia rate. Telemetry functions are of the most basic kind, and there is no diagnostic memory function.

The Cybertach 60 remains an economic option for a few particular clinical situations, for example paroxysmal atrial flutter, but has been largely rendered obsolete by the introduction of the Intermedics Intertach range of pacemakers which are considered in some detail below.

Intermedics Intertach

This unit incorporates a very wide range of programmable functions including the ability to use not only high rate but abrupt onset, rate stability and sustained high rate in a variety of combinations for accurate recognition of tachycardia. Accurately timed extrastimuli or sequences of extrastimuli in fixed or scanning mode are possible in response to tachycardia, and this response may be determined by the sensed rate in tachycardia. More than one termination algorithm may be programmed, so that the second acts as a back-up in the event of failure of the first. Alternatively, this system retains the option for external activation by patient or physician – which may, for example, allow for its use in cases of ventricular tachycardia.

A most useful feature of this system is the ability to perform non-invasive programmed stimulation (NIPS) using the programmer to communicate with and control timed stimulation by the implanted pulse generator. This allows repeated easy initiation of tachycardia during follow-up in order to test efficacy, to readjust programming to take account of variation in tachycardia properties, or to test the effects of changes in drug regimen.

There is a diagnostic memory function of some sophistication built into the pacemaker which provides a helpful objective guide to pacemaker function and efficacy during follow-up.

At the present time this pacing system represents the state of the art in tachycardia conversion pacing equipment, its major limitation being the lack of defibrillation back-up which restricts the safe application of Intertach to supraventricular arrhythmias.

Antitachycardia pacemakers have been used in conjunction with the implantable cardioverter–defibrillator (AICD) for malignant ventricular arrhythmias[51], but this application carries with it the risk of complex unwanted interaction between the two units and cannot be seen as the ideal solution to this problem.

Telectronics PASAR (programmable automatic scanning arrhythmia reversion)

This system has evolved through a series of increasingly flexible types to the presently available 4171 generator which uses a simple high rate criterion to identify tachycardia, responding with a timed sequence of up to seven extrastimuli in fixed, scanning or 'concertina' mode[52,53]. The initial coupling interval and the cycle length of the subsequent train of impulses is programmable, and the tachycardia recognition rate is variable within wide limits. There is bradycardia back-up at a rate of 60 bpm, and a limited memory function to allow the last successful termination sequence to be immediately reused on recognition of a new episode of tachycardia.

Major drawbacks with this system include the limited programmability of sensing and use of the crude rate criterion alone for tachycardia recognition. The success of an antitachycardia system, especially in the atrial position, depends heavily on the ability of the pacemaker to accurately sense tachycardia and to discriminate it from sinus rhythm[54]. Undersensing of the usually smaller atrial impulses during tachycardia will result in the failure of the pacer to terminate episodes of tachycardia, while sinus tachycardia (or far-field R-wave sensing) may result in inappropriate pacing which can actually initiate tachycardia, and this may exacerbate rather than relieve the clinical problem. A further notable omission from this system is a satisfactory method of tachycardia initiation for purposes of testing during follow-up. The use of scanning extrastimuli during sinus rhythm (only if faster than 65 bpm) is available, but is clumsy, time-consuming and frequently ineffectual.

Siemens-Elema Tachylog P43

This system is based on the the well proven circuitry of the Siemens 668 pacemaker, with the addition of sophisticated tachycardia sensing and termination options as well as a memory function[55]. It is designed primarily to operate in extrastimulus mode, and trains of up to 256 extrastimuli (the first 16 intervals independently programmable) can be introduced to terminate reciprocating tachycardias. Complex scanning modes are a feature of Tachylog – adaptive table scan, decremental and centrifugal geometric – aimed at seeking out a limited termination zone with the minimum of delay. The possibility of using the phenomenon of tachycardia reset to arrive rapidly at the termination zone gives an ingenious method of achieving this objective, but, because it automatically seeks out the vulnerable period of the paced chamber, may carry an increased risk of precipitating unwanted tachyarrhythmias.

Sensing of tachycardia can be programmed to depend not only on the crude high rate criterion but also on an abrupt change in rate. A deficiency in the Tachylog system appears to be a tendency for far-field ventricular signals to interfere with the accuracy of atrial sensing. Since antitachycardia pacemaker function depends critically on accurate sensing for satisfactory results, this must be seen as a serious problem – although it must be added that such mis-sensing depends also on lead characteristics and site of lead implantation, and other systems (notably PASAR) are also vulnerable on this point.

Tachylog has a memory facility for counting events (e.g. number of episodes of tachycardia detected) and builds up a priority list of successful termination patterns, so that these are then used in order of previous success when the next tachycardia is detected. This is designed to ensure the best chance of speedy termination of the episode.

The system also incorporates a triggered (SST) mode of pacing which provides a clever solution to the problem of non-invasive electrophysiology study for system testing during follow-up. In this mode the pacemaker will respond to external skin extrastimuli – delivered through skin electrodes by a programmed stimulator, for example – and allows for great flexibility in tachycardia study without the inconvenience of inserting intracardiac pacing wires. There is also an external magnet operated mode, which depends only on the high rate criterion being met, which permits antitachycardia operation only under direct supervision, or at the patient's discretion, if this is desired.

Tachylog suffers from an unreliable programmer/pacemaker communication link which can make programming sessions protracted and frustrating.

AUTOMATIC IMPLANTABLE CARDIOVERTER-DEFIBRILLATOR (AICD)

After a decade of development work, Mirowski and his colleages introduced this device into clinical trials in 1980[56]. AICD is a device designed to automatically sense and terminate malignant ventricular arrhythmias by the internal delivery of a 35 joule DC shock.

Indications

Patients so far considered for this form of treatment[57–60] have all survived at least one episode of life-threatening ventricular arrhythmia, unrelated to acute myocardial infarction, which has subsequently proved refractory to treatment with conventional antiarrhythmic drugs. The demonstrated ability of electrophysiological testing to predict those patients who are uncontrolled by drug therapy and remain at risk[61,62] should simplify this choice.

The majority of patients reported so far have had very severely impaired ventricular function[57], for the most part due to advanced coronary artery disease, although in 25% of them this was due to cardiomyopathy and in a few patients due to long QT syndrome.

The AICD requires a thoracotomy for implantation, but in one third to one half of reported patients this has been combined with other cardiovascular surgery, usually coronary bypass grafting or aneurysmectomy[57].

Patients perceive the internally delivered shocks as quite unpleasant, and in its present form the AICD stores enough energy for only between 100 and 150 shocks (including those required to test electrical integrity and efficacy of the unit), so that patients who are subject to very frequent episodes – once per week on average is a suggested maximum – are probably unsuitable for consideration for this treatment[58].

Equipment

This has evolved over the past 6 years through several stages and will certainly continue to do so[63]. In its present form (CPI Ventak AICD) the implanted unit has a volume of 200 cc and weighs 240 g. The capacitors charge to 700 V in approximately 8 s. The device can be activated and deactivated by the use of an external magnet, with alteration in mode confirmed by audio signals from a piezo-electric crystal located centrally within the implanted unit. Information regarding battery strength and number of shocks delivered can be telemetered to an external device called an Aidcheck-B.

The AICD is currently available with two different sensing modes. The AICD-BR uses bipolar ventricular endocardial sensing for rate measurement, and uses this alone to decide when to deliver a shock. Units with a choice of preset rate thresholds (120–200 bpm) are available from the manufacturer. The AICD-B version in addition uses the probability–density function – a mathematical derivation from the sensed waveform, which depends upon the proportion of time which the waveform spends off the baseline. This may help to prevent false sensing and shocking of supraventricular tachycardias, but may allow the unit to miss some narrower ventricular tachycardia[58,63,64].

The lead configuration used by the present versions of the AICD requires:

(1) A bipolar right ventricular endocardial lead or dual screw-in epicardial leads, for rate sensing. The AICD does not at this time feature a bradycardia support pacing mode, although this is shortly to become available.

351

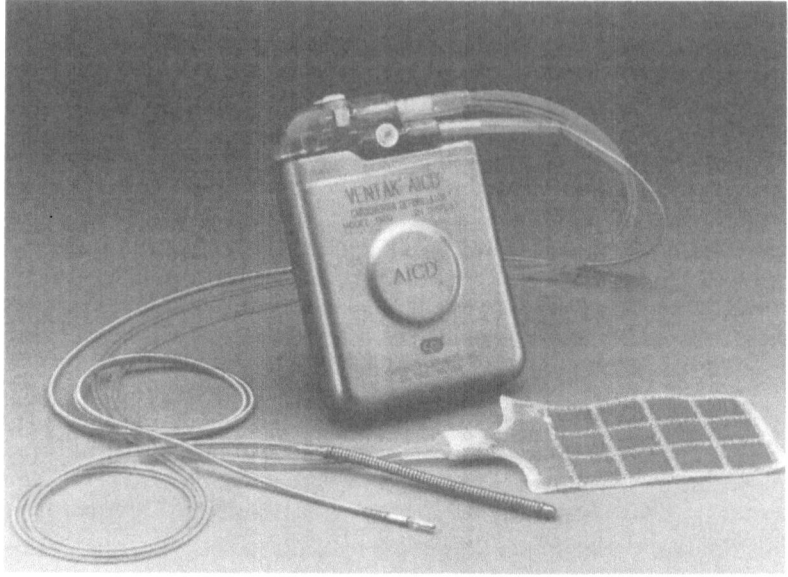

Figure 20.4 Implantable apparatus involved in the automatic implantable defibrillator (Ventak AICD). Shown are the pulse generator, the bipolar right ventricular sensing lead, the epicardial patch electrode and the superior vena cava coil electrode

(2) A pair of 10 or 20 sq cm titanium mesh flat 'patch' epicardial electrodes (which must be placed at thoracotomy) or alternatively one such patch electrode with a superior vena caval 10 sq cm titanium coil 'spring' electrode. These are used for the probability–density sensing function and for delivery of the defibrillating shocks (Figure 20.4).

The function of the implanted unit can be controlled by the application of an external magnet with confirmation of mode change (e.g. inactive to active mode) by audio signal from a centrally situated piezoelectric crystal within the implanted pulse generator[58]. However, interrogation of the unit for measurement of charge-time (an indicator of battery status) and number of shocks delivered to the patient, requires the use of Aidcheck-B interrogation device.

At implantation of the AICD a manually adjustable external cardioverter/defibrillator (ECD) is needed to check the defibrillation threshold of the spring/patch electrode arrangement, which clearly must be low enough for the AICD to reliably terminate VT/VF with margin of latitude to allow for changing chronic thresholds.

Clinical experience

Between 1980 and 1986 experience of AICD implants in over 700 patients was reported, with large individual series from Stanford, USA[58] and Baltimore, USA[57,65]. The Baltimore experience suggests an accuracy of identification of serious ventricular arrhythmias by the AICD of 98%, though other operators have reported less satisfactory results[66,67], particularly with the earlier AID models. In this group of severely ill patients the one year expected mortality was estimated at 48%, and actually found to be 22.9% after AICD implantation, with only 8.5% sudden deaths – presumed to be arrhythmic in origin[57]. These data are uncontrolled, but give reasonable grounds for supposing that the AICD is capable of extending the lifespan of some carefully chosen patients with an extremely poor outlook due to malignant ventricular arrhythmias.

As would be expected in relation to any major surgical procedure in such an ill group of patients, operative deaths (0.6%), perioperative deaths (5%) and complications have been reported[57,65]. These include infection of the pulse generator pocket, subcutaneous bleeding requiring transfusion, superior vena cava thrombosis, pneumothorax, haemopneumothorax, pericarditis, lead fracture, lead dislodgement, failure of sensing and unwanted discharges. The prevalence of supraventricular and ventricular arrhythmias in the immediate postoperative period has led to the suggestion that the AICD should be put into the inactive mode for several days after implant as a routine measure[58].

Problems that remain with AICD

This is a new and rapidly evolving treatment technique, and at the time of writing serious problems remain, many of which will be resolved within the next few years.

The large size of the AICD is a serious drawback, but with the advent of fully integrated circuitry and improved battery technology the size can be expected shortly to approach that of pacemakers of 10–12 years ago.

The expected lifespan of each AICD unit was designed to approach 3 years, but in practice has proved to be 18–24 months[66]. This again can be expected to improve before long.

The present lead configuration is far from ideal, and in particular the requirements for thoracotomy in these often very ill patients is less than ideal, as is the necessity for epicardial lead placement[68], giving all the problems with thresholds, wire fractures and pericarditis which will be only too tediously familiar to those involved in the early phases of cardiac pacing. A fully transvenous lead configuration will undoubtedly be a prior condition for the maturation of this extremely promising method of arrhythmia treatment.

Allied to this problem is that of mis-sensing, which has been improved in the current generation of AICD and will undoubtedly improve further

353

with the increasing programmability of these units[57,58]. With the present equipment, patients are still liable to be subjected to unwanted and unpleasant discharges, due mostly to misinterpretation of atrial fibrillation[66].

A bradycardia support pacing mode will soon be available in the AICD, and the fact that 15% of AICD patients have also received permanent pacemaker implantation attests[57] to the need for this facility to be routinely incorporated. The present arrangement of implanting two units can lead to mutual interference and is clearly suboptimal. It is anticipated that future generations of AICD will incorporate burst overdrive and extrastimulus tachycardia termination options and perhaps a transvenous low energy cardioversion facility[69].

A final, and not inconsiderable, drawback with the AICD is the very large expense involved, currently approximately £15 000 sterling for equipment for a first implantation. On top of this there is of course a large investment in operator time and expertise in the process of clinical work-up and follow-up.

These factors may be expected to improve more or less quickly, but will ensure for the present that AICD treatment is confined to small numbers of carefully selected patients in academic institutions which are generously endowed with personnel and funds for such work.

References

1. Abilgaard, C. P. (1775). Tentamina electrica in animalibus instituta. *Societatis Medicae Havniensis Collectenea*, **2**, 157
2. Prevost, J. L. and Batelli, F. (1899). La Mort par la courants electriques – Courants alternatifs a haute tension. *J. Physiol. Path. Gen.*, **1**, 427
3. Mines, G. R. (1913). On dynamic equilibrium in the heart. *J. Physiol.*, **46**, 23
4. Beck, C. S., Pritchard, W. S. and Fell, H. S. (1947). Ventricular fibrillation of long duration abolished by electric shock. *J. Am. Med. Assoc.*, **135**, 985
5. Lown, B., Amarasingham, R. and Neuman, J. (1962). New method for terminating cardiac arrhythmias. Use of synchronised capacitor discharge. *J. Am. Med. Assoc.*, **182**, 548
6. Durrer, D., Schoo, L., Schuilenburg, R. M. and Wellens, H. J. J. (1967). The role of premature beats in the initiation and termination of supraventricular tachycardia in the Wolff–Parkinson–White syndrome. *Circulation*, **36**, 644
7. Coumel, P., Cabrol, C., Fabiato, A., Gourgon, R. and Slama, R. (1967). Tachycardia permanente par rhythme reciproque. *Arch. Mal. Coeur*, **60**, 1830
8. Ryan, G. F., Easley, R. M., Zaroff, L. I. and Goldstein, S. (1968). Paradoxical use of a demand pacemaker in treatment of supraventricular tachycardia due to the Wolff–Parkinson–White syndrome. *Circulation*, **38**, 1037–43
9. Moss, A. J. and Rivers, R. J. (1974). Termination and inhibition of recurrent tachycardias by implanted pervenous pacemakers. *Circulation*, **50**, 942–7
10. Spurrell, R. A. J., Nathan, A. W., Bexton, R. S., Hellestrand, K. J., Nappholz, T. and Camm, A. J. (1982). Implantable automatic scanning pacemaker for termination of supraventricular tachycardia. *Am. J. Cardiol.*, **49**, 753–60
11. Sowton, E. (1984). Clinical results with the tachylog antitachycardia pacemaker. *Pacing. Clin. Electrophysiol.*, **7**, 1313–17
12. Griffin, J. C. and Sweeney, M. (1984). The management of paroxysmal tachycardias using the Cybertach 60. *Pacing Clin. Electrophysiol.*, **7**, 1291–5
13. Mirowski, M., Reid, P. R. and Mower, M. M. (1980). Termination of malignant

ventricular arrhythmias with an implanted automatic defibrillator in human beings. *N. Engl. J. Med.*, **303**, 322–4

14. Mirowski, M., Reid, P. R. and Mower, M. M. (1984). Clinical performance of the implantable cardioverter–defibrillator. *Pacing Clin. Electrophysiol.*, **7**, 1345–50

15. Zoll, P. M., Linenthal, A. J. and Zarsky, L. R. N. (1960). Ventricular fibrillation. Treatment and prevention by external electric currents. *N. Engl. J. Med.*, **262**, 105

16. Sowton, E. (1964). The use of artificial pacemaking in cardiac resuscitation. *Proc. R. Soc. Med.*, **57**, 368

17. Klassen, G. A., Broadhurst, C., Peretz, D. I. and Johnson, A. L. (1963). Cardiac resuscitation in 126 medical patients using external cardiac massage. *Lancet*, **1**, 1290

18. Sowton, E., Leatham, A. and Carson, P. (1964). The suppression of arrhythmias by artificial pacemaking. *Lancet*, **2**, 1098

19. Keren, A., Tzivoni, D., Gohlman, J., Corcos, P., Benhorin, J. and Stern, S. (1981). Ventricular pacing in atypical ventricular tachycardia. *J. Electrocardiol.*, **14**, 201

20. Zipes, D. P., Wallace, A. G., Sealy, W. and Floyd, W. L. (1969). Artificial atrial and ventricular pacing in the treatment of arrhythmias. *Ann. Intern. Med.*, **70**, 885

21. Kastor, J. A., DeSanctis, R. W., Harthorne, J. W. and Schwartz, G. H. (1967). Transvenous atrial pacing in the treatment of refractory ventricular irritability. *Ann. Intern. Med.*, **66**, 939

22. Moss, A. J., Rivers, R. J., Griffiths, L. S. C., Carmel, J. A. and Millard, E. B. (1968). Transvenous left atrial pacing for the control of recurrent ventricular fibrillation. *N. Engl. J. Med.*, **278**, 928

23. Zipes, D. P., Festoff, B. and Schaal, S. F. (1968). Treatment of ventricular arrhythmia by permanent atrial pacemaker and cardiac sympathectomy. *Ann. Intern. Med.*, **68**, 591

24. DeFrancis, N. A. and Giordano, R. P. (1968). Permanent epicardial atrial pacing in the treatment of refractory ventricular tachycardia. *Am. J. Cardiol.*, **22**, 742

25. Lichstein, E., Chadda, K. and Fenig, S. (1972). Atrial pacing in the treatment of refractory ventricular tachycardia associated with hypokalaemia. *Am. J. Cardiol.*, **30**, 550

26. Camm, A. J., Ward, D. E., Washington, H. G. and Spurell, R. A. J. (1979). Intravenous disopyramide phosphate and ventricular overdrive pacing in the treatment of paroxysmal ventricular tachycardia. *Pacing Clin. Electrophysiol.*, **2**, 395

27. Shaw, D. B. and Whistance, A. W. T. (1986). Clever pacemakers. *Cardiovasc. Med.*, **12**, 843–52

28. Frye, R. L., Collins, J. J. and DeSanctis, R. W. (1984). Guidelines for permanent pacemaker implantation. *Circulation*, **70**, 331A–339A

29. O'Keefe, D. B., Wainwright, R. J. and Curry, P. V. L. (1981). Pacemaker treatment for ventricular tachycardia. *Pacing Clin. Electrophysiol.*, **4**, 63

30. Rosenqvist, M., Brandt, J. and Schuller, H. (1986). Atrial versus ventricular pacing in sinus node disease: a treatment comparison study. *Am. Heart J.*, **111**, 292–7

31. Sutton, R. and Citron, P. (1979). Electrophysiological and haemodynamic basis of application of new pacemaker technology in sick sinus syndrome and atrioventricular block. *Br. Heart J.*, **41**, 600

32. Narula, O. S. (1971). Atrioventricular conduction defects in patients with sinus bradycardia. *Circulation*, **44**, 1096

33. O'Keeffe, D. B. and Geddes, J. S. (1983). Atrial pacing: Intracardiac conduction assessed by His bundle electrograms acquired from the permanent atrial electrode at implantation. *Pacing Clin. Electrophysiol.*, **6**, 949–52

34. Curzi, C. F., Massacci, C. and Viola, C. (1985). Actuarial survival curves and causes of death in patients treated with permanent VVI pacing. In Gomez, F. P. (ed.) *Cardiac Pacing.* (Madrid: Grouz)

35. Westveer, D. C., Stewart, J. R., Goodfleish, R., Gordon, S. and Timmis, G. C. (1984). Prevalence and significance of ventriculoatrial conduction. *Pacing Clin. Electrophysiol.*, **7**, 784–9

36. Coumel, C., Cabrol, C., Fabiota, A., Gourgon, R. and Slama, R. (1967). Tachycardia permanente par rhythme reciproque. *Arch. Mal. Coeur*, **60**, 1830

37. Akhtar, M., Gilbert, C. J., Al-Nouri, M. and Schmidt, D. (1979). Electrophysiological mechanisms for modification and abolition of atrioventricular junctional tachycardia with simultaneous and sequential atrial and ventricular pacing. *Circulation*, 60, 1443

38. Levy, S., Berkovits, B., Mandel, W., Broustet, J-P., Obel, I. W. P. and Bricaud, H. (1980). Refractory supraventricular tachycardia: Successful therapy with double-demand sequential pacemaker. *Am. J. Cardiol.*, 45, 457

39. Suppression and prevention of tachycardia by pacemakers. In Camm, A. J. and Ward, D. E. (eds.) *Pacing for Tachycardia Control*, pp. 43–57. (Frome, London: Butler and Tanner)

40. Spurrell, R. A. J. and Sowton, E. (1976). Pacing techniques in the management of supraventricular tachycardia. Part 2. *J. Electrocardiol.*, 9, 89

41. Sung, R. J., Styperek, J. L. and Castellanos, A. (1979). Complete abolition of the re-entrant supraventricular tachycardia zone using a new modality of cardiac pacing with simultaneous atrioventricular stimulation. *Am. J. Cardiol.*, 45, 72

42. Ogawa, S., Dreifus, L. S., Shenoy, P. N., Brockman, S. K. and Berkovits, B. V. (1978). Haemodynamic consequences of atrioventricular and ventriculoatrial pacing. *Pacing Clin. Electrophysiol.*, 1, 8

43. Haft, J. I., Kosowsky, B. D., Lau, S. H., Stein, E. and Damato, A. N. (1967). Termination of atrial flutter by rapid electrical pacing of the atrium. *Am. J. Cardiol.*, 20, 239

44. Ryan, G., Easly, R. M., Zaroff, L. I. and Goldstein, S. (1968). Paradoxical use of a demand pacemaker in treatment of supraventricular tachycardia due to the Wolff–Parkinson–White syndrome. *Circulation*, 38, 1037

45. Fisher, J. D., Kim, S. G., Matos, J. A. and Waspe, L. E. (1984). Pacing for ventricular tachycardia. *Pacing Clin. Electrophysiol.*, 7, 1278–90

46. Fisher, J. D., Mehra, R. and Furman, S. (1978). Termination of ventricular tachycardia with bursts of rapid ventricular pacing. *Am. J. Cardiol.*, 41, 94–102

47. Fisher, J. D., Kim, S. G., Furman, S. and Matos, J. A. (1982). Role of implantable pacemakers in control of recurrent ventricular tachycardia. *Am. J. Cardiol.*, 49, 194–206

48. Harzler, G. O. and Maloney, J. D. (1977). Programmed ventricular stimulation in management of recurrent ventricular tachycardia. *Mayo Clin. Proc.*, 52, 731–41

49. Leonard, R. F., Braun, T. E. and Levy, A. M. (1978). Initiation of uterine contractions by disopyramide during pregnancy. *N. Engl. J. Med.*, 299, 84–5

50. Griffin, J. C. and Sweeney, M. (1984). The management of paroxysmal tachycardias using the Cybertach-60. *Pacing Clin. Electrophysiol.*, 7, 1291–5

51. Luderitz, B., Gerckens, U. and Manz, M. (1986). AICD and antitachycardia pacemaker: combined use in ventricular tachyarrhythmias. *Clin. Prog. Electrophysiol. and Pacing.*, 4, (Suppl.), 29

52. Nathan, A., Hellestrand, K., Bexton, R., Nappholz, T., Spurrell, R. A. J. and Camm, A. J. (1982). *Pacing Clin. Electrophysiol.*, 4, 582

53. Spurrell, R. A. J., Nathan, A. W. and Camm, A. J. (1984). Clinical experience with implantable scanning tachycardia reversion pacemakers. *Pacing Clin. Electrophysiol.*, 7, 1296–300

54. Pless, B. D. and Sweeney, M. B. (1984). Discrimination of supraventricular tachycardia from sinus tachycardia of overlapping cycle length. *Pacing Clin. Electrophysiol.*, 7, 1318–24

55. Sowton, E. (1984). Clinical results with the tachylog antitachycardia pacemaker. *Pacing. Clin. Electrophysiol.*, 7, 1313–17

56. Mirowski, M., Reid, P. R., Mower, M. M. *et al.* (1980). Termination of malignant ventricular arrhythmias with an implanted automatic defibrillator in human beings. *N. Engl. J. Med.*, 303, 322

57. Mirowski, M., Reid, P. R., Mower, M. M., Watkins, L. and Platia, E. W. (1984). Clinical performance of the implantable cardioverter–defibrillator. *Pacing Clin. Electrophysiol.*, 7, 1345–50

58. Winkle, R. A., Stinson, E. B., Echt, D. S., Mead, R. H. and Schmidt, P. (1984).

Practical aspects of automatic cardioverter/defibrillator implantation. *Am. Heart J.*, **108**, 1335–46

59. Marchlinski, F. E., Flores, B. T. and Buxton, A. E. (1986). The automatic implantable cardioverter-defibrillator: Efficacy, complications, and device failures. *Ann. Intern. Med.*, **104**, 481–8

60. Echt, D. S., Armstrong, K., Schmidt, P., Oyer, P., Stinson, E. B. and Winkle, R. A. (1985). Clinical experience, complications, and survival in 70 patients with the automatic implantable cardioverter/defibrillator. *Circulation*, **71**, 289–96

61. Horowitz, L. N., Josephson, M. E. and Farshidi, A. (1978). Recurrent sustained ventricular tachycardia. 3. Role of electrophysiology study in selection of antiarrhythmic regimens. *Circulation*, **58**, 986

62. Mason, J. W. and Winkle, R. A. (1980). Accuracy of ventricular tachycardia-induction study for predicting long term efficacy and inefficacy of antiarrhythmic drugs. *N. Engl. J. Med.*, **303**, 1073

63. Mower, M. M., Reid, P. R. and Watkins, L. (1984). AICD structural characteristics. *Pacing Clin. Electrophysiol.*, **7**, 1331–7

64. Winkle, R. A., Bach, S. M. and Echt, D. S. (1983). The AICD local ventricular bipolar sensing to detect ventricular tachycardia and fibrillation. *Am. J. Cardiol.*, **52**, 256

65. Veltri, E. P., Mower, M. M., Guarnieri, T. and Mirowski, M. (1986). Clinical efficacy of the automatic implantable defibrillator: 6 year cumulative experience. *Circulation*, (Suppl.) Part II, **74**, II–109

66. Gabry, M. D., Brodman, R., Johnston, D., Frame, R., Fisher, J. D. and Furman, S. (1986). AICD longevity, shock delivery, patient survival. *Cardiac Pacing Electrophysiol.*, **4**, 29

67. Jordans, L., Waleffe, A., Derom, F., Fourny, J., Clement, D. L. and Kulbertus, H. (1986). Clinical performance of the AICD. The Belgian experience. *Cardiac Pacing Electrophysiol.*, **4**, 30

68. Watkins, L., Mirowski, M. and Mower, M. M. (1982). Implantations of the Automatic Defibrillator: The subxiphoid approach. *Ann. Thorac. Surg.*, **34**, 515–20

69. Zipes, D. P., Heger, J. J. and Miles, M. W. (1984). Early experience with an implantable cardioverter. *N. Engl. J. Med.*, **311**, 485–90

21
The high energy catheter ablation technique in the management of tachyarrhythmias

P. HOLT and E. BOYD

INTRODUCTION

Until recently the therapeutic choices open to patients with drug resistant paroxysmal tachyarrhythmias were pacemakers, which are inappropriate in some cases[1,2] or surgery with its associated morbidity and mortality[3,4]. The development of the high energy, direct current endocardial ablation technique marked the beginning of a new era in the management of drug resistant tachyarrhythmias.

The first endocardial ablation of His bundle conduction occurred inadvertently during an electrophysiology study of a patient with ventricular tachycardia[5]. External countershock was required and subsequently the patient had complete atrioventricular block, the shock having travelled via the His bundle catheter electrode.

Following this case report, animal studies by Gonzalez et al. showed that high energy direct current impulses from a standard defibrillator, via a catheter electrode to the His bundle, could produce permanent complete heart block with localized myocardial damage[6,7]. The technique was then applied clinically, and successful ablation of His bundle conduction in patients with paroxysmal supraventricular tachycardia was reported by Gallagher[8] and Scheinman[9].

Its potential in the management of patients with Wolff–Parkinson–White syndrome, and paroxysmal ventricular tachycardia was soon recognized. High energy impulses were delivered via catheter electrodes positioned in the coronary sinus, or right atrium in the former group, and the ventricles in the latter[10-14]. These developments in the endocardial ablation technique produced complications. Shocks delivered to the coronary sinus have produced coronary sinus rupture and thrombosis[10] and also circumflex artery lesions[15], while high energy impulses to the ventricles have resulted in arrhythmias, ventricular rupture, impaired ventricular function and sudden death[16-18].

Efforts to improve the safety and efficiency of this technique have

359

been directed at both the catheter electrodes[19,20], and energy delivery system[21,22]. In order for these efforts to be successful the biophysical effects produced by the delivery of high energy impulses via catheter electrodes must be understood, and the physical phenomenon responsible for the therapeutic effect identified.

This chapter is divided into three parts. The first describes these biophysical effects, the second presents the current clinical experience with the high energy ablation technique, and the third part discusses potential future developments.

BIOPHYSICAL EFFECTS

Physical effects

The high energy ablation (or fulguration) technique can be reproduced simply in the laboratory by immersing the back plate from a defibrillator, plus the distal end of a bipolar USCI catheter electrode, in a tank of normal saline. The distal pole of the electrode is connected to the cathodal output, and back plate to the anodal output of a standard defibrillator. If a high energy impulse is then delivered several phenomena will be noticed; first a flash of light around the catheter electrode, followed by gas bubbles in the surrounding fluid. These effects are accompanied by a loud report, and all occur extremely rapidly.

A system has recently been described which enables these effects to be investigated in more detail[23].

A plastic tank with side viewing-port was partially filled with Ringer's solution. The visual effects produced during energy delivery were initially recorded using 35 mm time exposures and videotape. Subsequently high speed cine film at 4000 frames/second was used. The voltage between the catheter electrode and back paddle, plus the current through the system, were measured and recorded on magnetic tape. During this study the pressure wave produced was measured by a piezoelectric crystal mounted on a back plate for mechanical support. Using this system the effects of low and high energies via different catheter electrodes can be evaluated.

The use of hearts from freshly killed sheep suspended in the tank of oxygenated Ringer's solution provided an even more graphic demonstration of the physical effects occurring during the ablation technique. Figure 21.1 shows single frames from a high speed cine film recorded when 50 J was delivered via the distal pole of a 6F USCI electrode positioned in the coronary sinus of a freshly killed sheep's heart. The time interval from impulse delivery is indicated under each frame. Following delivery of the 50 J shock a fireball is produced around the electrode tip. This can be seen extending laterally down the lumen of the coronary sinus. The initiation of this fireball resembles an explosion and is accompanied by a large positive pressure wave[23]. The effects of this positive pressure wave can be clearly seen on the free wall

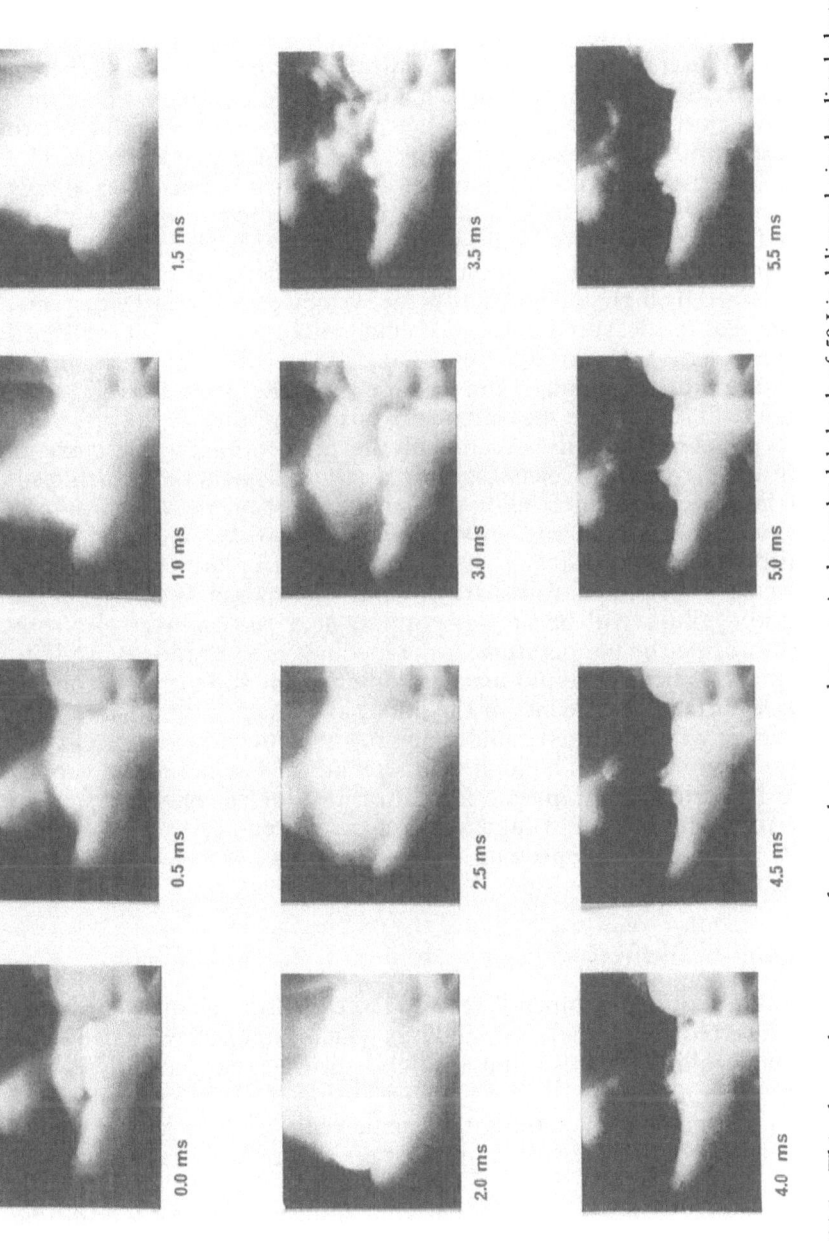

Figure 21.1 This shows the sequence of events that occur when a unipolar cathodal shock of 50 J is delivered via the distal electrode of a bipolar 6F USCI catheter electrode. The film was recorded at 4000 frames/second and the time postenergy delivery is indicated under each frame

of the coronary sinus, which expands. Following the initial 'explosive' energy delivery the flash of light condenses into a definite ball which further contracts into vapour and gas bubbles. This is accompanied by a negative phase in the pressure wave form, the effects of which can be seen in the indrawing of the free wall of the coronary sinus. If high energies are delivered in the same manner to the coronary sinus, then the initial positive pressure wave can produce distension sufficient to provoke rupture of the coronary sinus. This is illustrated in Figure 21.2 where 200 J was delivered. Figure 21.2a recorded 3.5 ms after energy delivery shows the fireball/vapour bubble escaping into the tank of saline. The hole produced is illustrated in Figure 21.2b.

Delivery of high energy impulses via a catheter electrode is also accompanied by high voltages across the system, and also large currents. The changes in measured current, voltage and pressure with increased energy are demonstrated in Figure 21.3. Other workers have attempted to measure pressure changes and found even higher values[24].

Reliable and accurate measurements of temperature at the electrode tip are difficult primarily because of the high voltages and currents present during the brief electrical impulse. Experiments in which electrode tips have been shielded by polytetrafluoroethylene (PTFE) tubing have resulted in fusion and erosion of the electrodes, indicating temperatures in excess of 1700 °C, the melting point of platinum. It is likely that even greater temperatures are present. The energy dissipated in the surrounding fluid will be at a maximum near the catheter electrode surface causing the temperature of the medium next to the electrode to rise rapidly. When the liquid reaches boiling point vapour forms on the electrode surface. As the last of the liquid in contact with the electrode vaporizes it will be heated rapidly due to the concentration of current in the remaining fluid. The high field strength in the last of the vapour film to be formed may initiate ionization producing plasma tracks in the surrounding vapour volume. Therefore, temperatures greater than 1700 °C are likely to be present since plasma temperatures are seldom less than 5000 °C.

Haematological effects

The presence of high temperatures and large pressure changes are likely to produce red cell damage. A study in which impulses were delivered to a small volume of fresh human blood showed that haemolysis and gas production occurred[25]. Recent work using fresh heparinized pigs' blood has attempted to quantify the haematological damage that occurs during delivery of high energy impulses[26]. Using a plastic tank and a gas collecting apparatus, cathodal and anodal shocks were delivered via the distal pole of a 6F USCI catheter electrode immersed in blood. Multiple shocks at energies of 10, 25, 50, 100, 200 and (in the case of cathodal impulses only) 400 J were delivered. The latter energy of 400 J could not be delivered with the electrode connected anodally since the gas col-

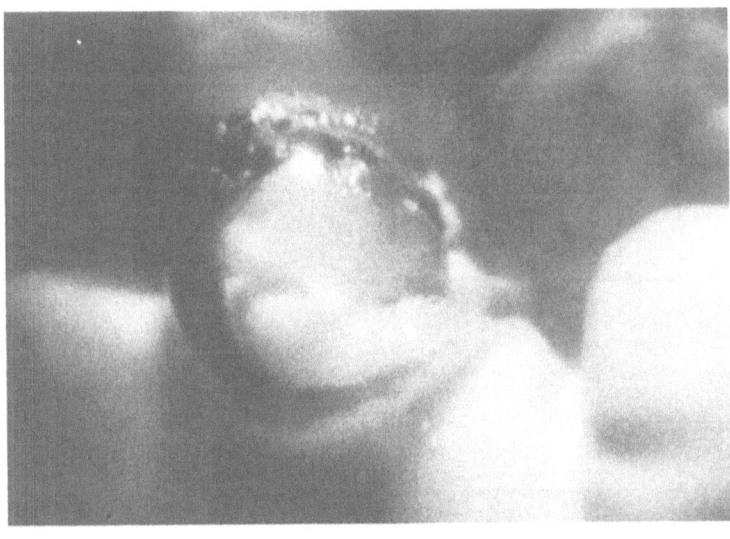

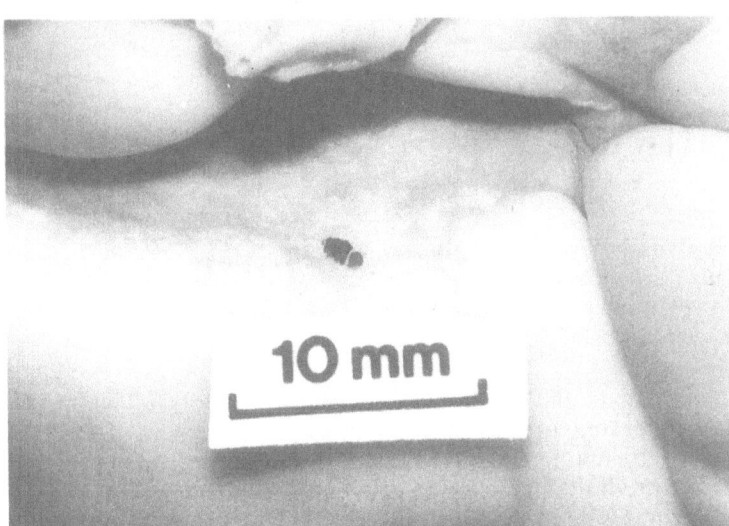

Figure 21.2(a)   This illustrates the effect of 200 J to the coronary sinus of a sheep's heart 3.5 ms after energy delivery. The gas bubble can be seen escaping into the surrounding saline. (b) The hole produced by a shock of 200 J

lecting apparatus could not withstand the higher shock waves produced. Haemolysis and gas production was measured for each energy value used.

The volume of gas liberated per single impulse at each energy value differed depending upon the polarity of the electrode. Using cathodal impulses the mean gas production over the energy range 10–50 J was

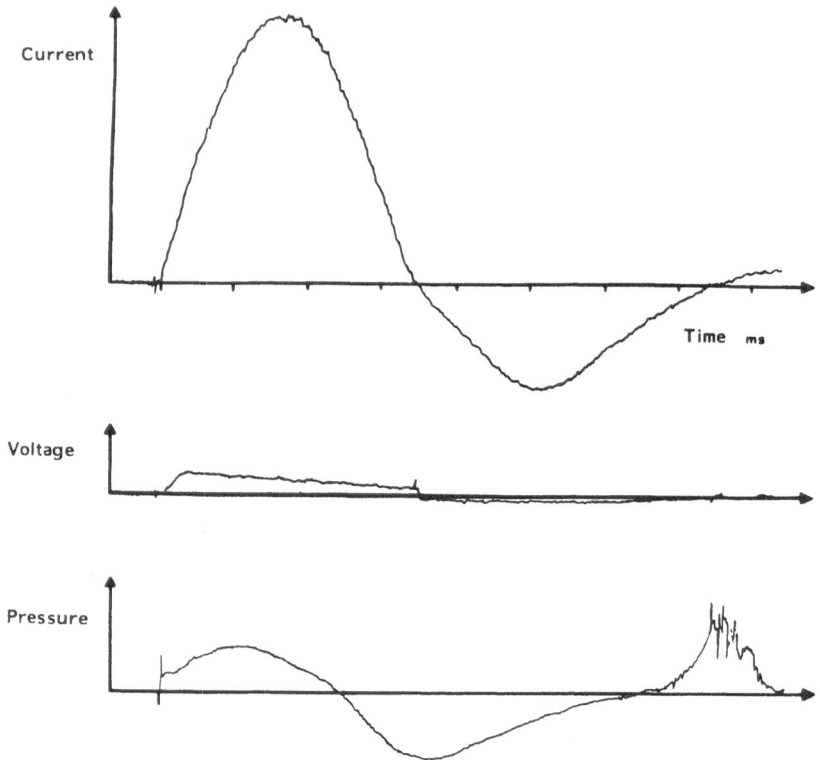

Figure 21.3 The current voltage and pressure effects produced when 400 J was delivered cathodally via the distal pole of 6F USCI catheter electrode immersed in a tank of Ringer's solution

$0.5\,\mu l/J$ falling to $0.24\,\mu l/J$ in the higher range of 100–400 J. Anodal impulses liberated greater gas volumes, at a rate of $4.25\,\mu l/J$ from energies of 10–200 J. Analysis of gas samples showed that they were composed predominantly of hydrogen and nitrogen, the figures for cathodal energy delivery being 50–68% for hydrogen and 20–40% for nitrogen. The corresponding figures for anodal energy delivery were 66–68% and 11–16%, respectively.

Haemolysis was also related to electrode polarity and amount of energy delivery. The haemolysis rate for cathodal energy delivery was $1.35\,\mu l/J$ and that for anodal electrodes $4.63\,\mu l/J$.

This experiment showed not only that gas and haemolysis occurred during delivery of high energy impulses to fresh whole blood, but also that cathodal energy delivery was safer than anodal since lower pressure waves were produced as well as less haematological damage. Therefore, cathodal energy delivery is preferable to anodal in clinical ablation procedures.

Time effects

Experiments in which shocks of 100 J were delivered to isolated perfused dog hearts failed to show any macroscopic endocardial lesion acutely[27]. A study was consequently performed in which energies of 50–400 J were delivered via one of three electrodes of different geometry to the right and left ventricles of eight healthy dogs[28]. Acute complications included sudden death from myocardial failure and ventricular arrhythmias. These were related to high energies especially via the USCI electrode. The major long term complication was the formation of an extremely thin walled right ventricular aneurysm at the site of 50 J delivered via the USCI electrode.

Those dogs dying acutely had little or no macroscopic evidence of endocardial injury, although circumscribed epicardial lesions were present. Histologically, cellular injury extending from immediately beneath the endocardium to the epicardium was demonstrated. This acute cellular injury consisted of loss of cell nuclei and contraction band necrosis with no rupture of cell membranes. The histological findings in those animals surviving for 5 months showed full thickness lesions composed of fibrous and adipose tissue. The results from this study suggested that low energies were safer than higher values, and that using active fixation electrodes would allow a more efficient delivery of these low energies.

There has been much speculation on which of the four physical effects produced by the high energy ablation technique, i.e. light, heat, pressure and high currents, is responsible for the therapeutic effect of interruption of conduction. Previous experiments on the cellular effects of defibrillation pulses[29–32], plus the histological effects reported above, and other studies[33] suggest that the high current intensities may be responsible.

CLINICAL APPLICATIONS OF THE HIGH ENERGY ENDOCARDIAL ABLATION TECHNIQUES

Since its first use in the ablation of His bundle conduction the high energy ablation technique has been employed to interrupt conduction in accessory atrioventricular pathways (both right and left sided) and also in ventricular tachycardia foci. Each of these clinical applications will be considered separately. In all cases the high energy ablation procedure is only offered to patients where drug therapy has proved totally ineffective or produced unacceptable side-effects.

His bundle ablation

The ablation of His bundle conduction may be performed in patients with drug-resistant paroxysmal supraventricular tachycardias. These include atrial fibrillation or flutter, and re-entry tachycardias involving dual atrioventricular nodal conduction or concealed accessory atrio-ventricular pathways.

When performing His bundle ablation, most workers introduce a temporary pacing electrode to the right ventricle, under local anaes-thesia, to provide pacing cover during the procedure. The catheter electrode to be employed (usually the 6F bipolar USCI electrode) is then inserted via the right femoral vein and positioned to obtain the maximum His bundle signal coupled with a good atrial electrogram. The indifferent electrode, or back plate, is positioned in the left scapular region. Under general anaesthesia the energy impulse is delivered as a unipolar shock via the distal electrode of the USCI catheter, which is connected to the cathodal output of a standard defibrillator. The back plate is connected to the anodal output of the defibrillator. Energy delivery is followed by complete heart block for which temporary pacing is usually required.

The site of origin of the escape rhythm varies. Ideally this should be a narrow complex rhythm with a rate around 60–65 bpm although this is not often achieved in practice. After the production of complete heart block most workers delay implantation of a permanent pacemaker for at least 24–48 hours to ensure that atrioventricular nodal conduction does not return. In order to improve exercise capacity a rate responsive or even DDD pacemaker[34] should be implanted following the production of permanent complete block.

Using the system described above with temporary catheter electrodes and a standard defibrillator the energies employed by different groups have varied considerably. Shocks have been delivered ranging in ampli-tude from 50 J by McComb[35], 150–300 J by Manz[36], 200–300 J by Gal-lagher[8], 300–400 J by Nathan[37] and 300–500 J by Scheinman[9]. The total energy delivered to a patient can be considerably higher than these figures would suggest, e.g. 11 shocks with a maximum energy of 350 J[37].

A worldwide voluntary registry has been organized by Scheinman et al.[38] and a recent report from the registry presented data from the first 209 consecutive patients undergoing His bundle ablation[39]. Chronic complete atrioventricular block was produced in 70%, 21% reverted to sinus rhythm but were symptomatically improved (13% with previously ineffective drug regimes). The procedure was ineffective in 9%. The early complications included transient ventricular arrhythmias immediately postablation in five patients and hypotension in four. Electromechanical dissociation occurred in one patient persisting only for a short period, and non-fatal cardiac tamponade was noted in another. Chronic com-plications were uncommon. A 2% incidence of sudden death has been reported 1–5 months after ablation, but all these patients had significant underlying heart disease.

Catheter ablation has abolished the need for His bundle ablative surgery and ushered in a new era in the management of drug-resistant supraventricular arrhythmias.

Ablation of accessory pathways

The extension of the catheter ablation technique into the management of patients with Wolff–Parkinson–White syndrome was initially very attractive. If successful it would have supplanted the need for surgery in those whose accessory atrioventricular pathways had short refractory periods. However, the delivery of high energy impulses, particularly in those with left sided accessory pathways where the catheter is positioned in the coronary sinus were fraught with complications including coronary sinus rupture and thrombosis[10] and circumflex artery lesions[15]. In the first 15 attempted coronary sinus ablative procedures reported to the registry four patients suffered coronary sinus rupture and one death occurred. Current recommendations on the use of the electrical ablation procedure in those with Wolff–Parkinson–White syndrome are based on the anatomical site of the accessory pathway.

Left free-wall accessory pathway

This procedure involved positioning the catheter electrode in the coronary sinus. Very accurate mapping of the position of the accessory pathway is required, and unipolar cathodal shocks are delivered via the mapping electrode closest to the pathway. A back plate acts as the indifferent pole. As can be seen from the data above this is an extremely hazardous procedure and should only be performed if the following conditions are fulfilled. Both the coronary sinus and circumflex coronary artery should be visualized using contrast medium. If the coronary sinus is small or irregular, or if the circumflex artery is a large dominant vessel, then energy delivery to the coronary sinus should not be attempted. Even if favourable anatomy is present energy delivery should not be attempted in the distal coronary sinus and should always be kept below 70 J (stored) energy. Such energy values are unlikely to completely abolish accessory pathway conduction but may modify it.

In view of the favourable surgical results with left free-wall accessory pathways this may be preferable to electrical ablation in this group of patients.

Posteroseptal pathways

Recently Morady et al.[40] described a technique for the ablation of this anatomical group of pathways. It must be stressed that this is only suitable for those patients where earliest retrograde atrial activation has been localized to the coronary sinus os. In this modified ablation technique a multipolar catheter electrode is introduced into the coronary sinus so that the distal electrodes are just outside the coronary sinus os. This distal electrode pair act as a joint cathode, the cathodal shock being delivered simultaneously through both. An external chest patch again acts as the anode. Great care must be taken to ensure that the electrical discharge is delivered just *outside* the coronary sinus. Again the coronary sinus anatomy should be determined prior to energy delivery.

Right sided accessory pathways

To date little experience has been reported on the electrical ablation of right free-wall accessory atrioventricular pathways. Mapping of the site of the accessory pathway can be performed on the ventricular or atrial side of the tricuspid valve ring. Of the two patients with right free-wall accessory pathways treated at Guy's Hospital one had mapping and energy delivery performed in the right ventricle and the other in the right atrium[41]. Manipulation of the catheter electrode for accurate mapping proved somewhat easier in the latter patient. Having located the accessory pathway, unipolar cathodal shocks were delivered from the adjacent electrode with a chest patch acting as the anode. The patient in whom energy was delivered to the right ventricle had complete ablation of conduction in the accessory pathway. The patient in whom the atrium was the site of energy delivery had considerable modification of accessory pathway conduction, although it was not completely abolished. However, two complications were encountered. Acutely, a small pericardial effusion occurred presumably due to production of a small self-sealing breach in the right atrial wall. Chronically, this patient experienced an increased frequency of episodes of paroxysmal atrial fibrillation. The stored energy value in this case was 200 J. As with left sided free-wall accessory pathways surgery is probably preferable to electrical ablation in this group of patients.

Figure 22.4 illustrates the modification in conduction demonstrated during right atrial pacing before and 4 hours after electrical ablation in one patient.

Ablation of ventricular tachycardia foci

The role of high energy electrical ablation technique in the treatment of patients with frequent or incessant, drug resistant ventricular tachycardia, is also open to discussion. The first report of ablation of ventricular tachycardia foci using this technique came from Hartzler[13]. Following his initial encouraging results other centres undertook the procedure. The method involves the use of multipolar catheter electrodes for endocardial mapping (earliest activation and pacemapping) of both ventricles. The catheter electrode is positioned against the endocardial area showing earliest activation, and shocks are delivered via the electrode with an external patch or back paddle as the indifferent. Most centres connect the cathodal output of the defibrillator to the catheter electrode, although some European centres[42] use anodal impulses.

Using this technique results have been mixed. Some report a favourable outcome while others have a less favourable experience.

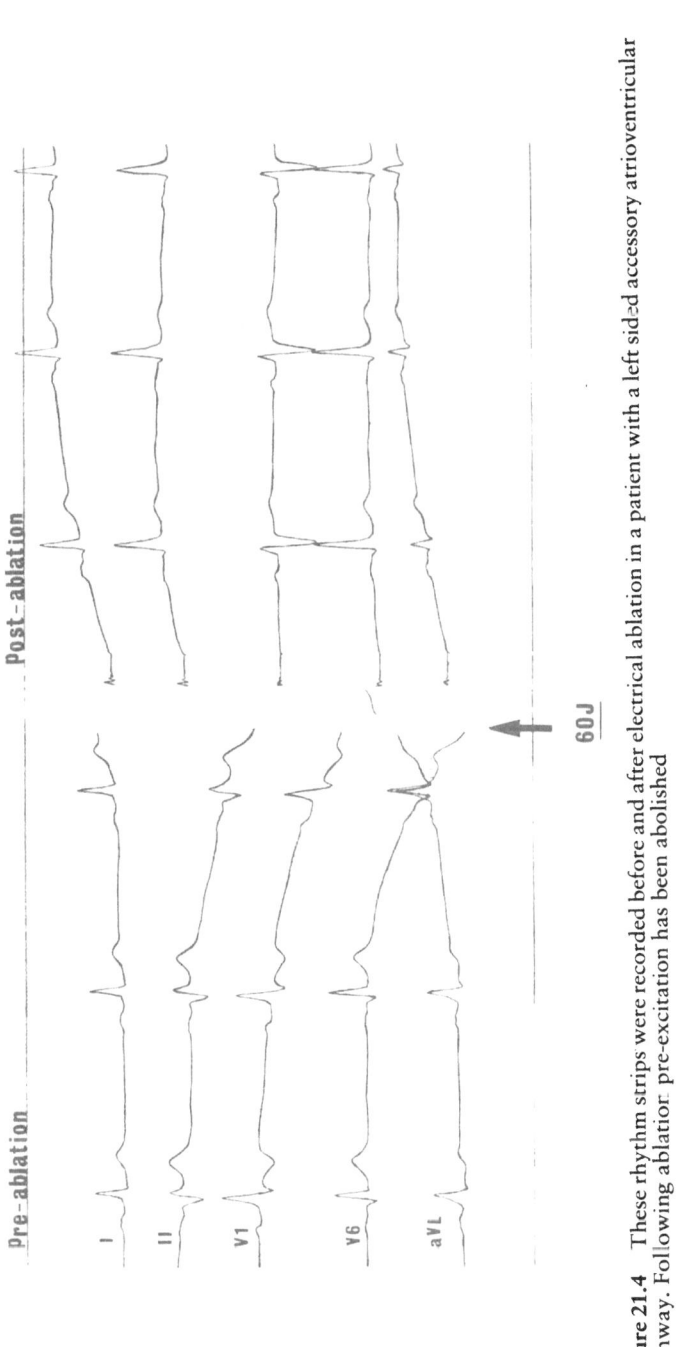

Figure 21.4 These rhythm strips were recorded before and after electrical ablation in a patient with a left sided accessory atrioventricular pathway. Following ablation pre-excitation has been abolished

Scheinman[39] in 12 patients with ventricular tachycardia, reported only three patients having long term arrhythmia control without drugs following electrical ablation. Serious side-effects have also been described including malignant ventricular arrhythmias within 1 week of ablation, impaired ventricular function, and electromechanical dissociation. In addition ventricular rupture and sudden death have also occurred. The energies used in these clinical procedures range from approximately 200 to 600 J as single or multiple impulses.

Results from animal experiments suggest that these complications are related to the energies used, high energies and multiple shocks being more likely to produce acute and long term complications identical to those described clinically. In an effort to reduce the energy requirements for the ablation of ventricular tachycardia we employed an active fixation electrode in a patient with a right ventricular arrhythmia. A single shock of 50 J via this electrode proved successful in producing long term arrhythmia control in this patient. Other workers have attempted to reduce energy requirements by using a second intracardiac catheter electrode as the indifferent pole[43].

At present, catheter ablation of ventricular tachycardia foci should be undertaken with great care, especially in those who have poor ventricular function since energy delivery can depress myocardial contractility still further, especially acutely[16].

FUTURE DEVELOPMENTS

In view of the deleterious effects of high energy impulses, attempts have been made to reduce the energy requirements for the catheter ablation technique. Initially these attempts were directed at the catheter electrodes. *In vitro* studies have shown that at low energies the shape of the emerging flash is dependent upon the electrode geometry. At low energies the active fixation electrodes have better 'directional' properties. Following animal studies the use of the Vitatron Helifix and Sorin S90 electrodes has allowed successful ablation of His bundle conduction using energies of 50 J and 10 J, respectively[19,28]. However, both these electrodes were designed for use with permanent pacing systems, and their torque characteristics render them very difficult to position accurately. Recently a method of fixing the smooth round electrode type has been devised using suction[20]. This is as yet an experimental lead, but it appears to allow successful His bundle ablation using energies of approximately 100 J. Catheter electrode designs continue to be investigated. No definitive solution has yet been achieved which combines efficiency of energy delivery, safety and easy manipulation which is essential for the accurate mapping required.

Another method of approach to reducing the energy requirements for ablation procedures is to modify the energy delivery system. Most units use the standard DC defibrillator to store and deliver the high energy electrical charge, the majority of which produce a damped sinusoidal current wave form. Laboratory tank studies have been performed to produce current wave forms that avoid the production of plasma arcing and, therefore, the generation of large pressure waves[22,44]. Further developments in this interesting field are awaited with interest[45].

Other energy sources such as radiofrequency devices[46] and lasers[47] are currently under evaluation, and may find a role in the non-surgical ablation of arrhythmogenic tissue.

CONCLUSIONS

The catheter ablation technique has proved valuable in the management of patients with drug resistant tachycardias. However, patients should be carefully selected and the role of other therapeutic options evaluated in view of the potential complications resulting from the delivery of high energy impulses. Future progress of the technique depends upon improving its safety by reducing the energy required for successful ablation (e.g. to less than 10 J). This may be achieved by modifying the catheter electrodes, energy delivery system, or both.

References

1. German, L. D. and Strauss, H. O. (1984). Electrical termination of tachyarrhythmias by discrete pulses. *Pacing Clin. Electrocardiol.*, 7, 514–40
2. Fisher, J. D., Kim, S. C., Burman, S. and Matos, J. A. (1982). Role of implantable pacemakers in control of recurrent ventricular tachycardia. *Am. J. Cardiol.*, 49, 194–206
3. Sealy, W. C., Gallagher, J. J. and Pritchett, L. C. (1978). The surgical anatomy of Kent bundles based on electrophysiological mapping and surgical exploration. *J. Thorac. Cardiovasc. Surg.*, 76, 804
4. Boineau, J. P. and Cox, J. L. (1982). Rationale for a direct surgical approach to control ventricular arrhythmias. *Am. J. Cardiol.*, 49, 381–90
5. Vedel, J., Frank, R., Fontaine, C. et al. (1979). Bloc auriculo–ventriculaire infra-Hisien definitif induit au cours d'une exploration endoventriculaire droite. *Arch. Mal. Coeur*, 72, 107
6. Gonzales, R., Scheinman, M., Margaretten, W. and Rubinstein, M. (1981). Closed-chest electrode-catheter technique for His bundle ablation in dogs. *Am. J. Physiol.*, (*Heart Circ. Physiol. 10*) 241, B283–287
7. Gonzales, R., Scheinman, M., Bharati, S. and Lev, M. (1983). Closed chest permanent atrioventricular block in dogs. *Am. Heart J.*, 105, 461–70
8. Gallagher, J. J., Svenson, R. B., Kassell, J. P., German, D. L., Hardy, G. H., Broughton, A. and Critelli, G. (1982). Catheter technique for closed chest ablation of the atrioventricular conduction system. *N. Engl. J. Med.*, 306, 194–200
9. Scheinman, M. M., Morady, F., Hess, D. S. and Gonzales, B. (1982). Catheter-induced ablation of the atrioventricular junction to control refractory supraventricular arrhythmias. *J. Am. Med. Assoc.*, 248, 851–5
10. Fisher, J. D., Brodman, R., Kim, S. C. et al. (1984). Attempted non-surgical electrical ablation of accessory pathways via the coronary sinus in the Wolff–Parkinson–White syndrome. *J. Am. Coll. Cardiol.*, 4, 685–94
11. Morady, F. and Scheinman, M. M. (1984). Transvenous catheter ablation of an accessory pathway in a patient with Wolff Parkinson White Syndrome. *N. Engl. J. Med.*, 310, 705–7
12. Ward, D., Drysdale, M. and Redwood, D. (1984). Interruption of anomalous atrioventricular conduction using a transvenous electrode catheter to deliver shocks in the coronary sinus. *Br. Heart J.*, 51, 686–7 (Abstr.)

13. Harzler, G. O. (1983). Electrode catheter ablation of refractory focal ventricular tachycardia. *J. Am. Coll. Cardiol.*, 2, 1107–13
14. Tonet, J. L., Fontaine, C., Frank, R. and Grosgogeat, Y. (1985). Treatment of refractory ventricular tachycardias by endocardial fulguration. *Circulation*, 72, III–388 (Abstr.)
15. Conde, A. X., Perez Gomez, F. and Harguindey, L. S. (1985). Endocardial ablation. In Perez Gomez, F. (ed.) *Cardiac Pacing Electrophysiology, Tachyarrhythmias*. pp. 1545–58. (Madrid: Pub. Editorial Group)
16. Abbott, J. A., Eldar, M., Segar, J. J., Ruder, M. A. *et al.* (1985). Non-invasive assessment of myocardial function following attempted catheter ablation of ventricular tachycardia foci. *Circulation*, 72, III–388 (Abstr.)
17. Schofield, P. M., Bowes, R. J., Lawrence, G., Prescott, M., Brooks, N. and Bennett, D. H. (1986). Impaired right ventricular function following transvenous fulguration of atrioventricular conduction. *Br. Heart J.*, 55, 506. (Abstr.)
18. Davies, D. W., Nathan, A. W. and Camm, A. J. (1986). Three deaths after attempted high energy catheter ablation of ventricular tachycardia. *Br. Heart J.*, 55, 506–7. (Abstr.)
19. Holt, P., Boyd, E. G. C. A., Crick, J. C. P. and Sowton E. (1985). Low energies and Helifix electrodes in the successful ablation of atrioventricular conduction. *Pacing Clin. Electrophysiol.*, 8, 639–45
20. Polgar, P., Bolnar, P., Worum, B., Bekassy, Sz., Kovacs, P. and Lorinerz, I. (1983). Closed chest ablation of the His bundle; a new technique using suction electrode catheter and D. C. shock. In Steinbach, K. (ed.) *Cardiac Pacing*, pp. 883–90. (Darstadt: Steinkopff Verlag)
21. Boyd, E. G. C. A., Holt, P. M. and Sowton, E. (1985). A modified energy delivery system for lower energy ablation. *Br. Heart J.*, 7, 651. (Abstr.)
22. Bardy, G. H., Coltorti, F., Rackson, M., Hanson, K., Greene, R. L. and Ivey, T. D. (1986). Multiple vs single pulses to avoid voltage breakdown and shockwave generation with catheter mediated electrical pulses. *J. Am. Coll. Cardiol.*, 7, 242A
23. Boyd, E. G. C. A. and Holt, P. (1985). An investigation into the electrical ablation technique and a method of electrode assessment. *Pacing Clin. Electrophysiol.*, 8, 815–24
24. Bardy, G. H., Coltorti, B., Rackson, M. M., Hanson, K., Greene, H. L. and Ivey, T. D. (1985). Current waveform modulation to avoid plasma-arcing and barotrauma with catheter mediated electrode discharges. *Circulation*, 72, (Suppl. III) III–474
25. Boyd, E. and Holt, P. (1985). Haematological and tissue effects of high energy ablation. *Br. Heart J.*, 53, 99 (Abstr.)
26. Holt, P. and Boyd, E. G. C. A. (1986). Haematological effects of the high energy endocardial ablation technique. *Circulation*, 73, 1029–36
27. Holt, P. M. and Boyd, E. G. C. A. (1984). Endocardial ablation: the background to its use in ventricular tachycardia. *Br. Heart J.*, 51, 687 (Abstr.)
28. Holt, P. and Boyd, E. G. C. A. (1986). Low energy ablation: the role of electrode geometry. *Br. Heart J.*, Abstr. (In press)
29. Jones, J. L., Lepeschkin, B., Jones, R. E. and Sush, S. (1978). Response of cultured myocardial cells to countershock-type electric field stimulation. *Am. J. Physiol.*, 253, H214–H222
30. Jones, J. L., Lepeschkin, B., Jones, R. and Rush, S. (1977). Cellular fibrillation appearing in cultured myocardial cells after application of strong capacitor discharges. *Am. J. Cardiol.*, 39, 273 (Abstr.)
31. Jones, J. L., Lepeschkin, B., Rush, S. and Jones R. (1978). Depolarisation induced arrhythmias following high intensity electric field stimulation of cultured myocardial cells. *Med. Instrum.*, 12, 54
32. Jones, J. L., Proskauer, C. C., Paull, W. K., Lepeschkin, E. and Jones, R. G. (1980). Ultrastructural injury to chick myocardial cells *in vitro* following 'Electrical Countershock'. *Circ. Res.*, 46, 387–94

33. Levine, J. H., Spear, J. F., Weisman, H. F., Kadish, A. H., Prood, C., Siu, C. O. and Moore, G. N. (1986). The cellular electrophysiologic changes induced by high energy electrical ablation in canine myocardium. *Circulation, 73*, 818–29

34. Schofield, P. M., Bowes, R. J., Brooks, N. and Bennett, D. H. (1986). Exercise capacity and spontaneous heart rhythm after transvenous fulguration of atrioventricular conduction. *Br. Heart J., 56*, 358–65

35. McComb, J. M., McGovern, B. A., Garen, H. and Ruskin J. W. (1985). Modification of atrioventricular conduction using low energy transcatheter shocks. *J. Am. Coll. Cardiol., 5*, 454. (Abstr.)

36. Manz, M., Steinbeck, G. and Luderitz, B. (1983). His bundel-ablation Bine Methode zur Behandling bedrohlicher supraventrikularer Herzrhythmusstorungen. *Ler Internist, 24*, 95–8

37. Nathan, A. W., Ward, D. B., Bennett, D. B., Bexten, R. S. and Camm, A. J. (1984). Catheter ablation of atrioventricular conduction. *Lancet, 1*, 1280–4

38. Scheinman, M. M., Evans-Bell, T., and the Executive Committee of the Percutaneous Mapping and Ablation Registry (1984). Catheter ablation of the atrioventricular function: a report of the Percutaneous Mapping and Ablation Registry. *Circulation, 70*, 1024

39. Scheinman, M. M. and Davis, J. C. (1986). Catheter ablation for treatment of tachyarrhythmias: present role and potential promise. *Circulation, 73*, 10–13

40. Morady, F., Scheinman, M. M., Winston, S. A., DiCarlo, L. A. Jr, Davis, J. C., Griffin, J. C., Ruder, M., Abbott, J. A. and Eldar, M. (1985). Efficacy and safety of transcatheter ablation of posteroseptal accessory pathways. *Circulation, 72*, 70

41. Holt, P., Boyd, E. and Sowton, E. (1986). Endocardial ablation of His bundle accessory pathway and ventricular tachycardia foci: comparison of safety and success. *Br. Heart J.*, Abstr. (In press)

42. Breithardt, G., Borggrefe, M., Karbenn, U., Schwartzmaler, J. and Rohner, D. (1985). Catheter ablation of ventricular tachycardia. *Eur. Heart J., 6*, (Suppl. 1) 19

43. Kadish, A. H., Spear, J. F., Prood, C., Levine, J. H. and Moore, G. K. (1986). Intercatheter energy delivery for ablation of ventricular myocardium. *J. Am. Coll. Cardiol., 7*, 237A

44. Bardy, G. H., Coltorti, F., Rackson, M., Hanson, K., Greene, B. L. and Ivey T. D. (1986). Catheter mediated electrical ablation: The relation between current and pulse width on voltage breakdown and shock wave generation. *J. Am. Coll. Cardiol., 7*, 99A

45. Cunningham, A. D., Rowland, E. and Rickards, A. F. (1986). A low energy power source for ablation and a new index for ablating devices. *Clin. Prog. Electrophysiol. Pacing, 4*, 125 (Abstr.)

46. Huang, S. K., Graham, A. R., Wharton, K., Odell, R. C. and Marcus, F. I. (1986). Closed chest catheter dessication of the ventricular myocardium using radiofrequency energy. *Pacing Clin. Electrocardiol., 9*, 288 (Abstr.)

47. Svenson, R. H., Gallagher, J. J., Selle, J. C., Sealy, W. C. *et al.* (1986). Successful intraoperative Nd: YAG laser ablation of ventricular tachycardia. *J. Am. Coll. Cardiol., 7*, 237A

22
Surgery for the treatment of tachycardias

A. W. NATHAN

INTRODUCTION

Surgery offers the possibility of a cure for some arrhythmias whereas all other therapies can only provide, at best, amelioration of tachycardias. The only obvious exception to this statement is of course catheter ablation which is a development of surgical techniques. Even in cases where a complete cure cannot be effective, the effects of some arrhythmias can be controlled by surgical techniques where other techniques have failed or are inappropriate.

The range of tachycardias that can be treated surgically are extensive and include the following:

Sinus node re-entrant tachycardia
Atrial tachycardia
Atrial flutter
Atrial fibrillation
Atrioventricular junctional ectopic tachycardia
Atrioventricular nodal re-entrant tachycardia
Atrioventricular re-entrant tachycardia (concealed or overt accessory
     pathway/Wolff–Parkinson–White syndrome)
Atrioventricular re-entrant tachycardia (long R–P')
Ventricular tachycardia
Ventricular fibrillation

The principles of arrhythmia surgery are either directly to ablate or to divide an abnormal focus or pathway, or to indirectly exclude the focus or create AV block for some supraventricular arrhythmias. This chapter describes actual surgical techniques for arrhythmias, but recently catheter ablation techniques have been developed and, in some cases, these complement or even supersede open surgery.

The indications for surgery are several and vary according to the arrhythmia. They include arrhythmias refractory to medical and device therapy, primary therapy for life-threatening arrhythmias and patient preference. Arrhythmia surgery may also be performed at the time of other cardiac surgery.

PRE-OPERATIVE EVALUATION

All patients must be carefully evaluated before being considered for arrhythmia surgery. This evaluation must include the general state of health, the assessment of myocardial function, and establishing whether or not other heart disease is present, as well as studying the arrhythmia itself, as the success or otherwise of surgery depends on all these factors.

The extent of such an evaluation will of course somewhat depend on the arrhythmia being treated. For example, most patients with junctional tachycardias or the Wolff–Parkinson–White syndrome will have an otherwise normal heart with no other heart disease, and they are likely to be young and fit. On the other hand, patients with ventricular tachyarrhythmias almost invariably have other heart disease which is actually the cause of their arrhythmias, most will have impaired myocardial function and the majority will be of an older age group and less fit. Thus most patients with ventricular tachycardias will require coronary and ventricular angiography whereas such a procedure is rarely necessary in those with junctional tachycardias. Similarly, patients with junctional tachycardias rarely need any other heart surgery performed, but those with ventricular tachycardia, for example due to ischaemic heart disease, may well need additional procedures such as aneurysmectomy or coronary grafting.

Virtually all patients undergoing arrhythmia surgery require pre-operative electrophysiological study. The main aim of this study is to precisely delineate the mechanism causing the symptomatic arrhythmia, and also to ensure that other mechanisms of arrhythmias are not present in the patient. The precise arrhythmia focus or position of any accessory pathway must be carefully established during the electrophysiological study, and it is our practice to cine-radiographically record the position of the mapping electrodes at the relevant mapped sites during the electrophysiological study.

In patients with AV accessory pathways it is usual to delineate both the anterograde and retrograde activation sequences, because multiple pathways may be present, one more prominent in the anterograde direction and the other retrogradely. It is certainly best to map during tachycardia, but mapping during atrial and ventricular pacing should also be performed. In patients with ventricular arrhythmias electrical activation mapping during tachycardia is the prime method of mapping. It is always useful to have a 12 lead ECG of the clinical presenting arrhythmia for comparison, as multiple morphologies of tachycardia may be induced during electrophysiological study. However, it is still not established what the full therapeutic significance is of non-clinical arrhythmias. Pace-mapping can also be performed, comparing the morphology of a paced complex and the clinical tachycardia. Mapping can also be performed looking for late potentials and fractionated activity, especially during sinus rhythm, which may indicate the site of origin of tachycardia, although several areas of late potentials may be mapped and not all of these are necessarily related to the mechanism of the clinical tachycardia. Whether all areas containing such late potentials should be treated or not is still controversial.

SINUS NODE AND ATRIAL ARRHYTHMIAS

These arrhythmias may be treated directly by resection of a specific focus or indirectly by exclusion procedures, or by inducing AV block.

Pathological sinus tachycardia is a rare arrhythmia, and can be difficult to treat. Yee et al.[1] describe a refractory case of sinus tachycardia, thought to be due to enhanced sinus node automaticity, treated by subtotal right atrial exclusion. In this case, a transverse right atrial transmural incision was made to divide the right atrium into a superior excluding cuff containing the SA node region, and an inferior segment in continuity with the rest of the heart. The patient initially did well with a junctional pacemaker of 60–70 beats per minute, increasing to 105 beats per minute on exercise; the patient did not require an artificial cardiac pacemaker. Two more patients were operated upon[2], but all three now have problems with either atrial fibrillation or atrial tachycardia.

In 1973 Coumel et al.[3] described the excision of part of the left atrium for the treatment of atrial tachycardia; other authors have described additional cases[4-7] due to several aetiologies including tumours[8]. Guiraudon et al.[2] described the successful use of cryosurgery for resistant re-entrant atrial tachycardia, and a similar experience has been reported by Gallagher et al.[9] and Bredikis et al.[10]. Atrial tachycardias requiring such surgery are more common in children[10] where localized atrial disease may be present. In adults diffuse atrial disease is more common, and excision or ablation of one focus may be successful but further abnormal foci may develop.

Atrial arrhythmias sometimes present in patients with symptoms and signs of cardiac failure, mimicking dilated cardiomyopathy. Although cardiomyopathy may be the cause of the arrhythmia in some cases, an incessant tachycardia may actually cause cardiac failure and successful surgical treatment may return cardiac function to normal[7].

Atrial flutter is thought to be a re-entrant arrhythmia, and Klein et al.[11] have attempted cryoablation of the focus in two patients with flutter. The wavefront originated in the coronary sinus region in both, and although their first patient had late atrial fibrillation the second did well. Atrial fibrillation may be a difficult arrhythmia to control. Guiraudon et al.[12] have attempted to insulate the AV node and the sinoatrial node from the rest of the fibrillating atria, and have tried to prevent atrial fibrillation by critically reducing the atrial mass; the left atrium is isolated and a thin strip of atrium including the SA and AV nodes is isolated from the rest of the atrial tissue. Early follow-up data are encouraging.

In refractory cases, surgical creation of complete AV block offers another approach to the treatment of atrial arrhythmias, providing that there are no other anterograde atrioventricular connections, such as an accessory pathway in patients with the Wolff–Parkinson–White syndrome. Giannelli et al.[13] deliberately created AV block in a patient with intractable atrial tachycardia who was also undergoing aortic and mitral valve replacement. The surgical technique consisted of a ligature around the area of the AV node and His bundle together with a small incision into this area. Slama et al.[14], in the same year, described two patients with atrial arrhythmias, both of whom were successfully treated with a ligature placed around the AV node and His bundle regions. Harrison et al.[15] described a similar operation to produce AV block using a cryosurgical technique, but this still required open heart surgery. Bredikis[16] has successfully used a cryosurgical method without bypass, inserting the mapping and cryoprobes through small atriotomies with purse-string sutures to prevent leaks. More recently, electrical catheter ablation techniques have been developed, and by and large these have superseded the surgical approach, although surgery is still required very occasionally for patients who have failed catheter ablation.

JUNCTIONAL ARRHYTHMIAS

AV 'nodal' tachycardias

AV junctional ectopic tachycardia is very rare and when surgical therapy is thought to be necessary, abolition of atrioventricular conduction is probably indicated. Until recently the technique of complete interruption of AV conduction was the only surgical method available for patients with AV nodal re-entrant tachycardia[17]. Patients with this arrhythmia are often young and otherwise fit, and even with dual chamber pacemakers may be haemodynamically impaired after such physiologically drastic surgery. If drugs are not appropriate, antitachycardia pacemakers may be used in some patients, but there are still patients who require surgical therapy. Recently, two types of surgical methodology have been devised to achieve a cure for such arrhythmias, preserving normal AV conduction and sparing the need for pacing.

Ross et al.[18] have devised two variations of an operation to prevent AV nodal re-entrant tachycardia. Their observations have led them to believe that there are at least two anatomically distinct types of tachycardia. In the commoner type A the earliest activation during tachycardia is antero-medial to the AV node consistent with exit from the conduction system in the region of the central fibrous body. This type is associated with a short conduction time for the retrograde limb ($\leqslant 40$ ms). In type B the earliest activation is posterior to the AV node and the retrograde conduction time is longer than in type A (> 40 ms).

After mapping the earliest site of atrial activation during tachycardia, the coronary sinus is dissected from the fat in the posterior space to expose the wall of the left atrium, the artery to the AV node, the central fibrous body and the tendon of Todaro. In the type A patients the earliest activation is at the apex of the triangle of Koch. In these patients the right atrial wall is carefully reflected anteriorly to expose the central fibrous body and the tendon of Todaro, divided at its insertion in to the central sinus body. The central fibrous body anteromedially to the node and the left atrial wall medial to the tendon are scraped clean, and the dissection continues posteriorly along the left margin of the pyramidal space as far as the coronary sinus, but preserving the posterior approaches to the AV node.

In the type B patients, with earliest activation along the posterior part of the triangle of Koch near the coronary sinus, the free wall of the right ventricular is dissected clean from the tricuspid annulus to the epicardium up to the lateral limits of the AV node and beneath it into the interventricular groove. The inferior wall of the coronary sinus is dissected clean to the epicardium from its mouth, continuing medially to the left atrial wall. The medial approach of the AV node is left intact.

Tachycardia induction was prevented in all patients at post-operative electrophysiological study in the patients reported. The AH time was mildly increased but the HV interval unchanged. One to one AV conduction was possible at rates faster than tachycardia rates in all patients. Dual AV nodal pathways remained in some patients, but slow antegrade pathway conduction was absent in most patients post-operatively.

Whilst most modern authorities have considered AV nodal re-entrant tachycardias to be due to dual AV node conduction totally within the AV node, these data from Ross et al. have suggested that a portion of the atrium is an essential part of the tachycardia circuit, although non-specific trauma to the AV node cannot be totally excluded[19]. Guiraudon[2] has successfully operated on a patient with AV nodal tachycardia using a different surgical technique, freeing the AV node and its fibrous sheath from the surrounding tissue.

Cox et al.[20] have used a completely different technique, first performed in animals, in patients with AV nodal re-entry[21]. Using a direct cryosurgical technique, monitoring AV conduction during atrial pacing, nine separate 3 mm cryolesions at $-60\,^{\circ}C$ for 2 minutes are made at sites around the triangle of Koch in the lower atrial septum.

Post-operatively, all patients have had single AV conduction pathways without tachycardia, and without any need for pacing.

Pre-excitation syndromes and related tachycardias

Patients with ventricular pre-excitation (e.g. the Wolff–Parkinson–White syndrome) may be at risk from rapid ventricular rates during atrial fibrillation as well as from macro-re-entrant tachycardias. Abolition of

AV nodal conduction has been performed in some patients to prevent atrioventricular re-entrant tachycardia[17,22], but it is a sub-optimal procedure because not only is permanent pacing necessary in most patients but the risk of rapid conduction still remains.

In 1964 Cartwright et al.[23] and in 1967 Lillehei et al.[24] reported the inadvertent interruption of Kent bundles in patients undergoing tricuspid valve replacement for Ebstein's anomaly associated with the Wolff–Parkinson–White syndrome. In 1968 Cobb et al. reported the first operation to deliberately divide a Kent pathway[25]. Since then a variety of surgical techniques have been used, and these include the use of epicardial and endocardial surgery on both the beating and non-beating heart. Dissection and cryoablation are both recognized techniques[17,25-31]. Particular care is needed with septal pathways as vital structures such as the coronary sinus, the atrioventricular valves, atrial septum, the membranous interventricular septum and His bundle lie close to these pathways. Initial attempts at an epicardial approach[26] met with limited success as only superficial accessory pathways were ablated, but Guiraudon et al.[31] described an effective epicardial closed heart technique that does not necessarily require bypass in all patients.

Of course it is not only patients with the overt Wolff–Parkinson–White syndrome who may require surgery. There are many patients who have concealed accessory pathways and in whom surgery may be indicated. The approach to the accessory pathways depends on their location. Most are epicardial region but some are endocardial, especially in the right free wall location. The atria and ventricles are adjacent to each other but separated by the annulus fibrosus along the entire circumference of the mitral and tricuspid orifices, except where the left atrium is attached to the aortic right anteriorly. In terms of the position of pathways across the AV ring it is appropriate to divide their locations into four areas, the left free wall, right free wall, anterior septum and posterior septum. Left free wall pathways traverse the AV groove in proximity to the parietal portion of the mitral annulus, and right free wall pathways traverse the AV groove in proximity to the tricuspid annulus. The remaining pathways are septal, and the dividing point between the anterior and posterior septal pathways is the atrial extension of the membranous septum, anatomically related to the right fibrous trigone. An intermediate subset probably exists[32,33], and in some hands surgery to these intermediate pathways may carry an increased risk of complete heart block as these pathways are close to the His bundle.

For pathways other than those in the anterior septal region the epicardial approach devised by Guiraudon[32,34] is probably the most popular at present due to its relative simplicity, safety and effectiveness. Careful mapping is of course required in all patients. In those with left free wall pathways the left atrioventricular fat pad is mobilized, cleanly dissecting the coronary sinus and the left atrial wall. Accessory pathway conduction almost always disappears during dissection, but for additional efficacy, cryosurgery is also applied at the region of interest,

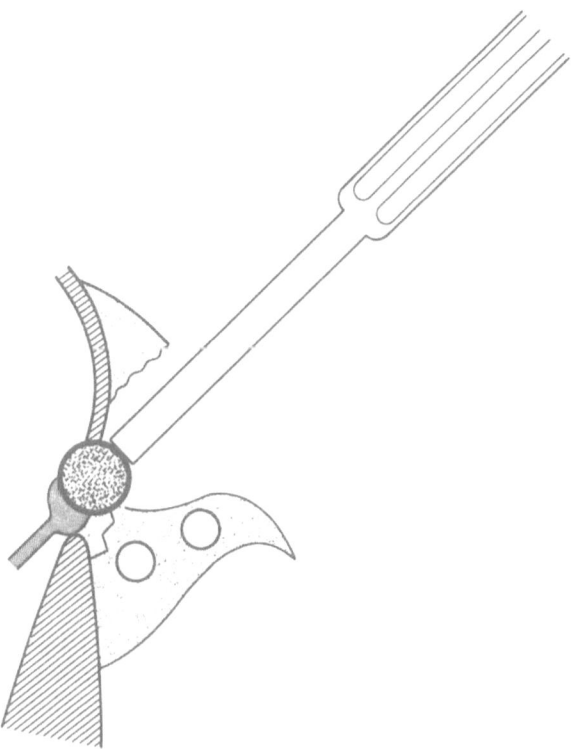

Figure 22.1   Section through heart showing diagrammatically Guiraudon's operation for left free wall accessory pathways. The coronary sinus and coronary artery have been retracted back in their fat pad and a cryolesion is being made. (Reproduced from Ward, D. E. and Camm, A. J. *Clinical Electrophysiology of the Heart*, Edward Arnold, 1987, with permission)

with the coronary sinus and coronary artery being kept away from the iceball (Figure 22.1). Posterior septal pathways[35] are treated by a similar approach as these pathways attach on to the posterior superior process of the left ventricle which is part of the right atrial-left ventricular coronary sulcus. Right-sided pathways are approached by dissection of the right AV fat pad, which is characterized by the presence of cardiac veins that may open directly into the right atrium. Some of the right-sided pathways may lie endocardially; cryoablation may, therefore, be more important than with left-sided pathways. Occasional right-sided wall pathways cannot be treated by this approach because of their endocardial location, these then require an endocardial approach. Cardiopulmonary bypass is used for most patients, although some right-sided posterior septal pathways can be approached without bypass using a conventional median sternotomy. Left lateral pathways can be treated without bypass if a left thoracotomy is used, although many surgeons do not find this the most favourable. At St Bartholomew's

Hospital, all patients are cannulated for bypass particularly as some tachycardias are extremely badly tolerated haemodynamically.

The original Duke University techniques, devised by Sealy and his colleagues and evolved by Cox[36,37], are still in widespread use although perhaps require slightly more complex surgery. Initially, very localized dissections were performed, but because of the variability of accessory pathway location together with the presence of multiple accessory pathways in some patients, together with the increasing safety of prolonged cardiac standstill with cardioplegic arrest, more extensive dissections are now employed.

The surgical approach for left free wall pathways is similar to that for a mitral valve replacement, with entry through an incision in the posterior interatrial groove. Following this, an incision is begun just above the mitral annulus and is extended anteriorly to the left fibrous trigone and posteriorly to the junction of the free wall with the septum. Right free wall pathways are approached via a similar technique from the right atrium, although a more limited dissection is usually used. These posterior septal pathways are approached by a very complex dissection of a pyramidal space bounded anteriorly by the insertion of the atrial extension of the membranous septum into the right fibrous trigone and posteriorly by the epicardium overlying the crux of the heart. The floor is the interventricular septum and the posterior superior process of the left ventricle. The lateral walls are formed by the diverging walls of the right atrium and the left atrium. The boundaries of this space are extensively dissected, especially the external aspect of the posterior medial mitral annulus. Technically this approach is much more demanding than Guiraudon's approach. Anterior septal pathways are by far the least common of all accessory pathways and must always be approached endocardially. The various methods of performing this dissection are essentially similar, involving the dissection of the right ventricular side of the atrial extension of the membranous septum.

Gallagher et al.[28] first described the use of cryosurgery for treating accessory pathways. Extensive use of this method has been made by the St Bartholomew's Hospital group[38] for left and right free wall pathways. The appropriate atrium is opened as for valve replacement and with the beating heart, using aortic perfusion, the pathway is mapped and the cryoprobe applied at the mapped position (Figures 22.2 and 22.3). Bredikis et al.[39,40] have used a cryosurgical method inserting a cryoprobe via limited atriotomies with purse-string sutures around them, without the use of cardiopulmonary bypass.

All the various approaches have their advantages and disadvantages, and although much has been made of the differences between the various approaches all are almost invariably successful and safe. The surgical approach used, therefore, becomes a simple matter of the preference of individual surgeons and cardiologists.

Lin et al.[41] have suggested that total atriotomy facilitates ablation of all accessory pathways in patients with multiple pathways. These

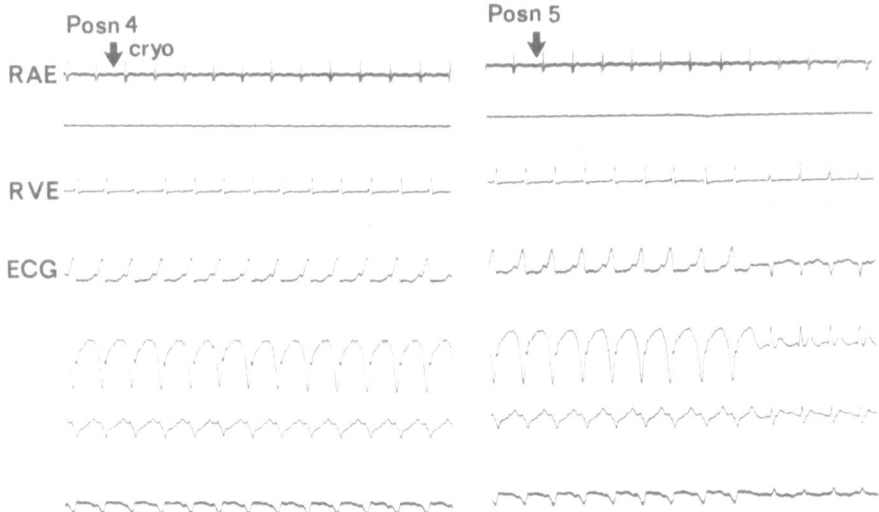

Figure 22.2 Cryomapping in a patient with an accessory pathway. In the left hand panel, the cryoprobe is being applied at position 4 without any effect but in position 5, after only a few seconds, pre-excitation is lost. The paper speed is 25 mm/s, RAE = right atrial electrogram, RVE = right ventricular electrogram

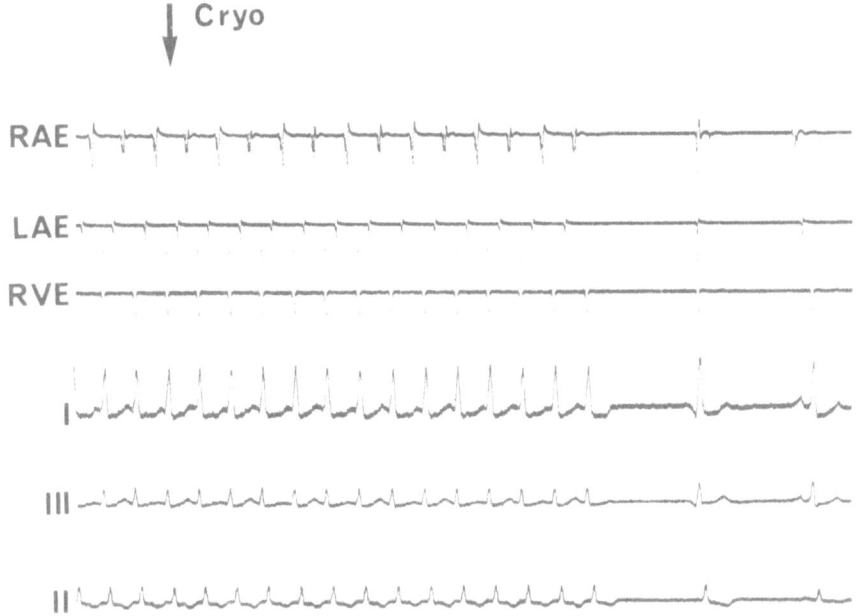

Figure 22.3 Cryothermy being used to ablate a left lateral accessory pathway. The cryoprobe has been applied during tachycardia. Tachycardia terminates in the retrograde (VA) direction and cryothermy is applied for a further 2 minutes. Abbreviations and paper speed as before. LAE = left atrial electrogram

pathways may not all be manifest at the time of either electrophysiological study or surgery because the presence of one pathway may obscure the presence of others. However, particularly when using the Guiraudon technique in which cardioplegia is not used and the heart remains beating throughout the procedure, multiple pathways are usually appreciated as one pathway may become manifest when another is divided. These additional pathways can then be tackled as necessary.

Left thoracic sympathectomy has been used for occasional patients with tachycardias due to accessory pathways[42], but this approach is of unproven efficacy.

Long-term results of surgery for accessory pathways are excellent. Prystowsky et al.[43] have reviewed 357 patients who have had accessory pathway surgery over an 18-year-period at Duke University. Surgical mortality was 4% (five patients intra-operatively, nine patients post-operatively) with five of these patients having other heart disease present. The quality of life was markedly improved with 93% having less frequent hospitalizations, 92% of patients being satisfied with surgery (75% completely and 17% incompletely), and 98% would recommend the surgery to others. Antiarrhythmic medication, necessary in all patients pre-operatively, was necessary in 23% of patients post-operatively. New atrial fibrillation was seen in only 2%. Fifty-two per cent of patients reported an arrhythmia post-operatively, but only 37% of these patients take antiarrhythmic drugs and episodes are usually short-lived.

Fischell et al.[44] examined 45 patients who had had surgery for accessory pathways. One patient had failed surgery and had recurrent tachycardias, and one other had a late recurrence of a delta wave without arrhythmias. Four others had frequent palpitations due to ventricular premature beats (three patients) and sinus tachycardia (one patient). Seventeen patients had occasional 'skipped beats', and 12 of 13 patients whose arrhythmias had limited employment before surgery returned to ʷork.

Sharma et al.[45] examined 50 consecutive patients who had surgery for the Wolff–Parkinson–White syndrome, 19 of whom had atrial fibrillation before surgery. Although three patients had atrial fibrillation the month following surgery, during a mean follow-up period of 1.9 years only one patient, who also had an associated cardiomyopathy, had recurrent atrial fibrillation. They considered that successful accessory pathway ablation prevents further atrial fibrillation, suggesting that re-entrant tachycardia or ectopy mediated by the accessory pathway is the mechanism of spontaneous atrial fibrillation in the majority of patients with the Wolff–Parkinson–White syndrome.

As stated by Cox[46] surgery for the Wolff–Parkinson–White syndrome is certainly no longer experimental and should be offered to the following patients:

- those with medically refractory re-entrant tachycardia who have an accessory pathway.
- patients with spontaneous atrial fibrillation who are at risk from sudden death because of the rapid conduction capabilities of the pathway.
- patients who require drug therapy but who are intolerant of this therapy.
- young otherwise healthy patients with symptoms requiring more than minimal medical therapy.

Although catheter ablation techniques are being developed for the treatment of accessory pathways and are sometimes effective, the problem of accurately apposing a catheter close to a pathway and then safely delivering sufficient energy to destroy it, while not damaging other cardiac structures, has yet to be resolved.

VENTRICULAR TACHYARRHYTHMIAS

Ventricular tachycardias usually carry a high mortality unless adequately treated. Drugs often fail to control ventricular tachycardias and other methods of treatment such as surgery may be necessary. There are many causes of ventricular tachycardia (Table 22.1) and there are many different ways of treating such arrhythmias.

Operative mapping

Accurate mapping is particularly important for patients with ventricular tachycardia. Pre-operative catheter mapping is useful both to enable more rapid operative mapping, because of the prior knowledge of the area of interest, and also to guide resection in patients in whom tachycardia cannot be induced at surgery.

At operation, electrical activation mapping is the most common method used[47-52], and overall seems to be the most reliable. Because most ventricular tachycardias originate in the endocardium or sub-endocardial region, endocardial mapping is to be preferred. Epicardial mapping may help at the beginning of an operation particularly with reference to where the ventriculotomy should be made. Occasional transmural mapping may be needed.

Miller et al.[53] have shown that most tachycardias spread in a centrifugal manner from the site of origin, usually within a 6 cm area, although a minority (10%) of tachycardias have a continuous loop of activation, for example around an aneurysm. It has been suggested that morphologically distinct tachycardias usually arise from a single site[54], but Waspe et al.[55] examined a number of patients with multiple tachycardia morphologies and found that some patients had different morphologies with sites of origins that were identical or were within 3 cm, whilst in others the sites were widely separated.

Cryomapping may be a useful adjunct to activation mapping. Cryo-

Table 22.1   Causes of ventricular tachycardia

Ischaemic heart disease
Cardiomyopathies – hypertrophic
– congestive
– restrictive
Right ventricular dysplasia
Myocarditis
Mitral valve prolapse
Long QT syndrome
Cardiac tumours
Pericardial disease
Trauma
Iatrogenic – drugs
– pacemakers
Idiopathic

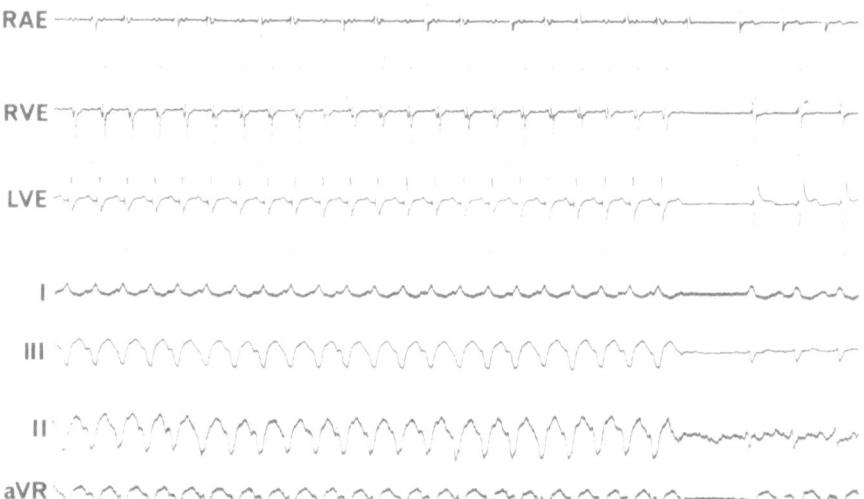

Figure 22.4   Cryomapping of left ventricular tachycardia. The cryoprobe is applied during stable tachycardia and 6 seconds later tachycardia terminates. Further surgery to this area resulted in a successful outcome. Abbreviations and paper speed as before. LVE = left ventricular electrogram

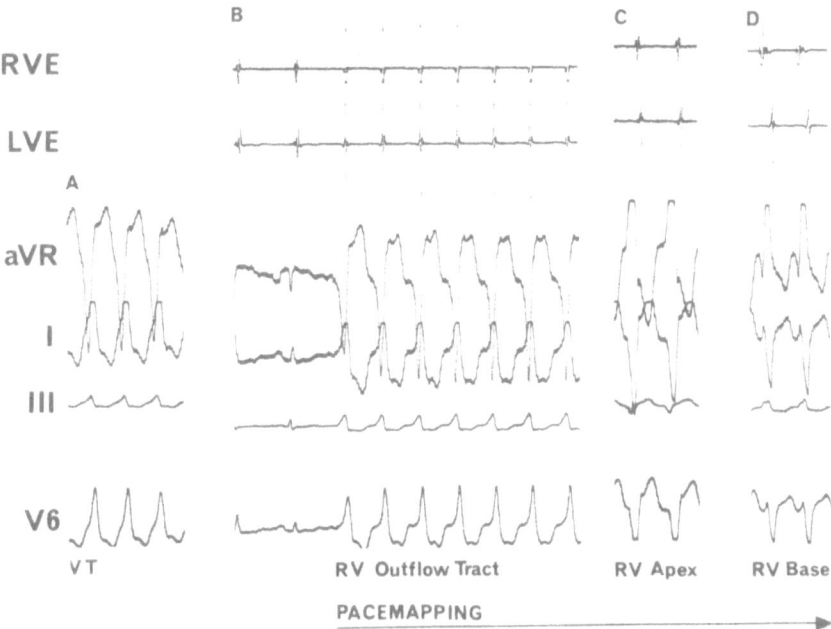

Figure 22.5 Operative endocardial pacemapping. An example of spontaneous tachycardia is shown in panel A. Panel B shows sinus rhythm followed by pacing at a similar rate to tachycardia at a site in the right ventricular outflow tract. The morphology is almost identical to that of tachycardia and is quite unlike that obtained from pacing at other sites, including the right ventricular apex (panel C) or base (panel D). Ablative surgery at the point mapped in panel B was curative. Paper speed and abbreviations as before. VT = spontaneous ventricular tachycardia

thermy at the site of origin (Figure 22.4) can terminate an arrhythmia if it is due to a micro-re-entrant mechanism[56]. In macro-re-entrant tachycardias the late diastolic loop must be cooled in order to effect termination[56], but this effect is usually temporary unless prolonged and deep cryothermy is used. As well as being shown to be effective in canine experiments the technique has been used in man[57].

The main disadvantage of the techniques described above is that tachycardia must be induced and preferably sustained in order for mapping to be performed. Two techniques exist which do not depend on tachycardia induction.

Mapping during sinus rhythm can be used to detect abnormal areas evidenced by delayed or fragmented activity. Richards et al.[58] found this useful as did Wiener et al.[59], but Kienzle et al.[60] found that fragmentation was not always related to the site of earliest activation and in any case tended to overestimate the amount of tissue requiring excision. Pacemapping (Figure 22.5) is a simple technique, where the ventricle is paced to mimic the tachycardia morphology, but may occasionally be misleading particularly because of changes in orientation of the heart and chest wall[61-63]. To speed mapping, and in particular to enable mapping of non-sustained tachycardias, a number of devices have been suggested. These include multi-polar 'sock' electrodes for epicardial mapping[64] and multi-polar endocardial balloon electrodes for endocardial use[65]. Using computer techniques multi-site acquisition and processing is enhanced, as is display[66], but such systems are not widely used at the present time.

Surgical techniques

For ventricular tachycardias not associated with ischaemic heart disease a number of measures have been described. These have included bundle branch resection in patients with bundle branch tachycardias[67], mitral valve replacement for arrhythmias in association with mitral valve prolapse[68,69] and isolation or resection of cardiac tumours which may be causing arrhythmias[70,71].

Simple ventriculotomy has been used (Figure 22.6), particularly for patients with right ventricular arrhythmias[71] but is generally unsuccessful, presumably because of the relatively large area of abnormal

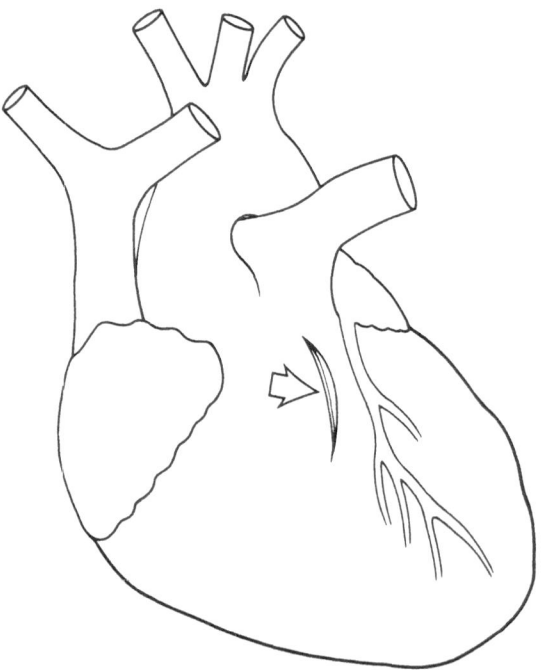

Figure 22.6   Diagram showing a simple right ventricular ventriculotomy

heart involved in an arrhythmia circuit – cutting one limb of the circuit may merely cause tachycardia to re-route elsewhere.

An entity that has been increasingly recognized is ventricular dysplasia which is thought to be a form of cardiomyopathy originating in the right ventricle, but sometimes spreading through the septum to the left. This condition is associated with a high incidence of malignant ventricular arrhythmias and surgical therapy may be necessary. Initially, simple ventriculotomy was attempted for this condition[71], but because the condition tends to be diffuse and also progressive a more radical approach is usually required. Guiraudon et al.[72] pioneered the technique of total disconnection of the right ventricular free wall for this condition, and Cox et al.[73] have also used this type of procedure.

The commonest cause of ventricular tachycardia is coronary artery disease, often following myocardial infarction, particularly when an aneurysm or scar is present. Early reports suggested that in such cases tachycardia control could be achieved with coronary artery bypass grafting alone[74–76], but recent studies have shown that this form of treatment is rarely effective[77]. Similarly, although aneurysmectomy with or without revascularization has been suggested as being effective therapy for ventricular tachycardias[78–80] other reports are pessimistic about its value[77,81,82]. Buda et al.[81] reported an overall mortality of 37.5% in patients treated by revascularization with or without aneurysmectomy for ventricular tachycardia, with 50% of the survivors having to take antiarrhythmic therapy. Mason et al.[82] later re-examined these patients, comparing the results of 32 patients who had left ventricular aneurysmectomy for ventricular tachycardia with 18 who had activation sequence mapping with map directed surgery. The former group had an arrhythmia recurrence rate of 50%, whereas the latter group had a much lower recurrence rate of only 11%. Sami et al.[83] also had poor results with non-guided aneurysmectomy, with a 20% mortality. Only three of their eight survivors had no evidence of ventricular tachycardia without the additional use of antiarrhythmic drugs, and two of these suffered from palpitations due to ventricular premature beats.

The reason for these failures is that the focus of a tachycardia is rarely actually within an aneurysm or scar (Figure 22.7), as this tissue is dead, but is usually in the border areas surrounding such lesions[84,85]. Several methods have been devised to resect or isolate sufficient tissue to ablate such arrhythmias. Although full thickness myocardial resection has been performed[51,58] it involves unnecessary resection of contractile tissue as the vast majority of foci are within the endocardium. Therefore, a number of different approaches have been devised to ablate or isolate the offending myocardium. Guiraudon et al.[84] have described an isolation procedure – the encircling endocardial ventriculotomy – designed to exclude the entire diseased area (Figure 22.8). However, the survival of residual myocardium distal to this incision may be jeopardized[86], and except for foci on vital structures such as papillary muscles (which retain sufficient blood supply to remain viable) the technique probably does not represent an ideal solution.

It seemed logical to attempt resection of the endocardium (Figure 22.9), and this technique was first described by Josephson *et al.* in 1979[87]. Miller *et al.*[88], working with Josephson, reviewed the first 100 patients who had undergone mapping guided endocardial resection at their institution. There were 91 survivors of surgery with 200 morphologically distinct types of tachycardia. 66% of patients were cured by surgery alone and a further 25% were cured by surgery with additional anti-arrhythmic drug therapy. There were four late sudden deaths and four patients continued to have episodes of ventricular tachycardia. The factors associated with failure included disparate sites of tachycardia origin, multiple morphologies of spontaneous tachycardia, the absence of a discreet left ventricular aneurysm and an inferior wall site of origin of tachycardia. Other groups have attempted endocardial resection without mapping using only visual guidance, removing all visually scarred endocardium[89]. This may be effective in many patients, but there is no doubt that in some patients the mapped site of origin is distinct from any visible scar. A number of other groups have reported results using endocardial resection, usually with mapping. McGiffin *et al.*[90]

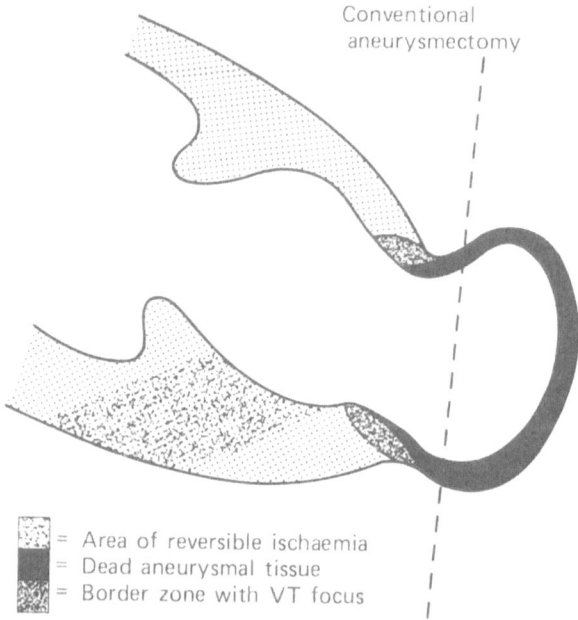

Figure 22.7 Diagrammatic section through heart in a patient who has a left ventricular aneurysm. The dead aneurysmal tissue is shown together with an area of reversible ischaemia which is remote from the actual border zone which has the ventricular tachycardia focus

390

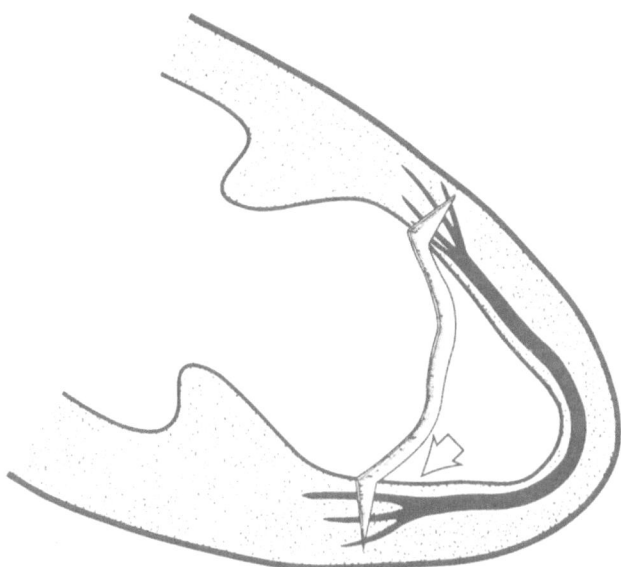

Figure 22.8 Diagram showing a section through the heart with an encircling endocardial ventriculotomy. The tachycardia focus is arrowed and is in the border zone

treated 123 patients with a 3-year survival of 46%, only 41% were alive without recurrence of VT at 3 years. Garan *et al.*[91] treated 36 patients with endocardial resection following mapping, with a mortality rate of 17%. All patients discharged from hospital were alive at the end of the follow-up period, but 12 required antiarrhythmic drug therapy at discharge, and two had a non-fatal sustained ventricular tachycardia after discharge. Patients with ventricular tachycardia following an inferior infarct show a worse prognosis than others. To address this problem, Josephson's group[92] have treated such patients using focal endocardial cryoablation of the annular isthmus as well as endocardial resection and they have achieved considerably improved results.

Endocardial resection is not thought to have any long-term adverse effect on ventricular function. Martin *et al.*[93] have examined this in detail, with very favourable results.

Cryosurgery (Figure 22.10) has been used by a number of authors[94,95] as both the sole ablative technique and also as an adjunct. Cryosurgery is attractive because collagen and fibroblasts are relatively resistant to cryothermal injury, and this enables treated areas to retain their strength and show resistance to rupture or aneurysm formation. Holman *et al.*[96] have shown that regional myocardial bloodflow in the regions surrounding and below the cryolesions is preserved, and that histologically there is a clear demarcation between damaged and normal tissue. Plumb *et al.*[97] treated 12 consecutive patients with cryosurgery.

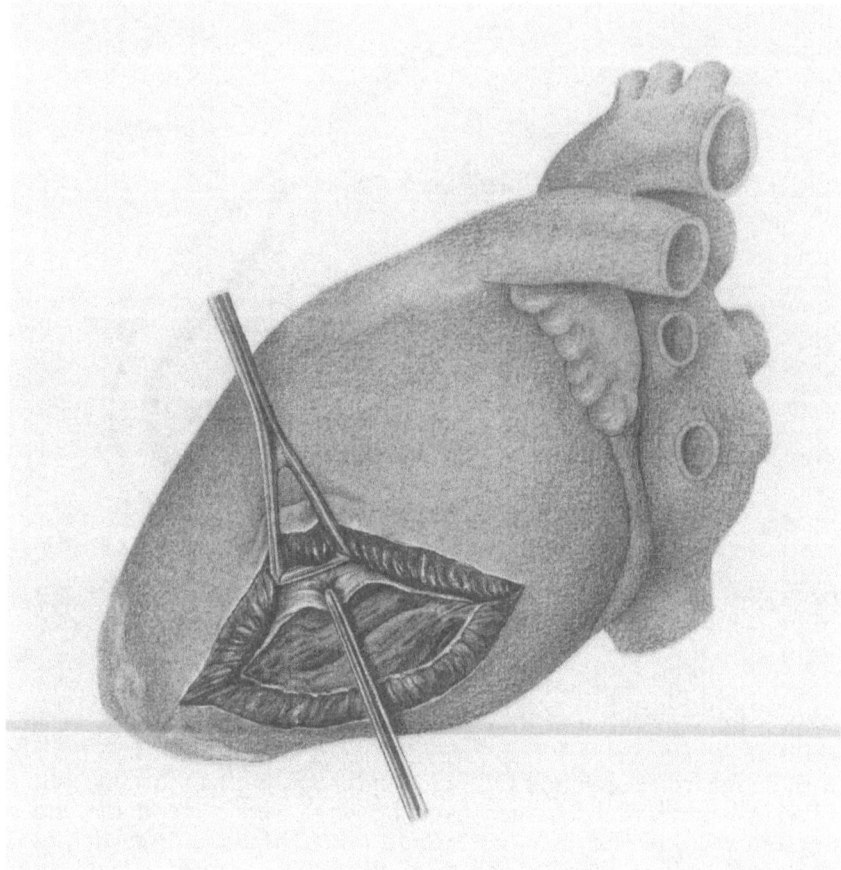

Figure 22.9 This demonstrates the technique of ventricular endocardial stripping and resection. The posterior aspect of the heart is shown

Although one patient died, 11 were treated satisfactorily with only one requiring additional antiarrhythmic drug therapy. There was no evidence of deterioration of left ventricular function. Guiraudon et al.[98] used a technique of encircling endocardial cryoablation with a series of overlapping cryolesions. Ventricular tachycardia could not be induced in either of the patients described, and both were sent home without antiarrhythmic medication. Krafchek et al.[99] used cryothermia from both sides of the interventricular septum in five patients with septal foci; all five were successfully treated although one patient had a postoperative recurrence and died later from congestive heart failure.

Tachycardias arising from the area of the papillary muscle, particularly the posterior papillary muscle, have certainly presented a problem, and cryosurgery in particular has been used. However, Kron *et al.*[100] noted papillary muscle scarring in 15 patients from a series of 46 undergoing map directed endocardial resection. Eleven patients had ventricular tachycardia with a site of origin on a scarred papillary muscle, whereas in four another site of origin was implicated. Six patients underwent papillary muscle scar resection (five with mitral valve replacement) and six underwent papillary muscle cryothermy. All six patients who underwent resection were alive and free of arrhythmia at follow-up, but five of the six patients treated by cryoablation alone had ventricular tachycardia during follow-up.

Cautery (diathermy) has been used for treating ventricular arrhythmias, but has the disadvantage that heat denatures collagen and destroys fibroblasts thus weakening the heart. In addition, it certainly cannot be used to effect a reproducible reversible state of dysfunction for mapping.

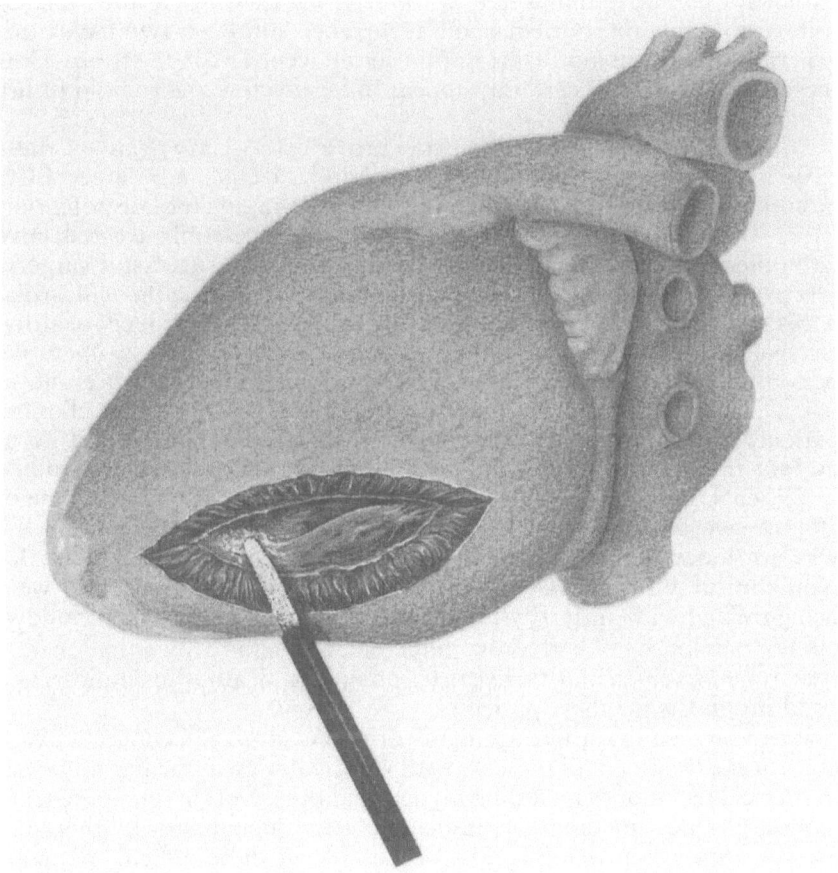

Figure 22.10   This is a diagram showing endocardial ventricular cryoablation. As with the previous illustration the posterior aspect of the heart is shown

There are of course limitations to the surgical management of patients with ventricular tachycardia. Patients in the first few weeks following acute myocardial infarction are particularly high risk candidates for surgery[101], but the risk of surgery in such patients is probably acceptable[102–104] bearing in mind their prognosis without surgery.

A new technique which is gaining popularity is the use of laser therapy for tachyarrhythmias, a subject that has been recently reviewed by Saksena and Gadhoke[105]. Downar et al.[106] have used an excimer laser in animal hearts and have shown sharp demarcation between the region of injury and normal tissue. Svenson et al.[107] have used an Nd-YAG laser photocoagulator to treat five patients. Following lasing, delayed potentials were abolished and ventricular tachycardia could not be induced post-operatively. Mesnildrey et al.[108] have used a similar type of laser to treat 22 patients using encircling thermo-exclusion. Nineteen patients were arrhythmia-free without drug therapy at the time of follow-up. Only one patient had a recurrence, although two have died; generally there was no deterioration in left ventricular function. Thus these laser techniques certainly appear to be effective and to hold future promise.

Follow-up and meticulous postoperative care is important in these patients. In the early post-operative period careful ambulatory ECG monitoring and telemetry is essential, signal averaging for late potentials is also valuable as many patients who are successfully treated have late potentials present before surgery but not after successful surgery. Electrophysiological assessment is also important, using either epicardial wires placed at the time of surgery, or using standard endocardial electrodes. The absence of inducible tachycardia in the post-operative period is a good predictor of clinical freedom from recurrence and in particular freedom from sudden death. However, in some of these patients non-clinical ventricular tachycardia can be induced and Borggrefe et al.[109] have examined the clinical significance of this. They studied 75 patients undergoing surgery, with a mortality of 6.6%. Sixty-nine of 70 post-operative survivors underwent electrophysiological testing. VT was not inducible in 41 patients, but clinical VT was inducible in 13. Non-clinical VT was induced in 15 patients of whom only two were being treated with antiarrhythmic drugs. However, at 2 years of follow-up no patient who had only inducible non-clinical VT had had a spontaneous ventricular tachycardia or sudden death, thus indicating a good prognosis for these patients.

It can be seen that there are many different surgical techniques available for the treatment of patients with ventricular tachycardia. Advances in surgical techniques including myocardial preservation, mapping techniques, and new methods of surgical ablation including laser therapies are constantly improving results obtainable in these difficult patients. There is still a significant operative mortality but many are not treatable in any other way. Even the advent of the implantable cardioverter/defibrillator has not negated the need for surgery in many patients; there are a considerable number who suffer from such frequent and debilitating attacks of tachycardia that an implantable device would not be appropriate.

References

1. Yee, R., Guiraudon, G. M., Gardener, M. J., Gulamhusein, S. S. and Klein, G. J. (1984). Refractory paroxysmal sinus tachycardia: management by subtotal right atrial exclusion. *J. Am. Coll. Cardiol.*, **3**, 400–4
2. Guiraudon, G. M., Klein, G. J., Sharma, A. D., Yee, R. and McLellan, D. G. (1986). Surgical treatment of supraventricular tachycardia: a five-year experience. *PACE*, **9**, 1376–80
3. Coumel, P., Aigueperse, J., Perrault, M.-A., Fantoni, A., Slama R. and Bouvrain, Y. (1973). Reperage et tentative d'exerese chirurgicale d'un foyer ectopique auriculaire gauche avec tachycardie rebelle: evolution favourable. *Ann. Cardiol., Angeiol.* *(Paris)*, **22**, 189–99
4. Gillette, P. C., Garson, A. Jr, Colley, D. A. and McNamara, D. G. (1981). Definitive surgical treatment of atrial automatic ectopic focus tachycardias. *Circulation*, **64**, IV–225
5. Russell, P. A., Johnson, D. C., Denniss, A. R. and Uther, J. B. (1982). Surgical management of right atrial tachycardia. *Am. J. Cardiol.*, **49**, 994
6. Iwa, T., Ichihashi, T., Hashizume, Y., Ishida, K. and Okada, R. (1985). Successful surgical treatment of left atrial tachycardia. *Am. Heart J.*, **109**, 160–2
7. Olsson, S. B., Blomstrom, P., Sabel, K.-G. and William-Olsson, G. (1984). Incessant ectopic atrial tachycardia: successful surgical treatment with regression of dilated cardiomyopathy picture. *Am. J. Cardiol.*, **53**, 1465–6
8. Josephson, M. E., Spear, J. F., Harken, A. H., Horowitz, L. N. and Dorio, R. J. (1982). Surgical excision of automatic atrial tachycardia: anatomic and electrophysiologic correlates. *Am. Heart J.*, **104**, 1076–85
9. Gallagher, J. J., Cox, J. L., German, L. D. and Kasell, J. H. (1984). Non-pharmacologic treatment of supraventricular tachycardia. In Josephson, M. E. and Wellens, H. J. J. (eds.). *Tachycardias: Mechanisms, Diagnosis, Treatment*, pp. 271–85. (Philadelphia: Lea and Febiger)
10. Bredikis, J. J., Bukauskas, R. I., Lekas, J. J., Sakalauskas, J. J., Bredikis, A. J., Laurushonis, K. A., Putelis, R. A. and Turkevichius, G. S. (1986). Surgery in tachycardia treatment. *PACE*, **9**, 1403–6
11. Klein, G. J., Guiraudon, G. M., Sharma, A. D. and Milstein, S. (1986). Demonstration of macrore-entry and feasibility of operative therapy in the common type of atrial flutter. *Am. J. Cardiol.*, **57**, 587–91
12. Guiraudon, G. M., Campbell, C. S., Jones, D. L., McLellan, D. G. and MacDonald, J. L. (1985). Combined sino-atrial node atrio-ventricular isolation: a surgical alternative to His bundle ablation in patients with atrial fibrillation. *Circulation*, **72**, III–220
13. Giannelli, S. Jr, Ayres, S. M., Gomprecht, R. F., Conklin, E. F. and Kennedy, R. J. (1967). Therapeutic surgical division of the human conduction system. *J. Am. Med. Assoc.*, **199**, 155–60
14. Slama, R., Blondeau, P., Aigueperse, J., Cachera, J., Degeorges, M. and Albou, E. (1967). Creation chirurgical d'un bloc auriculoventriculaire et implantation d'un stimulateur dans deux cas de troubles du rythme irreductibles. *Arch. Mal. Coeur*, **60**, 406–22
15. Harrison, L., Gallagher, J. J., Kasell, J., Anderson, R. H., Mikat, E., Hackel, D. B. and Wallace, A. G. (1977). Cryosurgical ablation of the AV node–His bundle: a new method for producing AV block. *Circulation*, **55**, 463–70
16. Bredikis, J. (1985). Cryosurgical ablation of atrioventricular junction without extracorporeal circulation. *J. Thorac. Cardiovasc. Surg.*, **90**, 61–7

17. Sealy, W. C., Anderson, R. W. and Gallagher, J. J. (1977). Surgical treatment of supraventricular tachyarrhythmias. *J. Thorac. Cardiovasc. Surg.*, 73, 511–22
18. Ross, D. L., Johnson, D. C., Denniss, A. R., Cooper, M. J., Richards, D. A. and Uther, J. B. (1985). Curative surgery for atrioventricular junctional ('AV Nodal') reentrant tachycardia. *J. Am. Coll. Cardiol.*, 6, 1383–92
19. Scheinman, M. M. (1985). Atrioventricular nodal or atriojunctional reentrant tachycardia? *J. Am. Coll. Cardiol.*, 6, 1393–4
20. Cox, J. L. and Cain, M. E. (1987). Discrete cryosurgical ablation of atrioventricular node reentry tachycardia in patients. *J. Am. Coll. Cardiol.*, 9, 249A
21. Holman, W. L., Ikeshita, M., Lease, J. G., Ferguson, T. B., Lofland, G. K. and Cox, J. L. (1984). Alteration of antegrade atrioventricular conduction by cryoablation of peri-atrioventricular nodal tissue. *J. Thorac. Cardiovasc. Surg.*, 88, 67–75
22. Edmonds, J. H. Jr, Ellison, R. G. and Crews, T. L. (1969). Surgically induced atrioventricular block as treatment for recurrent atrial tachycardia in Wolff–Parkinson–White Syndrome. *Circulation*, 39, I–105–I–111
23. Cartwright, R. S., Smeloff, E. A., Cayler, C. G., Fong, W. Y., Huntley, A. C., Blake, J. R. and McFall, R. A. (1964). Total correction of Ebstein's anomaly by means of tricuspid replacement. *J. Thorac. Cardiovasc. Surg.*, 47, 755–61
24. Lillehei, C. W., Kalke, B. R. and Carlson, R. G. (1967). Evolution of corrective surgery for Ebstein's anomaly. *Circulation*, 35, I–111–I–118
25. Cobb, F. R., Blumenschein, S. D., Sealy, W. C., Boineau, J. P., Wagner, G. S. and Wallace, A. G. (1968). Successful surgical interruption of the bundle of Kent in a patient with Wolff–Parkinson–White syndrome. *Circulation*, 38, 1018–29
26. Sealy, W. C., Hattler, B. G., Blumenschein, S. D. and Cobb, F. R. (1969). Surgical treatment of Wolff–Parkinson–White syndrome. *Ann. Thorac. Surg.*, 8, 1–11
27. Gallagher, J. J., Gilbert, M., Svenson, R. H., Sealy, W. C., Kasell, J. and Wallace, A. G. (1975). Wolff–Parkinson–White syndrome: the problem, evaluation, and surgical correction. *Circulation*, 51, 767–85
28. Gallagher, J. J., Sealy, W. C., Anderson, R. W., Kasell, J., Millar, R., Campbell, R. W. F., Harrison, L., Pritchett, E. L. C. and Wallace, A. G. (1977). Cryosurgical ablation of accessory atrioventricular connections: a method for correction of the pre-excitation syndrome. *Circulation*, 55, 471–9
29. Sealy, W. C. and Gallagher, J. J. (1981). Surgical problems with multiple accessory pathways of atrioventricular conduction. *J. Thorac. Cardiovasc. Surg.*, 81, 707–12
30. Sealy, W. C. and Gallagher, J. J. (1981). Surgical treatment of left free wall accessory pathways of atrioventricular conduction of the Kent type. *J. Thorac. Cardiovasc. Surg.*, 81, 698–706
31. Guiraudon, G. M., Klein, G. J., Gulamhusein, S., Jones, D. L., Yee, R., Perkins, G. and Jarvis, E. (1983). Surgical correction of the Wolff–Parkinson–White syndrome: a new closed-heart technique. *J. Am. Coll. Cardiol.*, 1, 687
32. Guiraudon, G. M., Klein, G. M., Sharma, A. D., Jones, D. L. and McLellan, D. G. (1986). Surgery for Wolff–Parkinson–White syndrome: further experience with an epicardial approach. *Circulation*, 74, 525–9
33. Gallagher, J. J., Selle, J. G., Sealy, W. C., Fedor, J. M., Svenson, R. H. and Zimmern, S. H. (1986). Intermediate septal accessory pathway (IS–AP): a subset of pre-excitation at risk for complete heart block/failure during WPW surgery. *Circulation*, 74, II–387
34. Klein, G. J., Guiraudon, G. M., Perkins, D. G., Jones, D. L., Yee, R. and Jarvis, E. (1984). Surgical correction of the Wolff–Parkinson–White syndrome in the closed heart using cryosurgery: a simplified approach. *J. Am. Coll. Cardiol.*, 3, 405–9
35. Guiraudon, G. M., Klein, G. J., Sharma, A. D., Jones, D. L. and McLellan, D. G. (1986). Surgical ablation of posterior septal accessory pathways in the Wolff–Parkinson–White syndrome by a closed heart technique. *J. Thorac. Cardiovasc. Surg.*, 92, 406–13
36. Gallagher, J. J., Sealy, W. C., Cox, J. L., German, L. D., Kasell J. H., Bardy G. H. and Packer, D. L. (1984). Results of surgery for pre-excitation caused by accessory

atrioventricular pathways in 267 consecutive cases. In Josephson, M. E. and Wellens, H. J. J. (eds.) *Tachycardias: Mechanisms, Diagnosis, Treatment*, pp. 259–69. (Philadelphia: Lea and Febiger)

37. Cox, J. L., Gallagher, J. J. and Cain, M. E. (1985). Experience with 118 consecutive patients undergoing operation for the Wolff–Parkinson–White Syndrome. *J. Thorac. Cardiovasc. Surg.*, **90**, 490–501

38. Nathan, A. W., Bexton, R. S., Edmondson, S. J., Rees, G. M., Spurrell, R. A. J. and Camm, A. J. (1984). Surgical treatment of supraventricular arrhythmias. *Br. Heart J.*, **51**, 104–5

39. Bredikis, J., Bukauskas, F., Zebrauskas, R., Sakalauskas, J., Loschilov, V., Nevsky, V., Bredikis, A. and Liakas, R. (1985). Cryosurgical ablation of right parietal and septal accessory atrioventricular connections without the use of extracorporeal circulation: a new surgical technique. *J. Thorac. Cardiovasc. Surg.*, **90**, 206–11

40. Bredikis, J. and Bredikis, A. (1985). Cryosurgical ablation of left parietal wall accessory atrioventricular connections through the coronary sinus without the use of extracorporeal circulation. *J. Thorac. Cardiovasc. Surg.*, **90**, 199–205

41. Lin, H.-T., Lawrie, G., Magro, S., Krafchek, J., Beckman, K., Robertson, N. and Wyndham, C. (1987). Total atriotomy improves results of transection of multiple accessory pathways. *J. Am. Coll. Cardiol.*, **9**, 100A

42. Mitsui, T., Yamagushi, I., Koishizawa, T., Terada, Y., Kuga, K. and Hori M. (1986). Left thoracic sympathectomy for treatment of refractory re-entrant tachycardia in concealed Wolff–Parkinson–White syndrome. *Am. J. Cardiol.*, **57**, 995–7

43. Prystowsky, E. N., Pressley, J. C., Gallagher, J., Lowe, J. E., Sealy, W., Cox, J., Pritchett, E., Pryor, D. and German, L. D. (1987). The quality of life and arrhythmia status after surgery for Wolff–Parkinson–White syndrome: an 18-year perspective. *J. Am. Coll. Cardiol.*, **9**, 100A

44. Fischell, T. A., Stinson, E. B., Derby, G. C. and Swerdlow, C. D. (1987). Long-term follow-up after surgical correction of Wolff–Parkinson–White syndrome. *J. Am. Coll. Cardiol.*, **9**, 283–7

45. Sharma, A. D., Klein, G. J., Guiraudon, G. M. and Milstein, S. (1985). Atrial fibrillation in patients with Wolff–Parkinson–White syndrome: incidence after surgical ablation of the accessory pathway. *Circulation*, **72**, 161–9

46. Cox, J. L. (1985). The status of surgery for cardiac arrhythmias. *Circulation*, **71**, 413–17

47. Guiraudon, G., Frank, R. and Fontaine, G. (1974). Interet des cartographies dans le traitement chirurgical des tachycardies ventriculaires rebelles recidivantes. *Nouv. Presse Med.*, **3**, 321

48. Gallagher, J. J., Oldham, H. N., Wallace, A. G., Peter, R. H. and Kasell, J. (1975). Ventricular aneurysm with ventricular tachycardia: report of a case with epicardial mapping and successful resection. *Am. J. Cardiol.*, **35**, 696–700

49. Gallagher, J. J., Kasell, J. H., Cox, J. L., Ideker, R. E. and Smith, W. M. (1982). Techniques of intraoperative electrophysiologic mapping. *Am. J. Cardiol.*, **49**, 221–40

50. Spurrell, R. A. J., Yates, A. K., Thornburn, C. W., Sowton, G. E. and Deuchar, D. C. (1975). Surgical treatment of ventricular tachycardia after epicardial mapping studies. *Br. Heart J.*, **37**, 115–26

51. Wittig, J. H. and Boineau, J. P. (1975). Surgical treatment of ventricular arrhythmias using epicardial, transmural, and endocardial mapping. *Ann. Thorac. Surg.*, **20**, 117–26

52. Josephson, M. E., Horowitz, L. N., Spielman, S. R., Greenspan, A. M., VandePol, C. and Harken, A. H. (1980). Comparison of endocardial catheter mapping with intraoperative mapping of ventricular tachycardia. *Circulation*, **61**, 395–404

53. Miller, J. M., Harken, A. H., Hargrove, W. C. and Josephson, M. E. (1985). Pattern of endocardial activation during sustained ventricular tachycardia. *J. Am. Coll. Cardiol.*, **6**, 1280–7

54. Josephson, M. E., Horowitz, L. N., Farshidi, A., Spielman, S. R., Michaelson, E. L. and Greenspan, A. M. (1979). Recurrent sustained ventricular tachycardia. 4. Pleomorphism. *Circulation*, 59, 459–68

55. Waspe, L. E., Brodman, R., Kim, S. G., Matos, J. A., Johnston, D. R., Scavin, G. M. and Fisher, J. D. (1985). Activation mapping in patients with coronary artery disease with multiple ventricular tachycardia configurations: occurrence and therapeutic implications of widely separate apparent sites of origin. *J. Am. Coll. Cardiol.*, 5, 1075–86

56. Gessman, L., Endo, T., Egan, J. and Maroko, P. R. (1983). Dissociation of the site of origin from the site of cryotermination of ventricular tachycardia. *Circulation*, 68, III–146

57. Gallagher J. D., Del Rossi, A. J., Fernandez, J., Maranhao, V., Strong, M. D., White, M. and Gessman, L. J. (1985). Cryothermal mapping of recurrent ventricular tachycardia in man. *Circulation*, 71, 733–9

58. Richards, D. A., Denniss, A. R., Johnson, D. C. and Uther, J. B. (1983). Mechanism of cure of ventricular tachycardia by mapping directed surgery. *J. Am. Coll. Cardiol.*, 1, 687.

59. Wiener, I., Mindich, B. and Pitchon, R. (1984). Fragmented endocardial electrical activity in patients with ventricular tachycardia: a new guide to surgical therapy. *Am. Heart J.*, 107, 86–90

60. Kienzle, M. G., Falcone, R. A., Kempf, F. C., Miller, J. M., Harken, A. H. and Josephson, M. E. (1983). Intraoperative endocardial mapping: relation of fractionated electrograms in sinus rhythm to endocardial activation in ventricular tachycardia – surgical implications. *J. Am. Coll. Cardiol.*, 1, 582

61. Curry, P. V. L., O'Keefe, D. B., Pitcher, D., Sowton, E., Deverall, P. B. and Yates, A. K. (1979). Localisation of ventricular tachycardia by a new technique – pace-mapping. *Circulation*, 60, II–25

62. Waxman, H. L. and Josephson, M. E. (1982). Ventricular activation during ventricular endocardial pacing. I. Electrocardiographic patterns related to the site of pacing. *Am. J. Cardiol.*, 50, 1–10

63. Josephson, M. E., Waxman, H. L., Cain, M. E., Gardener, M. J. and Buxton, A. E. (1982). Ventricular activation during ventricular endocardial pacing. II. Role of pacemapping to localize origin of ventricular tachycardia. *Am. J. Cardiol.*, 50, 11–22

64. Worley, S. J., Ideker, R. E., Mastrototaro, J., Smith, W. M., Vidaillet, H. Jr, Chen, P.-S. and Lowe, J. E. (1987). A new sock electrode for recording epicardial activation from the human heart: one size fits all. *PACE*, 10, 21–31

65. de Bakker, J. M. T., Janse, M. J., Van Capelle, F. J. L. and Durrer, D. (1983). Endocardial mapping by simultaneous recording of endocardial electrograms during cardiac surgery for ventricular aneurysm. *J. Am. Coll. Cardiol.*, 2, 947–53

66. Ideker, R. E., Smith, W. M., Wolf, P., Danieley, N. D. and Bartram, F. R. (1987). Simultaneous multichannel cardiac mapping systems. *PACE*, 10, 281–92

67. Spurrell, R. A. J., Sowton, E. and Deuchar, D. C. (1973). Ventricular tachycardia in 4 patients evaluated by programmed electrical stimulation of heart and treated in 2 patients by surgical division of anterior radiation of left bundle-branch. *Br. Heart J.*, 35, 1014–25

68. Cobbs, B. W. Jr and King, S. B. III. (1974). Mechanism of abnormal ventriculogram (VGM) and ECG associated with prolapsing mitral valve (PMV). *Circulation*, 50, III–7

69. Krikler, D. (1980). Ventricular tachycardia and ventricular fibrillation. In Mandel, W. J. (ed.). *Cardiac Arrhythmias: their Mechanisms, Diagnosis, and Management*, pp. 320–341. (Philadelphia: J B Lippincott)

70. Engle, M. A., Ebert, P. A. and Redo, S. F. (1974). Recurrent ventricular tachycardia due to resectable cardiac tumour: report of two cases in two-year-olds in heart failure. *Circulation*, 50, 1052–7

71. Fontaine, G., Guiraudon, G., Frank, R., Fillette, F., Cabrol, C. and Grosgogeat, Y. (1982). Surgical management of ventricular tachycardia unrelated to myocardial ischemia or infarction. *Am. J. Cardiol.*, 49, 397–410

72. Guiraudon, G. M., Klein, G. J., Gulamhusein, S. S., Painvin, G. A., Del Campo, C., Gonzales, J. C. and Ko, P. T. (1983). Total disconnection of the right ventricular free wall: surgical treatment of right ventricular tachycardia associated with right ventricular dysplasia. *Circulation*, 67, 463–70

73. Cox, J. L., Bardy, G. H., Damiano, R. J. Jr, German, L. D., Fedor, J. M., Kisslo, J. A., Packer, D. L. and Gallagher, J. J. (1985). Right ventricular isolation procedures for nonischemic ventricular tachycardia. *J. Thorac. Cardiovasc. Surg.*, 90, 212–24

74. Ecker, R. R., Mullins, C. B., Grammer, J. C., Rea, W. J. and Atkins, J. M. (1971). Control of intractable ventricular tachycardia by coronary revascularization. *Circulation*, 44, 666–70

75. Bryson, A. L., Parisi, A. F., Schechter, E. and Wolfson, S. (1973). Life-threatening ventricular arrhythmias induced by exercise: cessation after coronary bypass surgery. *Am. J. Cardiol.*, 32, 995–9

76. Tilkain, A.-G., Pfeifer, J. F., Barry, W. H., Lipton, M. J. and Hultgren, H. N. (1976). Effect of coronary bypass surgery on exercise-induced ventricular arrhythmias. *Am. Heart J.*, 92, 707–14

77. Ricks, W. B., Winkle, R. A., Shumway, N. E. and Harrison, D. C. (1977). Surgical management of life-threatening ventricular arrhythmias in patients with coronary artery disease. *Circulation*, 56, 38–42

78. Couch, O. A. (1959). Cardiac aneurysm with ventricular tachycardia and subsequent excision of aneurysm: case report. *Circulation*, 20, 251–3

79. Graham, A. F., Miller, D. C., Stinson, E. B., Daily, P. O., Fogarty, T. J. and Harrison, D. C. (1973). Surgical treatment of refractory life-threatening ventricular tachycardia. *Am. J. Cardiol.*, 32, 909–12

80. Loop, F. D., Effler, D. B., Navia, J. A., Sheldon, W. C. and Groves, L. K. (1973). Aneurysms of the left ventricle: survival and results of a ten-year surgical experience. *Ann. Surg.*, 178, 399–405

81. Buda, A. J., Stinson, E. B. and Harrison, D. C. (1979). Surgery for life-threatening ventricular tachyarrhythmias. *Am. J. Cardiol.*, 44, 1171–7

82. Mason, J. W., Stinson, E. B., Winkle, R. A., Oyer, P. E., Griffin, J. C. and Ross, D. L. (1982). Relative efficacy of blind left ventricular aneurysm resection for the treatment of recurrent ventricular tachycardia. *Am. J. Cardiol.*, 49, 241–8

83. Sami, M., Chaitman, B. R., Bourassa, M. G., Charpin, D. and Chabot, M. (1978). Long-term follow-up of aneurysmectomy for recurrent ventricular tachycardia or fibrillation. *Am. Heart J.*, 96, 303–8

84. Guiraudon, G., Fontaine, G., Frank, R., Escande, G., Etievant, P. and Cabrol, C. (1978). Encircling endocardial ventriculotomy: a new surgical treatment for life-threatening ventricular tachycardias resistant to medical treatment following myocardial infarction. *Ann. Thorac. Surg.*, 26, 438–44

85. Horowitz, L. N., Harken, A. H., Kastor, J. A. and Josephson, M. E. (1980). Ventricular resection guided by epicardial and endocardial mapping for treatment of recurrent ventricular tachycardia. *N. Engl. J. Med.*, 302, 589–93

86. Borggrefe, M., Breithardt, G., Ostermeyer, J. and Bircks, W. (1983). Long-term efficacy of endocardial encircling ventriculotomy for ventricular tachycardia: complete versus partial incision. *Circulation*, 68, III–176

87. Josephson, M. E., Harken, A. H. and Horowitz, L. N. (1979). Endocardial excision: a new surgical technique for the treatment of recurrent ventricular tachycardia. *Circulation*, 60, 1430–9

88. Miller, J. M., Kienzle, M. G., Harken, A. H. and Josephson, M. E. (1984). Subendocardial resection for ventricular tachycardia: predictors of surgical success. *Circulation*, 70, 624–31

89. Gardner, M. J., Landymore, R. W., Johnstone, D. E. and Kinley, C. E. (1985). Visually-directed endocardial resection for recurrent ventricular tachycardia: long-term results and effect on LV function. *Circulation*, 72, III–221

90. McGiffin, D. C., Kirklin, J. K., Plumb, V. J., Waldo, A. L., Blackstone, E. H. and Kirklin, J. W. (1986). Survival and relief of life-threatening ventricular tachycardia after direct operations. *Circulation*, 74, II–460

91. Garan, H., Nguyen, K., McGovern, B., Buckley, M. and Ruskin, J. N. (1986). Perioperative and long-term results after electrophysiologically directed ventricular surgery for recurrent ventricular tachycardia. *J. Am. Coll. Cardiol.*, **8**, 201–9

92. Hargrove, W. C., III, Miller, J. M., Vassallo, J. A. and Josephson, M. E. (1986). Improved results in the operative management of ventricular tachycardia related to inferior wall infarction. *J. Thorac. Cardiovasc. Surg.*, **92**, 726–32

93. Martin, J. L., Untereker, W. J., Harken, A. H., Horowitz, L. N. and Josephson, M. E. (1982). Aneurysmectomy and endocardial resection for ventricular tachycardia: favorable hemodynamic and antiarrhythmic results in patients with global left ventricular dysfunction. *Am. Heart J.* **103**, 960–5

94. Camm, J., Ward, D. E., Cory-Pearce, R., Rees, G. M. and Spurrell, R. A. J. (1979). The successful cryosurgical treatment of paroxysmal ventricular tachycardia. *Chest*, **75**, 621–4

95. Klein, G. J., Harrison, L., Ideker, R. F., Smith, W. M., Kasell, J., Wallace A. G. and Gallagher, J. J. (1979). Reaction of the myocardium to cryosurgery: electrophysiology and arrhythmogenic potential. *Circulation*, **59**, 364–72

96. Holman, W. L., Ikeshita, M., Lease, J. G., Ungerleider, R. M. and Cox, J. L. (1983). Regional myocardial blood flow within and surrounding cardiac cryolesions. *J. Am. Coll. Cardiol.*, **1**, 687

97. Plumb, V. J., McGiffin, D. C., Kirkin, J. K., Henthorn, R. W., Epstein, A. E. and Waldo, A. L. (1985). Cryosurgery for ventricular tachycardia. *J. Am. Coll. Cardiol.*, **5**, 409

98. Guiraudon, G. M., Klein, G. J., Vermeulen, F. E., Yee, R. and Van Hemel, N. M. (1983). Encircling endocardial cryoablation: a technique for surgical treatment of ventricular tachycardia after myocardial infarction. *Circulation*, **68**, III–176

99. Krafchek, J., Lawrie, G. M. and Wyndham, C. R. C. (1986). Cryoablation of arrhythmias from the interventricular septum: initial experience with a new biventricular approach. *J. Thorac. Cardiovasc. Surg.*, **91**, 419–27

100. Kron, I. L., DiMarco, J. P., Nolan, S. P. and Lerman, B. B. (1986). Resection of scarred papillary muscles improves outcome after surgery for ventricular tachycardia. *Ann. Surg.*, **203**, 685–90

101. Marchlinski, F. E., Waxman, H. L., Buxton, A. E. and Josephson, M. E. (1983). Sustained ventricular tachyarrhythmias during the early postinfarction period: electrophysiologic findings and prognosis for survival. *J. Am. Coll. Cardiol.*, **2**, 240–50

102. Miller J. M., Marchlinski, F. E., Harken, A. H., Hargrove, W. C. and Josephson, M. E. (1985). Subendocardial resection for sustained ventricular tachycardia in the early period after acute myocardial infarction. *Am. J. Cardiol.*, **55**, 980–4

103. DiMarco, J. P., Lerman, B. B., Kron, I. L. and Sellers, T. D. (1985). Sustained ventricular tachyarrhythmias within 2 months of acute myocardial infarction: results of medical and surgical therapy in patients resuscitated from the initial episode. *J. Am. Coll. Cardiol.*, **6**, 759–68

104. Bourke, J., Tansuphaswadikul, S., Cowan, J. C., Hilton, C. J. and Campbell, R. W. F. (1987). Surgical management of ventricular arrhythmias within two months of myocardial infarction. *Br. Heart J.*, **57**, 63.

105. Saksena, S. and Gadhoke, A. (1986). Laser therapy for tachyarrhythmias: a new frontier. *PACE*, **9**, 531–50

106. Downar, E., Butany, J., Jares, A. and Stoicheff, B. P. (1986). Endocardial photoablation by excimer laser. *J. Am. Coll. Cardiol.*, **7**, 546–50

107. Svenson, R. H., Gallagher, J. J., Selle, J. G., Sealy, W. C., Zimmern, S. H., Fedor, J. M., Marroum, M.-C., Tatsis, G. P., Seifert, K. T. and Robicsek, F. (1986). Successful intraoperative Nd:YAG laser ablation of ventricular tachycardia. *J. Am. Coll. Cardiol.*, **7**, 237A

108. Mesnildrey, P., Laborde, F. and Piwnica, A. (1986). Surgery of ischemic ventricular tachycardia: a further experience with the ND-YAG laser beam. *Circulation*, **74**, II–134

109. Borggrefe, M., Podczek, A., Ostermeyer, J., Schwarzmaier, J. and Breithardt, G. (1987). Induction of non-clinical ventricular tachycardia after map-guided surgery for refractory ventricular tachyarrhythmias: incidence and clinical significance. *J. Am. Coll. Cardiol.*, **9**, 108A

23
Cardiopulmonary resuscitation

D. A. ZIDEMAN

There are three irregularities of the heart beat which result in no cardiac output and thus require immediate treatment if permanent damage is to be prevented. The three irregularities of rhythm are:

(1) Ventricular fibrillation,
(2) Asystole,
(3) Electromechanical dissociation.

Their management is described under the global term of cardio-pulmonary resuscitation.

Unlike the treatment of many other abnormal cardiac rhythms, the treatment or correction of these rhythms may not be immediately possible. Thus the priority becomes the maintenance of life by providing an artificially driven circulation by external chest compression and, if required, the maintenance of the oxygenation of blood by artificial respiration (expired air resuscitation). This is known as *basic life support*. Even the shortest of delays in the initiation of basic life support cannot be tolerated especially when this may be as a result of waiting for specific equipment and drugs to treat the particular arrhythmia. The use of equipment and drugs in resuscitation is known as *advanced life support*. Should these adjuncts be immediately available it may be more appropriate not to delay its implementation whilst establishing basic life support. The linking of basic and advanced life support is, therefore, of outstanding importance. It requires training, practice and experience to achieve the best results.

BASIC LIFE SUPPORT

Basic life support is classically described as an Airway, Breathing, Circulation sequence. It is used to maintain a flow of oxygenated blood to various vital organs of the body until a more definitive therapy, advanced life support, is available. In hospital this period may be short, if at all. In the out-of-hospital situation basic life support techniques may be carried out for prolonged periods of time. Cummins and Eisenberg[1]

403

examined the determinants of survival in nine studies of pre-hospital resuscitation. They found that the chance of survival was improved in witnessed arrests, where the emergency medical system (the ambulance/paramedic system) had been activated and in the early arrival (within 4 minutes) and implementation of advanced life support procedures. Tweed and Wilson[2] in another analysis of survival similarly found that the time to the initiation of basic life support was a highly significant factor. Furthermore, they found that the time to arrival of the emergency medical team and the immediate defibrillation of ventricular fibrillation was even more highly significant. Thus basic life support 'buys time' until the arrival of definitive therapy. Some authors believe that this time may be as short as 4–6 minutes, and that prolonged basic resuscitation produces similar results to no resuscitation[3].

Airway

In the unconscious victim of a cardiac arrest the muscles of the tongue, neck and pharynx relax resulting in the tongue and/or epiglottis obstructing the upper airway[4]. Furthermore, if respiratory efforts continue in the victim with a fully or a partially obstructed airway, then the negative inspiratory pressures created may suck the tongue or epiglottis into a position where they occlude the upper airway[5]. Guildner[6] showed that the best way of opening and monitoring the airway was to tilt the head, thus extending the head on the neck, and to support and lift the jaw to displace the tongue forward from the posterior pharyngeal wall. The upper airway should then be inspected and any vomit or foreign material carefully removed.

Breathing

Having opened the airway as described above, it is a simple matter to now check whether the victim is still breathing by looking for chest wall movement, by listening for breathing and by feeling over the mouth to see if these movements are effective. If there is no effective respiration then expired air ventilation must be commenced. Mouth to mouth, mouth to nose or mouth to stoma are all methods of expired air ventilation. Initially, two normal individual breaths should be given by the rescuer to the victim. With each breath the rescuer should observe the chest rise and fall thus confirming successful ventilation. High inspiratory pressures and gas flow rates, excessive inspiratory volumes or not allowing for expiration between breaths may result in gastric inflation and distension, and should be avoided[7].

Circulation

In basic life support the circulation is assessed by palpating a major pulse, preferably the carotid pulse. If there is no palpable pulse then the circulation is maintained by external chest compressions. These are performed on the lower third of the victim's sternum, two fingers breadth above the xiphisternum, with the heel of one hand superimposed on the other hand and stabilized by interlocking the fingers. Compressions should be 4–5 cm in depth and carried out at a rate of 80 compressions per minute. After 15 compressions the rescuer should give two expired air ventilations. If two rescuers are present then one should perform chest compression at a rate of at least 60 per minute whilst the second performs a single expired air ventilation after every fifth compression. The second rescuer should also check that the chest compressions are achieving a palpable pulse.

Chest compressions were originally described by Kouwenhoven and his colleagues in 1960[8], and have become part of conventional or standard cardiopulmonary resuscitation. They postulated that during compressions the heart was compressed between the sternum and the vertebral bodies of the spine. This has been described as the heart pump theory[9]. More recently, Maier and his colleagues[10] have used moderate force, brief duration chest compressions, performed at high rates and demonstrated higher stroke volumes and improved coronary blood flow. In 1976, Criley[11] found that vigorous coughing by a cardiac arrest victim was able to sustain consciousness for 92 seconds before defibrillation. He proposed that the rise in intrathoracic pressure that resulted from coughing provided a significant cerebral blood flow. Other authors[12,13] have taken this 'thoracic pump' theory further. In this theory it has been proposed that external chest compressions will raise the intrathoracic pressure thus increasing the pressure in all intrathoracic structures. This increased pressure is transmitted to the extrathoracic arteries as these vessels have relatively rigid walls. Veins on the other hand, which are relatively thin walled, collapse. This creates an extrathoracic arteriovenous pressure gradient and a resultant blood flow. The passive role of the heart, the heart as a conduit during CPR[14], was further supported by pressure-synchronized cineangiography in dogs[15] and 2D-echocardiography in man[16,17]. They demonstrated little change in cardiac chamber volume during external chest compressions; that the aortic and mitral valves open simultaneously during compressions; and that the pulmonary valve prevents retrograde blood flow by closing during compression and opening during relaxation. More recently, a preliminary report has challenged these findings by demonstrating motion of the heart valves and chamber compression during the initial 4 minutes of external chest compression[18].

Chandra and her colleagues converted the thoracic pump theory into a practical treatment schedule and applied it initially to dogs[19] and then to man[20]. They synchronized prolonged chest compressions, 60% downstroke, at a rate of 40/minute, with ventilation performed at high airway pressures of 70–110 mmHg. They alternated this synchronized compression ventilation CPR (New 'CPR') with conventional CPR every 30 seconds. Provided the high airway pressure was maintained they achieved an improvement in systolic pressure of 13 mmHg and a 250% increase in carotid blood flow using the 'New CPR'.

Interposed abdominal compression CPR[21] has also been tested as a method of augmenting intrathoracic pressure during cardiopulmonary resuscitation. A clinical trial in Milwaukee did not demonstrate any significant improvement in results over conventional methods[22]. Furthermore, Martin[23] has recently confirmed the fear of others[24] that there is a deterioration in myocardial perfusion pressure in patients undergoing synchronized compression and ventilation resuscitation. In Martin's study, no patient receiving 'New CPR' was successfully resuscitated. The newer methodologies need much more research in humans, including evaluation of survival, before they can be recommended.

ADVANCED LIFE SUPPORT

The use of equipment and drugs during resuscitation is called advanced life support. It is essential to initiate and continue basic life support until these adjuncts arrive and their use is established.

Airway management and ventilation

A detailed examination of this topic in this article is probably inappropriate. Endotracheal intubation is the definitive method of airway management. Not only does it guarantee an established airway, but it will also protect the airway from the aspiration of vomit. Hess and Baran[25] have shown that the alternative methods of mouth-to-mask and bag-valve-mask provide inadequate tidal volumes even in experienced hands.

Drug therapy

The administration of drugs during resuscitation requires the resuscitator to establish a reliable and safe intravenous route at an early stage. Cannulation of a central vein is the most ideal and access can be achieved via the internal or external jugular veins, subclavian or femoral vein. A recent study has shown that there is a significant delay in drugs reaching the heart, and a lower peak drug level when drugs are administered via a peripheral rather than a central route, even with effective chest compressions[26].

A more successful alternative is to administer drugs via the endotracheal tube[27]. This route is often considered preferable, especially when there is delay in establishing intravenous access. Lignocaine, atropine, adrenaline and isoprenaline can all be given by the endotracheal route, instillation being followed by 5–10 rapid ventilations. The intracardiac route must be considered a poor third, and is probably only indicated if the intravenous and endotracheal routes are not available. Sabin and his colleagues showed that using the left sternal edge approach, only 11% of intracardiac injections entered the left ventricle and in 25% the needle had lacerated the left anterior descending coronary artery[28].

SPECIFIC ARRHYTHMIA THERAPIES

Effective treatment of the arrhythmias of cardiac arrest requires the initiation of basic life support to be coordinated with specific arrhythmia therapies. Specific preplanned regimens have been recommended for the treatment of ventricular fibrillation, asystole and electromechanical dissociation. The advanced planning and practice of these treatments is essential in order to coordinate the resuscitation team and to allow the rapid establishment of an effective treatment policy with minimal delay.

Ventricular fibrillation (and pulseless ventricular tachycardia)

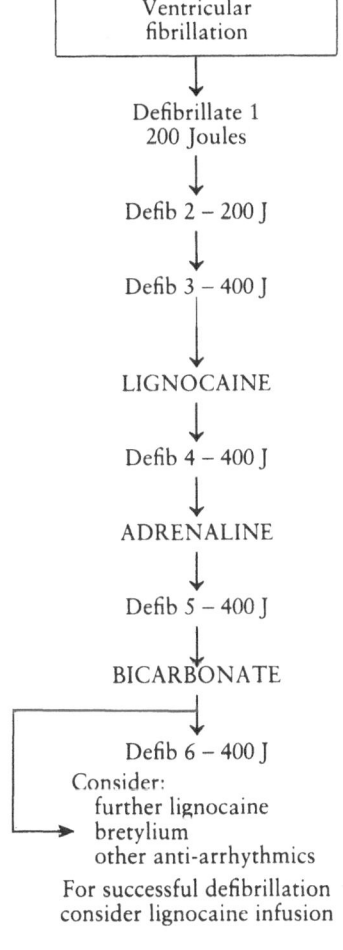

Ventricular fibrillation represents the total breakdown of ordered electrical conduction within the myocardium. The result is a heart with no cardiac output and a pulseless patient. It is the commonest of the pulseless rhythms in patients with ischaemic heart disease and although it may be heralded by the signs and symptoms of a myocardial infarction, heart failure or cardiogenic shock, it sometimes occurs without any warning causing sudden cardiac death.

The treatment of ventricular fibrillation is to convert it, as rapidly as possible, to a more ordered rhythm with a cardiac output. The definitive treatment is electrical defibrillation. Caldwell and his colleagues found that they successfully converted 23 patients in hospital with the mechanical intervention of either a cough or a chest thump[29]. These patients were pulseless in ventricular fibrillation or ventricular tachycardia. In the out-of-hospital patient, another study[30] found the chest thump a less useful technique. Of the 23 patients that were thumped for ventricular fibrillation none were converted, but 10 were later converted by electrical defibrillation. In the same study 15 of the 27 thumped for ventricular tachycardia changed rhythm, but only three changed to an improved rhythm, of which two were successfully resuscitated.

The importance of electrical defibrillation in the conversion of ventricular fibrillation is reflected in its repeated occurrence in the recommended treatment schedule (see scheme above). Defibrillation should be attempted as rapidly as possible with 200 joules of electrical energy. This initial defibrillation level was set following out-of-hospital[31] and in-hospital studies[32] showing that eventual survival and subsequent discharge was the same for those patients receiving 175 joule or 320 joule shocks. The lower level of energy was recommended as it seemed safer when considering that the higher level may cause myocardial damage. Following defibrillation external chest compressions must be continued until the 'recovery' of the ECG trace. Should fibrillation continue then a second shock of 200 joule and a third shock of 400 joule is recommended. It was originally believed that repeated electrical energy discharge across the thoracic cavity decreases transthoracic resistance[33]; thus defibrillating with the same energy would deliver more current to the heart. Kerber and his colleagues[34] have more recently found that transthoracic resistance varied considerably in humans, but that it was best related to chest size. Furthermore, they found that repeated shocks of the same energy level had minimal and unpredictable effects on the transthoracic resistance.

If ventricular fibrillation persists then the administration of lignocaine, either intravenously or via the endotracheal tube, may improve the response to the next defibrillation attempt. Lignocaine raises the ventricular fibrillation threshold, suppresses automaticity, decreases action potential amplitude and shortens the action potential duration and the effective refractory period in the Purkinje fibres[35]. Lignocaine has also been found, when given as a bolus or as a constant infusion, to raise the threshold for delivered energy to electrically defibrillate the heart[36].

If the heart does not respond to this initial therapy then it becomes necessary to improve the cardiac output and blood pressure which is being maintained by external chest compressions. 10 ml of 1 in 10 000 adrenaline (1.0 mg) administered via the intravenous or the endotracheal route will increase myocardial and central nervous system blood flow by stimulating α-adrenergic receptors[37]. It will also stimulate β-adrenergic receptors thus increasing inotropy and coarsening the ventricular fibrillation[38].

Should resuscitation continue for a prolonged period, or if there is inadequate ventilation or a period of prolonged hypoxia, then it is necessary to give sodium bicarbonate, 1 mmol/kg intravenously. Large doses of bicarbonate are detrimental as they can cause hypercarbia (by the metabolic conversion of bicarbonate to carbon dioxide), paradoxical cerebrospinal spinal fluid acidosis, hyperosmolarity and may inactivate simultaneously administered catecholamines[39]. Thus the administration of bicarbonate should not be considered routine, but should only be given if indicated, probably by the measurement of arterial pH and blood gases.

Bretylium tosylate has been reported as producing chemical defibrillation[40]. Bretylium releases noradrenaline from adrenergic nerve endings and blocks the reuptake mechanism. In electrophysiological terms it increases the action potential duration, prolongs the effective refractory period in the Purkinje cells and raises the ventricular fibrillation threshold[41]. Other antifibrillatory agents that may be considered useful are procainamide, verapamil and β-adrenergic blocking drugs such as propranolol. Administration of any of these must be accompanied by careful monitoring of the blood pressure as they may cause a precipitous fall in blood pressure.

The above recommendations for the treatment of ventricular fibrillation are the same for the treatment of pulseless ventricular tachycardia.

Asystole

Asystole is the cessation of electrical and mechanical ventricular activity. It is estimated that 10% of out-of-hospital cardiac arrests and 25% of in-hospital cardiac arrests are asystolic. As asystole has a worse prognosis than ventricular fibrillation and the distinction between them, and thus the appropriate treatment, is made by monitoring the ECG, it is essential when a flat ECG trace is obtained that the switches, connections and gain of the monitoring system are carefully checked.

Parasympathetic overactivity, especially in the presence of depressed sympathetic tone (e.g. ischaemia, infarction or β-blocker) may cause asystole by depression of the sinus and atrioventricular nodes. Thus atropine, a parasympathetic blocking drug, in a dose of 1 mg via the intravenous or endotracheal route has been recommended as being

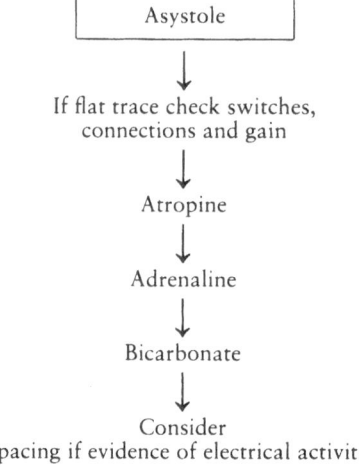

effective in asystole[42]. Ventricular fibrillation and tachycardia have been reported following the administration of atropine[43].

Further treatment of asystole depends on the maintenance of the circulation by external chest compressions together with the aid of the adrenergic stimulation of adrenaline. Sodium bicarbonate may be given to correct any serious acidosis that has occurred. In addition the pure β-adrenergic effects of isoprenaline on the myocardium and on the depressed nodes may be of use. The advent of transthoracic pacing, using large high impedance electrodes applied to the thoracic wall, has been reported as being effective in those patients in asystole but with 'P-wave activity'[44]. Others have shown the results of pacing in the out-of-hospital situation as disappointing and have not recommended its use[45].

Electromechanical dissociation

Electromechanical dissociation is the failure of the heart to pump blood despite organized electrical activity. It is usually seen as an in-hospital phenomenon; less than 3% of cardiac arrests occurring outside hospital are due to electromechanical dissociation. The prognosis for survival is very poor.

Before treating the pump failure, it is necessary to exclude the known physical causes: drugs, hypovolaemia, severe acidosis, or secondary to mechanical causes such as cardiac tamponade, pulmonary embolism, tension pneumothorax, intracardiac tumour or thrombus, myocardial rupture or exsanguination. It may also be seen as the final event in a prolonged ventricular fibrillation. The mechanism is not fully understood, but it is believed to be, in part, due to inadequate myocardial blood flow, intracellular acidosis and autonomic causes.

410

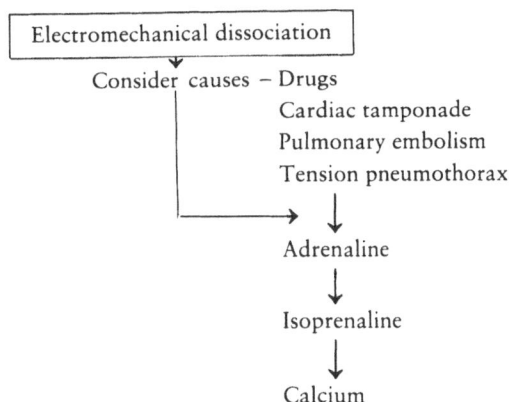

The treatment of electromechanical dissociation is initially to exclude the physical causes given above and then to support the circulation with adrenaline and isoprenaline. The α-adrenergic effects on the peripheral vascular resistance are particularly useful here as they improve perfusion pressure. In addition methoxamine, an α-adrenergic agonist, may be of use. Calcium chloride, 10 ml of a 10% solution, may be used to improve myocardial contraction but Dembo found that calcium may worsen coronary artery spasm and increase myocardial ischaemia[46]. The use of calcium channel blockers has not, as yet, been established in resuscitation.

CONCLUSION

The foregoing text has described the management of the arrhythmias associated with cardiac arrest and resuscitation. It is of great concern that recent studies have shown that doctors[47-49] and nurses[50] perform poorly when tested in their theoretical and practical knowledge of resuscitation. Perhaps regular formal training in resuscitation procedures would improve the management of this life and death medical emergency.

References

1. Cummins, R. O. and Eisenberg, M. S. (1983). Prehospital cardiopulmonary resuscitation. Is it effective? *J. Am. Med. Assoc.*, **253**, 2408–12
2. Tweed, W. A. and Wilson, E. (1984). Is CPR on the right track (Editorial). *Can. Med. Assoc. J.*, **131**, 429–33
3. Krause, G. S., Kumar, K., White, B. C., Aust, S. D. and Wiegenstein, J. G. (1986). Ischemia, resuscitation and reperfusion. Mechanisms of tissue injury and prospects for protection. *Am. Heart J.*, **111**, 768 80
4. Boidin, M. P. (1985). Airway patency in the unconscious patient. *Br. J. Anaesth.*, **57**, 306–10
5. Ruben, H., Elam, J. O. and Ruben, A. M. (1961). Investigation of upper airway problems in resuscitation. *Anaesthesiology*, **22**, 271–9

6. Guildner, C. W. (1976). Resuscitation – opening the airway. A comparative study of techniques for opening an airway obstructed by the tongue. *JACEP*, **5**, 588–90
7. Melker, R. (1985). Recommendations for ventilation during cardiopulmonary resuscitation. Time for change? *Crit. Care Med.*, **13**, 882–3
8. Kouwenhoven, W. B., Jude, J. R. and Knickerbocker, G. G. (1960). Closed-chest cardiac massage. *J. Am. Med. Assoc.*, **173**, 1064–7
9. Babbs, C. F. (1980). New versus old theories of blood flow during CPR. *Crit. Care Med.*, **8**, 191–5
10. Maier, G. W., Tyson, G. S. and Olsen, C. O. (1984). The physiology of external cardiac massage: High impulse cardiopulmonary resuscitation. *Circulation*, **70**, 86–101
11. Criley, J. M., Blaufuss, A. H. and Kissel, G. L. (1976). Cough-induced cardiac compression. Self induced form of cardiopulmonary resuscitation. *J. Am. Med. Assoc.*, **236**, 1246–50
12. Niemann, J. T., Rosborough, J., Garner, D. and Criley, J. M. (1979). The mechanism of blood flow in closed chest cardiopulmonary resuscitation. *Circulation*, **60**, (Suppl 2), 74
13. Rudikoff, M. T., Maughan, W. L., Effron M., Freund, P. and Weisfeldt. M .L. (1980). Mechanisms of blood flow during cardiopulmonary resuscitation. *Circulation*, **61**, 345–52
14. Criley, J. M., Niemann, J. T., Rosborough, J. P., Ung, S. and Suzuki, J. (1984). The heart is a conduit in CPR. *Crit. Care Med.*, **9**, 373–4
15. Niemann, J. T., Rosborough, J. T., Hausknecht, M., Gardner, D. and Criley, J. M. (1981). Pressure-synchronised cineangiography during experimental cardiopulmonary resuscitation. *Circulation*, **64**, 985–91
16. Werner, J. A., Green H. L., Janko, C. L. and Cobb, L. A. (1981). Visualisation of cardiac valve motion in man during external chest compression using two dimensional echocardiography. Implications regarding the mechanisms of blood flow. *Circulation*, **63**, 1417–21
17. Rich, S., Wix, H. L. and Shapiro, E. P. (1981). Clinical assessment of heart chamber size and valve motion during cardiopulmonary resuscitation by two dimensional echocardiography. *Am. Heart J.*, **102**, 368–73
18. Desmukh, H., Weil, M. H. and Swindall, A. (1985). Echocardiographic observations during cardiopulmonary resuscitation: A preliminary report. *Crit. Care Med.*, **13**, 904–6
19. Chandra, N., Rudikoff, M. T., Tsitlick, J. and Weisfeldt, M. L. (1979). Augmentation of carotid flow during cardiopulmonary resuscitation in the dog by simultaneous compression and ventilation with high airway pressure. *Am. J. Cardiol.*, **43**, 422
20. Chandra, M., Radikoff, M. T. and Weisfeldt, M. L. (1980). Simultaneous chest compression and ventilation at high airway pressure during cardiopulmonary resuscitation. *Lancet*, **1**, 175–8
21. Ralston, S. H., Babbs, C. F. and Niebauer, M. J. (1982). Cardiopulmonary resuscitation with interposed abdominal compression in dogs. *Anesth. Analg.*, **61**, 645–51
22. Mateer. J. R., Stueven, H. A., Thompson, B. M., Aprahamian, C. and Davin, J. (1985). Prehospital IAC–CPR versus standard CPR. Paramedic resuscitation of cardiac arrests. *Am. J. Emerg. Med.*, **3**, 143
23. Martin, G. B., Carden, D. L., Nowak, R. M., Johnston W. and Tomlanovich, M. C. (1985). Aortic and right atrial pressures during standard and simultaneous ventilation and compression CPR in human beings. *Ann. Emerg. Med.*, **14**, 497
24. Sanders, A. B., Ewy, G. A. and Taft, T. (1983). The importance of aortic diastolic blood pressure during cardiopulmonary resuscitation. *J. Am. Coll. Cardiol.*, **1**, 609
25. Hess, D. and Baran, C. (1985). Ventilatory volumes using mouth-to-mouth, mouth-to-mask and bag-valve-mask techniques. *Am.J. Emerg. Med.*, **3**, 292
26. Kahn, G. J., White, B. C. and Swetnam, R. E. (1981). Peripheral vs central circulation times during CPR: A pilot study. *Ann. Emerg. Med.*, **10**, 417–19
27. Greenberg, M. I. (1984). The use of endotracheal medication in cardiac emergencies. *Resuscitation*, **12**, 155–65

28. Sabin, H. I., Coghill, S. B., Khunti, K. and McNeil, G. O. (1983). Accuracy on intracardiac injections determined by a post-mortem study. *Lancet*, **2**, 1054–5
29. Caldwell, G., Millar, G., Quinn, E., Vincent, R. and Chamberlain, D. A. (1985). Simple mechanical methods for cardioversion: defence of the precordial thump and cough version. *Brit. Med. J.*, **291**, 627–30
30. Miller, J., Tresch, D., Horwitz, L., Thompson, B. M., Aprahamian C. and Davin, J. C. (1984). The precordial thump. *Ann. Emerg. Med.*, **13**, 791–4
31. Weaver, W. D., Cobb, L. A., Copass, M. K. and Hallstrom, A. P. (1982). Ventricular defibrillation – a comparative trial using 175 J and 320 J shocks. *N. Engl. J. Med.*, **307**, 1101–6
32. Kerber, R. E., Jensen, S. R. and Gascho, J. A. (1983). Determinants of defibrillation: Prospective analysis of 183 patients. *Am. J. Cardiol.*, **52**, 739–45
33. Dahl, C. F., Ewy, G. A. and Ewy, M. D. (1976). Transthoracic impedance to direct current discharge· Effect of repeated countershocks. *Med. Instrum.*, **10**, 151–5
34. Kerber, R. E., Grayzel, J., Hoyt, R., Marcus, M. and Kennedy, J. (1981). Transthoracic resistance in human defibrillation. *Circulation*, **63**, 676–82
35. Rosen, M. R., Hoffman, B. F. and Wit A. L. (1975). Electrophysiology and pharmacology of cardiac arrhythmias v cardiac antiarrhythmic effects of lidocaine. *Am. Heart J.*, **89**, 526–36
36. Babbs, C. F., Yim, G. K. W. and Whistler, S. J. (1979). Evaluation of ventricular defibrillation threshold in dogs by antiarrhythmic drugs. *Am. Heart J.*, **98**, 345–50
37. Redding, J. S. and Pearson, J. W. (1963). Evaluation of drugs for cardiac resuscitation. *Anesthesiology*, **24**, 203–7
38. Livesay, J. J., Follette, D. M. and Fey, K. H. (1978). Optimizing myocardial supply/demand balance with adrenergic drugs during cardiopulmonary resuscitation. *J. Thorac. Cardiovasc. Surg.*, **76**, 244–51
39. Bishop, R. L. and Weisfeldt, M. L. (1976). Sodium bicarbonate administration during cardiac arrest *J. Am. Med. Assoc.*, **235**, 506–9
40. Sanna, G. and Arcidiancono, R. (1973). Chemical ventricular defibrillation of human heart with bretylium tosylate. *Am. J. Cardiol.*, **32**, 982–7
41. Bacaner, M. (1968). Quantitative comparison of bretylium with other antifibrillatory drugs. *Am. J. Cardiol.*, **21**, 504–21
42. Myerburg, R. J., Estes, D. and Laman, L. (1984). Outcome of resuscitation from bradyarrhythmic or asystolic prehospital cardiac arrest. *J. Am. Coll. Cardiol.*, **4**, 1118
43. Cooper, M. J. and Abinader, E. G. (1979). Atropine induced ventricular fibrillation: Case report and review of the literature. *Am. Heart J.*, **97**, 225–8
44. Zoll, P. M., Zoll, R. H. and Falk, R. H (1985). External non-invasive temporary cardiac pacing: Clinical trials. *Circulation*, **71**, 937–44
45. Falk, R. H., Jacobs, L. and Sinclair, A. (1983). External non-invasive cardiac pacing in out-of-hospital cardiac arrest. *Crit. Care Med.*, **11**, 779–82
46. Dembo, D. H. (1981). Calcium in advanced life support. *Crit. Care Med.*, **9**, 358
47. Lowenstein, S. R., Hansbrough, J, F., Libby, L. S., Hill, D. M., Mountain, R. D. and Scoggin, C. H. (1981). Cardiopulmonary resuscitation by medical and surgical house officers. *Lancet*, **2**, 679–81
48. Casey, W. F. (1984). Cardiopulmonary resuscitation: a survey of standards among junior hospital doctors. *J. R. Suc. Med.*, **77**, 921–4
49. Skinner, D. V., Camm, A. J. and Miles, S. (1985). Cardiopulmonary resuscitation skills of preregistration house officers. *Br. Med. J.*, **290**, 1549
50. Evans, T. R. (1986). The inability of trained nurses to perform basic life support – Presented paper British Cardiac Society

Further reading

ABC of Resuscitation (1986). Evans, T. R. (ed.) (London: *British Medical Journal*)
Standards and Guidelines for Cardiopulmonary Resuscitation and Emergency Cardiac Care (1986). *J. Am. Med. Assoc.*, **255**, 2841–3044

Index